HANDBOOK OF
RELIGION
AND
MENTAL HEALTH

HANDBOOK OF
RELIGION
AND
MENTAL HEALTH

Edited by
HAROLD G. KOENIG
Department of Psychiatry
Duke University Medical Center

ACADEMIC PRESS
San Diego   London   Boston   New York   Sydney   Tokyo   Toronto

This book is printed on acid-free paper. ∞

Academic Press
a division of Harcourt Brace & Company
525 B Street, Suite 1900, San Diego, California 92101-4495, USA
http://www.apnet.com

Academic Press
24-28 Oval Road, London NW1 7DX, UK
http://www.hbuk.co.uk/ap/

Library of Congress Catalog Card Number: 98-84981

International Standard Book Number: 0-12-417645-3

PRINTED IN THE UNITED STATES OF AMERICA
98 99 00 01 02 03 BB 9 8 7 6 5 4 3 2 1

To Sir John Templeton
for his generous support of scientific research
on the relationship
between religion and mental health.

CONTENTS

SECTION I

HISTORICAL BACKGROUND

1

REFLECTIONS ON THE ROLE OF RELIGION IN THE HISTORY OF PSYCHIATRY

SAMUEL B. THIELMAN

2

ETHICS, RELIGION, AND MENTAL HEALTH

STEPHEN G. POST

SECTION II

A NEW RESEARCH FRONTIER

3

RESEARCH ON RELIGION AND MENTAL HEALTH: AN OVERVIEW OF EMPIRICAL FINDINGS AND THEORETICAL ISSUES

JEFFREY S. LEVIN AND LINDA M. CHATTERS

4

WHAT SOCIOLOGY CAN HELP US UNDERSTAND ABOUT RELIGION AND MENTAL HEALTH

ELLEN L. IDLER AND LINDA K. GEORGE

5

RELIGION AND PERSONALITY

ROBERT A. EMMONS

6

THE NEUROPSYCHOLOGY OF SPIRITUAL EXPERIENCE

ANDREW B. NEWBERG AND EUGENE G. D'AQUILI

7

FUTURE DIRECTIONS IN RESEARCH

MICHAEL E. MCCULLOUGH AND DAVID B. LARSON

SECTION III

RELIGION AND MENTAL FUNCTIONING

8

RELIGION AND COPING

KENNETH I. PARGAMENT AND CURTIS R. BRANT

9

RELIGION AND DEPRESSION

GARY J. KENNEDY

10

RELIGION AND ANXIETY: WHICH ANXIETY? WHICH RELIGION?

JAMES A. THORSON

11

RELIGION AND PSYCHOSES

WILLIAM P. WILSON

12

SPIRITUAL AND RELIGIOUS FACTORS IN SUBSTANCE USE, DEPENDENCE, AND RECOVERY

JENNIFER BOOTH AND JOHN E. MARTIN

SECTION IV

RELIGIOUS PERSPECTIVES
ON MENTAL HEALTH

13

RELIGION AND MENTAL HEALTH
FROM THE PROTESTANT PERSPECTIVE

H. NEWTON MALONY

14

RELIGION AND MENTAL HEALTH
FROM THE CATHOLIC PERSPECTIVE

NANCY CLARE KEHOE

15

RELIGION AND MENTAL HEALTH
FROM THE MORMON PERSPECTIVE

SALLY H. BARLOW AND ALLEN E. BERGIN

16

RELIGION AND MENTAL HEALTH
FROM THE UNITY PERSPECTIVE

GLENN R. MOSLEY

20

RELIGION AND MENTAL HEALTH
FROM THE MUSLIM PERSPECTIVE

SYED ARSHAD HUSAIN

21

RELIGION AND CULTURE IN PSYCHIATRY:
CHRISTIAN AND SECULAR PSYCHIATRIC THEORY
AND PRACTICE IN THE UNITED STATES

ATWOOD D. GAINES

SECTION V

CLINICAL APPLICATIONS

22

RELIGION AND PSYCHOTHERAPY

HAROLD G. KOENIG AND JOHN PRITCHETT

23

THE ROLE OF NONPARISH CLERGY IN THE MENTAL HEALTH SYSTEM

LARRY VANDECREEK, DAVID CARL, AND DUANE PARKER

24

MENTAL HEALTH PROFESSIONALS WORKING WITH RELIGIOUS LEADERS

ANDREW J. WEAVER

SECTION VI

EDUCATION OF MENTAL HEALTH PROFESSIONALS

25

INTEGRATING RELIGION INTO THE EDUCATION OF MENTAL HEALTH PROFESSIONALS

ELIZABETH S. BOWMAN

26

RELIGION AND ACADEMIA IN MENTAL HEALTH

DAN G. BLAZER

SUMMARY AND CONCLUSIONS

CONTRIBUTORS

Numbers in parentheses indicate the pages on which the authors' contributions begin.

Sally H. Barlow (225) Department of Psychology, Brigham Young University, Provo, Utah 84602.

Allen E. Bergin (225) Department of Psychology, Brigham Young University, Provo, Utah 84602.

Dan G. Blazer (379) Duke University School of Medicine, Durham, North Carolina 27705.

Jennifer Booth (175) San Diego State University, San Diego, California 92120.

Elizabeth S. Bowman (367) Department of Psychiatry, Indiana University School of Medicine, Indianapolis, Indiana 46202.

Curtis R. Brant (111) Department of Psychology, Baldwin–Wallace College, Berea, Ohio 44017.

David Carl (337) Department of Pastoral Care, Carolinas Medical Center, Charlotte, North Carolina 28232.

Linda M. Chatters (33) Department of Health Behavior and Health Education, School of Public Health, University of Michigan, Ann Arbor, Michigan 48109.

Eugene G. d'Aquili (75) Department of Psychiatry, Hospital of the University of Pennsylvania, Philadelphia, Pennsylvania 19104.

Robert A. Emmons (63) Department of Psychology, University of California at Davis, Davis, California 95616.

Atwood D. Gaines (291) Case Western Reserve University and School of Medicine, Cleveland, Ohio 44106.

Linda K. George (51) Department of Sociology and Center for the Study of Aging and Human Development, Duke University, Durham, North Carolina 27710.

Syed Arshad Husain (279) University of Missouri at Columbia, Columbia, Missouri 65212.

Ellen L. Idler (51) Department of Sociology and Institute for Health Care Policy and Aging Research, Rutgers University, New Brunswick, New Jersey 08903.

Nalini V. Juthani (271) Albert Einstein College of Medicine, New York, New York 10461.

Nancy Clare Kehoe (211) Harvard Medical School, Cambridge, Massachusetts 02139.

Gary J. Kennedy (129) Department of Geriatric Psychiatry, Albert Einstein College of Medicine, New York, New York 10461.

Harold G. Koenig (323, 391) Department of Psychiatry, Duke University Medical Center, Durham, North Carolina 27705.

David B. Larson (95) Duke University Medical Center, Durham, North Carolina 27705, and National Institute for Healthcare Research, Rockville, Maryland 20852.

Jeffrey S. Levin (33) National Institute for Healthcare Research, Rockville, Maryland 20852.

H. Newton Malony (203) Graduate School of Psychology, Fuller Theological Seminary, Pasadena, California 91101.

John E. Martin (175) San Diego State University, San Diego, California 92120.

Michael E. McCullough (95) National Institute for Healthcare Research, Rockville, Maryland 20852.

Glenn R. Mosely (245) Association of Unity Churches, Lee's Summit, Missouri 64081.

Andrew B. Newberg (75) Division of Nuclear Medicine, Department of Psychiatry, Hospital of the University of Pennsylvania, Philadelphia, Pennsylvania 19104.

Kenneth I. Pargament (111) Department of Psychology, Bowling Green State University, Bowling Green, Ohio 43403.

Duane Parker (337) Interfaith Healthcare Ministries, Rhode Island Hospital, Providence, Rhode Island 02903.

Stephen G. Post (21) Center for Biomedical Ethics, School of Medicine, Case Western Reserve University, Cleveland, Ohio 44106.

John Pritchett (323) Private Practice of Psychiatry, Charleston, South Carolina 29412.

Bruce W. Scotton (263) Department of Psychiatry, University of California at San Francisco, San Francisco, California 94140.

Samuel B. Theilman (3) Department of Psychiatry, Duke University Medical Center, Durham, North Carolina 27705.

James A. Thorson (147) Department of Gerontology, University of Nebraska at Omaha, Omaha, Nebraska 68182.

Larry VandeCreek (337) Department of Pastoral Care, The Ohio State University Medical Center, Columbus, Ohio 43210.

Andrew J. Weaver (349) Department of Psychology, University of Hawaii, and Hawaii State Hospital, Kaneohe, Hawaii 96744.

William P. Wilson (161) Duke University Medical Center, Durham, North Carolina 27705.

Michael R. Zedek (255) The Temple, Congregation B'nai Jehudah, Kansas City, Missouri 64131.

PREFACE

Religion has been one of the most powerful forces throughout human history. Yet the medical and mental health professions have generally not acknowledged that power. In fact, as demonstrated by Dr. Koenig and his collaborators in the *Handbook of Religion and Mental Health,* the links of spirituality and religion with disease and health and mental health are unavoidable. Rather than continue this avoidance, mental health professionals need to be better poised to make the best use of these connections to benefit patients.

This task (to which this *Handbook* is addressed) requires that the field look at ways to appropriately convey relevant, valid, and useful information to trainees and practitioners and to expand the science base in this area. With regard to education and clinical care, it is clear that the assessment of religious and spiritual issues should become an expected part of patient evaluation in all of medicine and especially mental health care, no different from the consideration of the patient's family and social context, the mental status examination, and the elucidation of patient preferences for particular treatment options. Importantly, efforts to expand the understanding of the role of spirituality and religion in health care should be made within the context of existing approaches, under a "both–and" paradigm rather than "either–or," with practitioners maintaining respect for their patients' beliefs. When individuals are educated about specific techniques and approaches, it is critical that they be given complete information about the evidence base (i.e., the strengths and weaknesses in the existing literature, the good and the bad impacts of interventions). Ideally, in the development of guidelines or other teaching tools, the specific evidence underlying the recommendations should be delineated with clarity. In essence, a systemic approach to educational issues is needed—from curriculum development, to model testing, to continuing medical education. This *Handbook* provides a very useful resource for attaining these ends.

The *Handbook* also makes clear that, although there is a great deal of support for the interconnection among religion, spirituality, and health, there is a need to learn much more about the mechanisms underlying these links as well as the outcomes of interventions for their targeted purposes. Because of this, efforts should be aimed at both enhancing the methodology for the field and expanding its infrastructure: to gain a better understanding of the impact and specificity of different elements of religiousness; to better ascertain the active ingredients of religion-informed approaches; and to develop frameworks for research on religious and spiritual issues in the context of development across the lifespan, from childhood and adolescence through adulthood and the elder years.

In summary, this book not only calls attention to the important connections among spirituality, religion, health, and mental health but also identifies important areas for future development. Dr. Koenig and the contributors to the *Handbook* have made it very clear that anyone involved in providing health and mental health care services, studying or evaluating public health interventions, or trying to improve quality and patient satisfaction in health care delivery systems cannot ignore the importance of these issues.

Harold Alan Pincus, M.D.
Deputy Medical Director
American Psychiatric Association
Office of Research

Acknowledgments

We are grateful to Niki Levy and Barbara McKinster at Academic Press for their assistance in putting this volume together. We also thank the John Templeton Foundation which provided funding support for this project (for Dr. Koenig).

INTRODUCTION

For reasons of intellectual integrity, psychiatry cannot afford to ignore or dismiss millennia of religious and philosophical thought about the very essence of human nature, reality and existence. Nor can it fail to acknowledge the lesson of history: that even the most secure seeming truth, religious or scientific, may be relative. To do either would be to risk the eventuality (which in some opinion may already have occurred) of psychiatry losing its human relevance and drifting out of touch with what people feel, believe and need.

—Turbott (1996)

The *Handbook of Religion and Mental Health* is a book for mental health professionals, religious professionals, and counselors that is designed to meet the need for information about how religious beliefs and practices relate to mental health and influence mental health care.

CONTENTS

In the chapters that follow, we seek to address a number of important and fundamental questions. What is the relationship between religion and mental health? There has been a virtual explosion of research during the past decade that has addressed this question for persons of different ages and life situations. What do these studies show, and what are some theoretical models that may help guide our understanding and future research? What have other disciplines such as sociology contributed to our understanding of religion's impact on mental health? What is the relationship between religion and personality and brain functioning? How do people use religion to help cope with or adjust to difficult life circumstances? Are all types of religious coping equally helpful or are some types more so than others? Is religious belief and practice helpful for specific mental disorders? How does one distinguish religious beliefs and practices from psychopathology? Does mental disorder itself disrupt or distort religious or spiritual beliefs?

In this religiously diverse society (Table 1), in which literally hundreds of different religious faiths flourish and guide their adherents through life, the mental health professional is likely to encounter many persons of different religious beliefs and backgrounds during the course of a routine practice day. How does one address the mental health needs of persons from diverse religious faith traditions, particu-

TABLE I.1 Religions in the United States and throughout the World

Religion	United States[a]	Worldwide[b]
Christian (total)	151,225,000	1,927,953,000
Catholic	60,280,454	968,025,000
Protestant	—	395,867,000
Baptist	36,481,698	—
Methodist	13,370,459	—
Lutheran	8,327,086	—
Church of God in Christ	5,499,875	—
Pentecostal churches[c]	4,822,253	—
Presbyterian	4,141,775	—
Christian Church/Church of Christ	2,725,616	—
Episcopalian	2,542,634	—
United Church of Christ	1,472,123	—
Disciples of Christ	929,725	—
Seventh Day Adventist	790,731	—
Eastern Orthodox	2,674,885	217,948,000
Mormon	4,889,279	—
Jehovah Witness	966,243	—
Anglican	—	70,530,000
Other Christian	—	217,948,000
Jewish	3,137,000	14,117,000
Muslim/Islamic	527,000	1,099,634,000
Unitarian/Universalist	502,000	—
Buddhist	401,000	323,894,000
Hindu	227,000	780,547,000
Native American	47,000	—
Scientologist	45,000	—
Baha'i	28,000	6,104,000
Taoist	23,000	—
New Age	20,000	—
Ekankar	18,000	—
Rastafarian	14,000	—
Sikh	13,000	19,161,000
Wiccan	8,000	—
Shintoist	6,000	2,844,000
Deity	6,000	—
Other unclassified	831,000	—

[a]From *Yearbook of American & Canadian Churches 1997* (may or may not include children), pp. 1, 252–258.
[b]From *The World Alamanac and Book of Facts 1997*, p. 646.
[c]Includes Pentecostals, Assemblies of God, and other Churches of God.

larly when the religious faith is different from one's own? What are the belief systems of Catholics, Protestants, fundamentalist Christians, Mormons, Unity church members, Jews, Buddhists, Hindus, and Muslims, and how do these beliefs and practices relate to mental health issues likely to be encountered during treatment?

Do psychiatric patients have spiritual needs that require the expertise of mental health professionals? Is addressing religious issues in the context of a mental health visit ethical and appropriate or is this a dimension of the person that mental health specialists should avoid? Should religious or spiritual issues be assessed in all patients, both religious and nonreligious? What are examples of specific interventions and how can these be applied in a sensitive way? When is it appropriate or necessary to refer such patients to clergy? What is the role of the chaplain and pastoral counselor in our mental health system? What are the risks and benefits of collaboration between mental health and religious professionals? What are the educational needs of mental health professionals in this area, and what is the best way of providing this training?

Addressing religious issues in treatment is particularly important because practice guidelines are encouraging all practitioners to recognize the patient's religious background and consider how it affects their mental illness. Likewise, professional training programs are now mandating trainees to consider religious and cultural factors when evaluating and treating patients. Thus, there is need for a sourcebook that both clinicians and educators can depend on to learn about the complex relationship between religion and mental health. This book contains carefully selected chapters written by experts from a wide range of disciplines, including biomedical ethics, public health, sociology, medicine, psychiatry, psychology, gerontology, theology, anthropology, pastoral care, and medical education.

BOOK STRUCTURE

This book contains six major sections that address each of the subject areas described previously. The first section presents a brief historical background that will give the reader some perspective on the relationship between religion and the mental sciences as it has evolved over the centuries. Section II examines research that has legitimized this field as a valid area for study and explores new frontiers and future directions in research that will help this field develop and mature. The third section delves into religion and mental functioning, exploring the role that religion plays in coping and providing an examination of specific disorders, such as depression, anxiety, psychosis, and substance abuse. Section IV examines specific religious belief systems and how they may impact on the mental health and mental health care of their adherents. The fifth section examines the integration of religion into clinical practice, describing specific techniques on how to do so and providing information about the important role that clergy play in the mental health care delivery system. The final section delves into how to educate and sensitize mental health professionals on religious issues so that they will be able to address the spiritual needs of patients, and this section ends with a discussion of religion's place in academic psychiatry.

OVERVIEW

Dr. Sam Thielman, a practicing psychiatrist and medical historian, begins Section I by taking us on a fascinating journey through time tracing the turbulent and often antagonistic relationship between religion and the mental sciences. Where did medicine and psychology originate from and why did they eventually separate and distance themselves from religion? What historical events set the stage for the growing conflict between religious and mental health professionals? What are the real facts about what happened during the Middle Ages (demonology, the Inquisition, and the persecution of mentally ill as possessed)? Where did the notion of moral treatment evolve from and where did it make its first appearance in the United States? What role did Sigmund Freud play in influencing the profession's views on religions? Ethicist Stephen Post from Case Western University then brings us into the twenty-first century by discussing the ethics of including religion in the clinician–patient relationship. He provides moving stories of people in the grips of hopelessness and chronic illness and the role that faith played in overcoming these circumstances. Dr. Post also addresses what it means to be a mental health professional and how the roots of both the impulse to care for others and professionalism have their origins within the religious traditions.

Jeffrey Levin and Linda Chatters begin Section II with an overview of research on the relationship between religion and mental health. They argue eloquently and forcefully that we should examine the effects of religious factors at all stages of health and illness (from the time when persons are mentally healthy to the appearance of preclinical signs of illness, the onset of overt clinical pathology, and recovery, healing, and reintegration following illness). Their brilliant research and many writings in this area have laid key theoretical foundations for a true "epidemiology of religion and health."

Sociologists Ellen Idler from Rutgers and Linda George from Duke masterfully examine the relationship between religion and mental health from the sociological perspective. They trace the history of sociology back to the research and writings of Emile Durkheim and Max Weber, showing how these pioneers stimulated interest and wrote extensively about the effects of religious belief and participation on individuals and society. For example, Durkheim is credited with one of the first scientific studies on the relationship between suicide and religious involvement, from which he developed important theories about the social functions of religion which continue to inform us today. A passage from the Gospel of Mark is used to cleverly illustrate the importance of social and religious factors in the healing of mind, body, and spirit.

We then move from an analysis at the social or group level to an examination of the individual person and his or her character. Personality psychologist Robert Emmons from the University of California at Davis explores what we can learn about religion from personality theory and vice versa. After overviewing the goals of personality psychology, Emmons discusses a three-tiered approach to the study of personality (dispositional traits, personal concerns, and life narratives) and then explores how each of these tiers can help us to better understand the religious lives of persons. He encourages increasing dialogue between personality psychologists and theologians as a way to enrich both fields of study.

Next, medical internists Andrew Newberg and Eugene d'Aquili from the University of Pennsylvania take us from the person level to the neuron level as they explore the neuropsychological bases for religious and spiritual experience in brain and central nervous system processes. These investigators trace spiritual experiences to activation of sympathetic and parasympathetic nervous systems which facilitate or inhibit discrete areas of the brain responsible for mental experience. They present hypotheses and models of how the capacity for religious and spiritual experience may have evolved from lower primates and examine how electroencephalograms and, recently, positive emission tomography and single photon emission computed tomography can be used to better study and visualize activation of brain structures during spiritual states. While this chapter may seem overly reductionistic to some readers, Newberg and d'Aquili are brilliant researchers on the cutting edge of their field, boldly going where few have gone before to help broaden our horizons.

Completing Section II, psychologist Michael McCullough and psychiatrist David Larson from the National Institute for Healthcare Research outline directions for future research on religion and mental health. They emphasize a need to build a knowledge base for scientific progress to occur and argue that this will best be accomplished by "specialization." Dimensions of future specialization are described in detail, underscoring areas of high priority.

Psychologists Kenneth Pargament and Curtis Brant begin Section III on religion and mental functioning by reviewing the coping literature and examining how specific religious behaviors might facilitate or hinder the coping process. They address the following questions: Is religion related to mental health outcomes following stressful life events? Is religious coping more helpful to some individuals than others? Is religious coping better suited for certain types of situations than others? and are there unique benefits to using religious forms of coping compared to nonreligious or secular forms of coping? They conclude that religion may be helpful, harmful, or irrelevant depending on the type of religious coping, the sample, the situation, and the time frame.

Next, religion's impact on specific mental pathologies—depression, anxiety, psychosis, and substance abuse—is addressed. Psychiatrist, researcher, and educator Gary Kennedy from Albert Einstein College of Medicine examines the high rate of religious activity among older adults in the United States and discusses how religious involvement may suppress, moderate, deter, or prevent the effects of stress that lead to depression. In particular, Kennedy focuses on the relationship between religious attendance, affiliation, and depressive symptoms, reviewing the results of a large epidemiologic study of persons living in the Bronx, New York. Kennedy's sample is especially important because it is composed of large numbers of Catholics (48%) and Jews (40%) living in the northeastern United States; this contrasts with most studies on this type conducted in largely Protestant samples living in the Midwest or the South.

Psychologist and University of Nebraska gerontologist James Thorson examines the relationship between anxiety, religious belief, and practice. He begins by providing a general review of the research on religion and anxiety, then focuses on death anxiety in particular, and finally expands his scope to examine differences in the relationship between religion and death anxiety in different cultures—one study examining the association in a predominantly Christian sample in the United States and the other study in a predominantly Muslim sample in Egypt. The reader will find these data fascinating and the discussion provocative.

William P. Wilson, a widely known and respected Duke psychiatrist and one of the first researchers in psychiatry to publish on religion and mental health in mainstream medical and psychiatric journals, examines the relationship between religion and the psychoses. First, he examines the influence of religion on the etiology and clinical presentation of schizophrenia, major affective disorders, and the organic mental disorders. Next, he explores the topic of demon possession and discusses how this may be distinguished from psychotic disorders such as schizophrenia or mania. Finally, he makes several suggestions on how spiritual therapy (from a Christian perspective) may facilitate healing in these patients.

Behavioral psychologists John Martin and Jennifer Booth from San Diego State University conclude this section by comprehensively reviewing what is known about the relationship between religion/spirituality and alcohol, drug, and cigarette abuse. They examine studies of adolescents, college students, and adults and studies of psychiatric inpatients and outpatients. They examine the positive and negative effects of religious attendance, private religious activities, other spiritual practices, and religious affiliation on different types of substance abuse. They take a critical look at the research that examines the effectiveness of Alcoholics Anonymous (AA) and other 12-step programs and compare them to secular recovery programs. In particular, they examine how important or unimportant the spiritual and religious dimensions of AA is in its effectiveness.

Section IV is a more clinical section composed of a series of chapters that examine the belief systems of a variety of major religious groups and how they might influence the presentation of mental disorders and their response to treatment. Newton Malony, psychologist and professor at Fuller Theological Seminary, begins this section by describing the Protestant Christian perspective. He first underscores the diversity of belief and emphasis within Protestantism and then outlines four Protestant types (fundamentalist, evangelical, traditional, and liberal) based on understanding of authority and criteria for religiousness. Dr. Malony then describes how each Protestant type might define "mental health" and what treatment each would expect from mental health professionals.

Religious professional, psychologist, and Harvard consultant Nancy Kehoe examines mental health from the Catholic perspective. She describes the education and religious formation of Catholics before and after the Second Vatican Council, the effects of the family on Catholic identity, and the effects of ethnicity on what it means to be Catholic. Just as Dr. Malony stresses the diversity within Protestantism, Dr. Kehoe also stresses that wide range of beliefs and commitment to those beliefs found within Catholicism. Finally, implications with regard to treatment modality, authority issues, fantasies and sins, religious messages, and countertransference issues are discussed.

Sally Barlow and Allen Bergin, professors of clinical psychology at Brigham Young University, provide a clear and concise description of the beliefs, practices, and values of Mormons and discuss how these might impact and influence psychological functioning and health. They passionately review the history and development of Mormonism, explore the difficulties that Mormons have had to endure to survive in the United States, examine the benefits and consequences of the close Mormon social system, explore special issues that Mormon women and unmarried members must face, review particular psychopathologies that may have been influenced by Mormon culture, and explore clinical issues that mental health professionals need to be aware of when working with Mormon patients.

Glenn Mosley, president and chief executive officer of the Association of Unity Churches, describes the Unity perspective on mental health, articulating the attitudes of Unity members toward medication, psychotherapy, and alternative treatments. Dr. Mosley underscores that alternative treatments are considered necessary, not optional, by many Unity members for recovery from mental health problems. Finally, he notes that the Unity philosophy strongly emphasizes the need to treat the whole person—spirit, mind, and body—and that prayer and meditation are essential for recovery.

Michael R. Zedek, rabbi of a large Jewish congregation in Kansas City, Missouri, briefly reviews the 4000-year-old history of Judaism, focusing on three major themes: God, Torah, and Israel. What does it mean culturally and spiritually to be a Jew? What has been the effect of world events during the past century on the way Jews look at health, illness, and death? What are some beliefs that distinguish an Orthodox from a conservative and a reformed Jew, and how might this impact their responses to mental health professionals? How might working with an Orthodox Jew's rabbi enhance the patient's receptivity to and effectiveness of psychotherapy and other mental health treatments? What are some basic differences in belief and worldview between Christians and Jews, and how might the clinician sensitively take these into account when working with Jewish patients.

Bruce Scotton, senior editor of *The Textbook of Transpersonal Psychiatry and Psychology* and associate professor of psychiatry at the University of California at San Francisco, examines the treatment of Buddhist patients. He succinctly reviews the basic tenets of Buddhist belief, resulting worldview, and psychological and behavioral tendencies of Buddhists and then provides a number of useful clinical pearls about assessing and treating Buddhist patients.

Nalini Juthani, associate professor of psychiatry at Albert Einstein College of Medicine, writes about treating Hindu patients. Dr. Juthani first briefly and clearly reviews basic information about the Hindu belief system and sacred texts and describes the six major elements of Hindu philosophy (Law of Karma, reincarnation, Dharma, guru, idol worship, and Ayurveda). She then examines 11 common practices of Hindu followers and how they might impact on the clinical evaluation and treatment of Hindu patients. She concludes her chapter by making recommendations on how to assess and treat Hindu patients in a way that both respects their belief system and enhances the clinician–patient relationship.

Syed Arshad Husain, professor and chief of child and adolescent psychiatry at the University of Missouri, Columbia, provides a skillful and ardent review of the historical background of Islam, the basic teachings of the Muslim faith, Muslim concepts of illness and wellness, and the role of prayer and spiritual therapies in healing. He profiles a Muslim patient and then discusses points to consider when evaluating a Muslim patient.

Taking a broad view of how cultural factors can influence the treatment of mental health problems of persons from diverse religious traditions, Atwood Gaines, professor of anthropology, nursing, psychiatry, and bioethics at Case Western Reserve University, examines religious and cultural aspects of professional (ethno) psychiatric theory and practice in the United States. Dr. Gaines stresses that with the advent of the anthropology of biomedicine, it has been discovered that cultural beliefs are just as prevalent and influential in "professional" medicine and psychiatry as they are in popular or folk health practices. Dr. Gaines focuses on the "core clinical functions" of psychiatry, such as help-seeking, the cultural construction of illness and clinical realities, the hermeneutic nature of clinical encounters, and the logic of therapeutic modalities. He concludes the chapter by considering some ethical implications of divergent beliefs for patient care in modern psychiatry.

Psychiatrists Harold Koenig and John Pritchett from Duke University begin Section V on clinical applications by exploring how the religious and spiritual beliefs of patients can be utilized in psychotherapy to achieve a more rapid and complete healing of emotional disorder. Various techniques, including taking a religious history and use of both prayer and scripture in psychotherapy, are described and sensitively discussed.

The next two chapters focus on the important role that clergy play in the mental health system and the need for greater collaboration between clergy and mental health professionals. First, chaplains Larry VandeCreek, David Carl, and Duane Parker examine the role of chaplains and nonparish clergy in the mental health system. They examine the chaplain's role in psychiatric inpatient facilities, the role of clergy as pastoral counselors, and the role of clergy as "mental health brokers" (performing as intermediaries or interpreters between religious congregations and the mental health system). Finally, they examine future directions that this ministry might take and how research might elucidate this effort.

Clergyman, psychologist, and prolific writer, Andrew Weaver, explores the important role that community clergy play as front-line mental health workers who provide nearly as much or more mental health services than do secular mental health professionals. He underscores the need for greater collaboration between mental health and religious professionals, discussing the barriers to collaboration and pointing out areas most fruitful for future linkages (depression and suicide among the elderly, elder abuse, family violence, psychological trauma, and working with populations of ethnic minorities, rural Americans, and adolescents).

Beginning Section VI, Elizabeth Bowman, well-known educator and associate professor of psychiatry at Indiana University School of Medicine, explores the integration of religion into the *education* of mental health professionals. After reviewing the literature on this topic, she examines why religion/spirituality should be taught, who should be taught, what should be taught, when it should be taught, and how it should be taught. In addition, Dr. Bowman discusses resistances likely to be encountered when attempting curricular integration and the rising interest and openness to religion and spirituality in society that are forcing changes in this area.

Finally, Dan G. Blazer, Duke University's dean of medical education, examines the response of academic psychiatry to the scientific study of religion and mental health. He examines the newest "empirical" approach to the study of religion and mental health, which he traces back to the initial work of Durkheim in the late 1800s. He then contrasts the empirical approach to the "humanistic," "postmodern," "pragmatic," "biological mechanistic," and "life cycle" approaches. Dr. Blazer stresses that the empirical approach which has proliferated in recent years at academic health centers is viewed as a partial approach at best by some (such as humanists) and a total erroneous approach by others (postmoderns). He concludes that the academician must recognize the considerable overlap in interests and methods across the approaches to studying religion and mental health and the need for more interdisciplinary conversation.

We conclude this volume with a summary and synthesis of the major take-home points. The *Handbook of Religion and Mental Health* will be useful to mental health and religious professionals alike as we strive to learn more about the religious or spiritual dimension of patients which we can no longer ignore. In his book, *Modern Man in Search of Soul,* Carl Jung (1933) stated, "Neurosis must be understood as the suffering of a human being who has not discovered what life means for him" (p. 260). As mental health professionals, we are often called on by our patients to help them to discover or rediscover new meaning for their lives. The struggle for meaning, purpose, and hope is not only a psychological endeavor but also a deeply spiritual one. I now invite you to read on and expand your understanding of the fascinating and complex relationship between religion and mental health.

REFERENCES

Jung, C. (1933). *Modern Man in Search of Soul.*

Turbott, J. (1996). Religion, spirituality and psychiatry: Conceptual, cultural and personal challenges. *Australian and New Zealand Journal of Psychiatry, 30,* 720–727.

SECTION

I

HISTORICAL

BACKGROUND

1

REFLECTIONS ON THE ROLE OF RELIGION IN THE HISTORY OF PSYCHIATRY

SAMUEL B. THIELMAN

Department of Psychiatry
Duke University Medical Center
Durham, North Carolina 27705

And almost every one when age,
Disease, or sorrows strike him,
Inclines to think there is a God,
Or something very like Him.
           —*Arthur Hugh Clough (1819–1861)*

Although the mental health literature of the twentieth century has often displayed a hostility toward religion, medical thinking about mental disorders of earlier times has often reflected a much more nuanced attitude toward religion and spirituality. Historically, Western medical writers have held a variety of views on the relationship between religion, spirituality, and madness. Plato, for example, wrote both of madness that was medically based and a madness resulting from a state of divine enthusiasm (Screech, 1980). The ancient Jews appear to have viewed madness in both natural and supernatural terms at various times (Rosen, 1968). Most Christian thinkers have seen no inherent contradiction between a medical view of madness and a Christian view that acknowledges the existence of supernatural forces at work in the world. Islam has a long tradition of compassion for those who are mad and a very complex view of the spiritual implications of madness (Dols, 1992).

Religions of Asia and Africa, on the other hand, tend to fuse ideas of demon possession and madness. Despite frequent claims to the contrary, medical explanations for madness have often coexisted with religious interpretations of madness in the world's great religions, and madness has not been seen by most religious adherents as a phenomenon that in itself explains spiritual states, religious belief, religious rituals, or the individual's awareness that a spiritual force beyond the self is influencing life. Though this chapter focuses on Christian thought about mental illness, other religious traditions undoubtedly have similarly complex views of madness.

ANCIENT WORLD

Religion and healing have been intertwined since earliest recorded history. Throughout history the role of the priest and physician have overlapped frequently and have in many cultures been difficult to separate. In the Bible, Exodus 13 and 14, priests are instructed to make determinations about the presence and management of leprosy. The medical literature of ancient Egypt and Babylon describe similar priestly roles. The relationship between spirituality and mental disease is somewhat more problematic than that of the relationship between spirituality and physical healing. When the faculty of reason is disrupted by dementia or by disease producing aberrant behavior there are often ambiguities that emerge. One has to look no further than the Bible to appreciate the multifaceted nature of the relationship between spirituality and mental health. For example in 1 Samuel 21:13, David (ca. 1000 BC) feigned madness to protect himself from the Philistine King Achish. The chronicler who wrote 1 Samuel makes clear that David was pretending to be mad and that the impact on King Achish was not one of fear but of derision, for Achish asks his court, "Do I lack madmen, that you have brought this fellow to play the madman in my presence?" (1 Samuel 21:15). However, the same book of the Bible records emotional turmoil of King Saul by saying that "the Spirit of the Lord departed from Saul, and an evil spirit from the Lord tormented him" (1 Samuel 16:14, Revised Standard Version), indicating that mental illness could be caused by an evil spirit sent by God.

PLATO

Early Christian thought was deeply influenced by Plato and Platonism, and Plato wrote at times about the relationship of the soul to mental health. In his work the *Timaeus* (fourth century BC/1977), Plato discussed the nature of diseases of the soul. Plato held that the soul consisted of three parts: The first part, composed of the faculties of reason and decision, was located in the head and was immortal. The part of the soul that experienced emotions was located in the heart. The part of the soul that experienced the physical appetites was located in the abdomen. In the *Timaeus,* Plato held that most instances of aberrant behavior could be attributed to bodily abnormality. Plato noted,

> It is generally true that it is unjust to blame overindulgence and pleasure as if wrongdoing were voluntary; no one wishes to be bad, but a bad man is bad because of some flaw in his physical makeup and failure as education, neither of which he likes or chooses. (p. 117)

He also asserted that humoral excess caused diseases of the soul and could lead to various sorts of mood instability, including irritability, depression, rashness, timidity, forgetfulness, and dullness. Mental disorders were multifactorial in origin; when individuals with flaws of temperament lived under bad forms of government, were offered inadequate education, and had inadequate upbringing, imbalance of the soul occurred. For Plato balance of the mind and body was essential to mental health. Plato (fourth century BC/1977) noted,

> When the mind is too big for the body its energy shakes the whole frame and fills it with inner disorders; the effort of study and research breaks it down, the stresses and controversies involved in teaching and argument, public or private, rack it with fever and bring on rheums which deceive most so-called physicians into wrong diagnosis. (p. 119)

For Plato, the principal safeguard against overemphasis of bodily or physical exercise was to avoid exercising the body without the mind or the mind without the body. He recommended that anyone engaged in mathematics or other strenuous intellectual pursuit should undertake physical training. Those who were involved in heavy physical exercise should engage in mental exercise and have cultural and intellectual interests (Plato, fourth century BC/1977, p. 119).

Plato's approach to mental life and spirituality becomes most interesting in his discussions of the charm because, at times, his discussion of the use of the charm contains parallels to current notions of the way words in therapy can be curative. These have been summarized and explored at some length by Pedro Lain Entralgo in his book *The Therapy of the Word in Classical Antiquity* (1958/1970). In Plato's early writings charm represents a magical force. In his later writings charm, or epode, represents a soothing table or soothing words. The charm, provided with medicine, provides more defective healing then simply bodily medicines alone. In Plato's view, it was a poor physician who treated only the body without attention to the epode, or charm, used to treat the soul (Lain Entralgo, 1958/1970). As a result, even though diseases of the soul might be caused by bodily humors, proper words were capable of healing.

THE CULT OF ASCLEPIUS

There were many gods of healing in the Roman Empire. Asclepius, however, was the god of the most widely practiced healing cult in the ancient world (Edelstein & Edelstein, 1945; Temkin, 1991; Temkin & Temkin, 1967). Asclepius is referred to in various ways in ancient literature; in the writings of Homer he is a mortal, but later Greek poets referred to him as the son of Apollo who had been raised by Cheiron, the centaur, who taught him how to cure disease. Shrines to Asclepius existed from at least the fifth century BC and Asclepian temples existed throughout ancient Greece and Rome (Edelstein & Edelstein, 1945; Temkin, 1991). The sick would come to the Asclepian temple, bringing offerings in the form of small images of the affected part. They would sleep in the temple, and healing took place during dreams in which Asclepius would come and provide a cure. Payment to Asclepius was made in the form of inscriptions and money. The cult of Asclepius existed in the ancient world side by side with Hippocratic medicine and Christianity. Galen, who was born in Pergamum, a center of the Asclepian cult, was a devotee of Asclepius. Like other sick people, the mad were taken to the Asclepian temples for cure (Simon, 1978, pp. 122–123).

Healing of all kinds in the ancient world generally seems to have taken place within a context that was religious. Though much has been made of the contrast between the naturalistic medicine and religious interpretations of disease, religious and medical views of disease in the ancient world were not mutually exclusive. Hippocratic medicine did, however, avoid supernatural interpretations of illness, including mental illness. This avoidance of pagan supernaturalism made Hippocratic medicine congenial to Christians and led to the acceptance of a natural origin of diseases of the body and mind by most early Christian writers. For the ancient philosophers of the West, as well as for early Christian writers, interpretation of the philosophical and spiritual meaning of mental disorders was inherently problematic.

Ancient writers, both Christian and pagan, lacked a precise vocabulary for describing various mental disorders and mood states. The fathers used many terms to describe discouragement or persistent sadness. Both Eastern and Western Christian writers at times used the word melagcolia (or melancholia), but this term referred to madness as often as it did to depression (Thielman & Thielman, 1997). Although the early Christians rejected Asclepius as a false god (Temkin, 1991, p. 118), many Christian writers found Hippocratic medicine congenial to Christian thought because its naturalistic approach focused on care of the body, eschewed the supernatural, and left the care of the soul to other philosophers. The medical authorities cited most frequently by the fathers (the Hippocratic writings and the writings of Soranus of Ephesus, Celsus, and Galen) held that persistent sadness proceeded from a disorder of black bile (Caelius Aurelianus, fifth century AD/1950, p. 561) and that both medicinal and psychological treatments could be used to relieve it.

Paradoxically, this lack of interest by the Hippocratic writers in problems of spirituality and the soul made Hippocratic medicine appealing to early Christian writers, who found the cult of Asclepius to be antithetical to the Christian view of Jesus Christ as the great physician and healer of mankind. The earliest Christian writers viewed Asclepius as being simply another pagan god to be avoided. He was condemned or ridiculed by Justin Martyr, Tertullian, Minucius Felix, and Tatian (Temkin, 1991, p. 118). By contrast, Christian writers often held the Hippocratic writers, Galen, Soranus of Ephesus, and Celsus, in high esteem.

Although some early Christians, such as Tatian, rejected the efforts of physicians, most early Christian writers after the third and fourth centuries AD seemed to value medical effort. References to physicians and their work are frequent in the writings of St. John Chrysostom. St. Augustine in particular refers often to Christ as the great physician, the healer of mankind. Of particular interest are the passages in which St. Augustine referred to Jesus himself as a healer of human souls. For Augustine, humans in their sin were like the madman, afflicted by a loss of reason and unable to accept the ministrations of the physician. Augustine viewed Christ as the physician who comes to the madman and as one who, despite resistance and even threat of physical harm, persists in efforts to heal. In using this analogy, Augustine tacitly indicated his acceptance of the validity of the efforts of the position of the body to heal diseases of mind. In his writings, as well as in those of other church fathers, we find indications of an understanding of the value of physical medicines in dealing with diseases of the mind.

Many of the church fathers wrote in ways that specifically acknowledged their acceptance of contemporary humoral physiology (Thielman & Thielman, 1997). Though the early Christian writers rarely wrote of "the four humors" per se, they did refer to humors in their writings. Their writings show there was a diversity of ideas about what humors represented and about their role in disease. They saw noxious humors as being evidence of disease and sometimes as causing disease. Jerome, writing in the fourth and fifth centuries, indicated an awareness of the Galenic synthesis of humoral theories (Jerome, ca. 400 AD/1994, p. 105), as did John Chrysostom, Jerome's contemporary, who wrote in Homily 10 from *On the Statues* that the body consisted of four "elements," namely, yellow bile, black bile, blood, and phlegm (Chrysostom, ca. 400 AD/1994, p. 105).

Beyond this implicit acceptance of the four humors, some fathers offered more specific theories about the effect of the body on the mind and soul. Gregory of Nyssa (ca. 330–395), one of the "Cappadocian Fathers" and a man widely read in Greek literature, observed in his treatise *On the Making of Man,* "Physicians declare that our intellect is also weakened by the membranes that underlie the sides being affected by disease . . . [and] they call the disease [caused by this weakening] frenzy, since the name given to those membranes is phrenes" (Gregory of Nyssa, fourth century/1994, p. 397). Gregory explained further that physicians believe that there is a compression and closing of the pores in grief, and as a result breathing becomes more labored; this is why people feel the need to groan during grief (Gregory of Nyssa, fourth century/1994, pp. 397–398). Gregory explained that this groaning depressed a region near the entrance to the stomach, causing bile to pour into the veins from excessive pressure, and created a jaundiced look.

Nemesius of Emesa (late fourth and early fifth century) wrote about the physiological effects of fear in his *On the Nature of Man* (fourth century/1955). This work looks to medical philosophy to explain a variety of mysteries about man and this mental and physical nature. In discussing emotions, Nemesius explained that fear causes a chilling of the extremities because the hot blood rushes to the heart, "just as a mob, when frightened, rushes to the rulers of the city" (pp. 360–361). He cited Galen to explain that fear produces an inflow of yellow bile into the stomach, producing a gnawing sensation that will be relieved by vomiting, and he observed that anger resulted from a heating of the blood around the heart. Nemesius seems to understand these changes in bile to be a result of the emotion as much as a cause of it, though he does not address the question of cause and effect. Humors and physiological explanations permeate the work.

The fathers exhibited not only an awareness of humoral physiology and the connection of the body with mental processes but also an interest in the physical basis of madness. Early Christian writings asserted repeatedly that the person who was mad was bereft of reason and was not responsible for his or her actions. Terms for madness were utilized most frequently by Christian writers as a means of describing the mind set of ecclesiastical opponents, but at times these writers referred to madness in passages that dealt directly with medical states of insanity or depression. Such references provide insight into Christian writers' understanding of states of mental disorder.

Early Christian writers certainly did not rely entirely on natural explanations for disease because the early church saw supernatural forces at work even where natural factors seemed to be the immediate cause of disease. The church father Origen (ca. 185–254) was particularly instrumental in formulating the demonological ideas of the early church. In his most important theological work, *De Principiis,* he observed that demons could completely take over the mind of an individual, thereby depriving the mind of the possessed of the power of understanding and emotion. He used the terms possession and insanity interchangeably and referred to Christ as having been a healer of the insane, although the New Testament records no instance of Christ healing anyone with mania (the term *mainetai* is used in the New Testament on five occasions, the most interesting of which is in John 10:20 when Jesus's opponents said "He has a demon and is out of his mind (mainomai)"). Matthew tells of Jesus healing the epileptics, which, in light of the Hippocratic view of epilepsy as a melancholic disease, has some relevance for understanding how the early church might have thought of melancholic diseases (Temkin, 1971, p. 54).

MEDIEVAL AND EARLY MODERN EUROPE

The views of the church toward mental illness and madness did not change significantly for a lengthy period of time. Kroll and Bachrach (1984) reviewed 57 descriptions of mental illness from pre-Crusade European literature and found that sin was mentioned as a cause of mental disorder in only 16% of the descriptions. Their review led them to conclude that medieval physicians did not heavily emphasize sin as a cause of insanity. Also, while medieval writers certainly considered demonic causation of mental illnesses possible or even probable, parallel naturalistic explanations were also used.

Renaissance medical literatures focused on naturalistic understandings and treatments of madness. Bartholomeus Anglicus (thirteenth century) observed in his work *De Proprietatibus Rerum* (1398/1975, p. 350) that mad patients should be entertained with musical instruments and should be kept occupied. Andrew Boorde, in his sixteenth-century health manual *A Breviary of Health* (1552, lxxvi), instructed those dealing with the mad to "kepe the pacient from musynge and studieng, and use myrth and mery communication."

Though many changes in medicine and science occurred during the time of the Renaissance and Reformation, ideas about mental illness remained fairly constant. One issue that the Reformers and Roman Catholics agreed on in the sixteenth century was that the devil existed and that he was supporting the opposite side very vigorously. Both Protestants and Catholics acknowledged the existence of demons and demonic possession. Abnormal mental states were sometimes (but not always) attributed to demons. Various writers also acknowledged both the existence of mental disorders related to bodily changes and those of a type of depression that was produced by bodily disease more than spiritual forces.

Melancholy was of interest to spiritual advisors. St. John of the Cross (1542–1591), whose *Dark Night of the Soul* described the purgation of the soul through the "night of the senses" and the "night of the spirit," advised Catholic confessors that some who come for confession are made much worse by instructions to retrace their sins. John of the Cross warned those receiving confession to be alert to the possibility that those who came to them might be suffering from melancholy more than the "dark night of the soul." Melancholy led to further despair and the dark night of the soul to spiritual growth. It was necessary for the confessor to determine the following of one who is in spiritual distress (John of the Cross, 1578/1962):

> Whether it be of sense or of spirit (which is the dark night whereof we speak), and how it may be known if it be melancholy or some other imperfection with respect to sense or to spirit. For there may be some souls who will think, or whose confessors will think, that God is leading them along this road of the dark night of spiritual purgation, whereas they may possibly be suffering only from some of the imperfections aforementioned.

EMERGING COMPLEXITIES OF THE EUROPEAN VIEW OF SPIRITUALITY AND MENTAL DISORDERS

Robert Burton, who coined the term "religious melancholy" in his classic work, *The Anatomy of Melancholy* (1621), attributed religious melancholy to a variety of causes, both natural and supernatural. Burton, however, was only one of many religious writers of the seventeenth century who wrote on topics relating to mental health. Another religious writer on melancholy, Timothy Rogers (1658–1728) was a Protestant minister who had suffered depression as a young man for a period of 2 years and continued to struggle with depression for years afterward. His book, *A Discourse Concerning Trouble of Mind* (1691), discounted the direct role of demons or the demonic in producing depression and emphasized instead the need for the sufferer of melancholia to receive compassionate and reassuring treatment by those with whom he or she came into contact. He wrote (as quoted in Hunter & McAlpine, 1963)

> Melancholy seizes on the Brain and Spirits, and incapacitates them for Thought or Action. . . . I pretend not to tell you what Medicines are proper to remove it, and I know of none; I leave you to advise with such as are learned in the Profession of Physick, and especially to have recourse to such Doctors as have themselves felt it. . . . Look upon those who are under this woful Disease of Melancholly with great pity and compassion. . . . Do not attribute the effects of meer Disease, to the Devil; though I deny not that the Devil has an hand in the causeing of several Diseases. . . . But notwithstanding all this, it is a very overwhelming thing to attribute every action almost of a Melancholy man to the Devil, when there are some unavoidable Expressions of sorrow which are purely natural, and which he cannot help. (pp. 248–250)

Rogers' sympathy toward sufferers of insanity and the manner in which he balanced spiritual, medical, and psychological concerns reflect a particular strain of thought within Christian writings that dealt with the complexities of mental disorders.

The scientific revolution of the seventeenth century and the social and intellectual ferment of the eighteenth century brought with them changes that affected thinking about madness at a variety of levels. The book of Johannes Weir (1515–1588), *De Praestigiis Daemonum* (1563), is usually cited as the first modern work to clearly assert that many who were thought to be possessed were suffering from madness. However, ideas of both physicians and religious thinkers from this period are complex. One very detailed study of Richard Napier, a seventeenth-century astrological physician, documented the intertwining of spiritual and medical thought in the treatment of madness in England during the time of the scientific revolution. Theologians, physicians, and the common people believed that mental disorders could be caused by either natural or supernatural forces (McDonald, 1981, p. 173).

Spiritual healers such as George Fox looked to God for healing of those under their care. The devil and the demonic forces often seemed to them to be behind many cases of madness, though people were less likely to see madness as a punishment from God than has sometimes been suggested (McDonald, 1981, pp. 173–175). McDonald, in his book *Mystical Bedlam,* described the practice of an astrological physician, Richard Napier. Napier used medicine, psychological healing, and astrological knowledge to treat the patients in his charge. Roy Porter described in a more general way the complex views of madness during the late seventeenth and eighteenth centuries (Porter, 1987). It was during this period that explicit references to the supernatural began to disappear from medical literature.

For instance, George Cheyne, in his book *The English Malady* (1733/1991) openly rejected explanations of nervous disorders that involved "witchcraft, enchantment, sorcery, and possession" (p. x). Cheyne was a religious person who wrote about both the difficulties that religious preoccupation could produce and the reassurance that religious study had to offer. He produced as evidence for his observations the positive effects of religious study on his own case of nervous distemper (Cheyne, 1733/1991, pp. 325–334). During the eighteenth century, physicians wrote a number of works about madness. Madness was also the subject of the writings of a number of clergy. Alexander Cruden, author of the best known concordance of the King James version of the Bible, suffered from a form of madness and wrote of his mistreatment in his book *The London Citizen Exceedingly Injured* (Porter, 1987, p. 270).

William Cowper (1731–1800), the author with John Newton of the *Olney Hymnal* and a secular poet of some notoriety, described at length his own early madness in a manuscript he called *Adelphi*. Although a member of the church in England, Cowper had not been particularly religious until this period, when he began to be quite preoccupied with negative religious ideas. Cowper apparently began to suffer some depressive symptoms in the early 1760s. He began to feel that God was reeking vengeance on him: "I saw plainly that God alone could deliver me, but was firmly persuaded that he would not and therefore omitted to ask it" (Cowper, 1772/1979, p. 17).

In November of that year, he went to an apothecary shop, "affecting as cheerful and unconstrained an air as I could" (Cowper, 1772/1979, p. 19). He asked for, and received, a vial of liquid laudanum that he intended to use to kill himself. Cowper lapsed into deeper depression and eventually was hospitalized at the Collegium Insanorum, a privately run asylum near St. Albans in England. There, Nathaniel Cotton (1705–1788), a physician trained by Hermann Boorhaave at Leyden, won his confidence. Cowper nonetheless continued to worry about spiritual matters, believing that Satan was tormenting him with thoughts of despair. Cotton, who was himself a devout man, apparently continued to watch Cowper quite closely. Eventually, Cowper improved and wrote of how

> much sweet communion I had with him [Dr. Cotton] concerning the things of our salvation. He visited me every morning while I stayed with him, which was near twelve months after my recovery, and the Gospel was always the delightful theme of our conversation. A sweet calm and serenity of mind succeeded this season of triumph. (pp. 40–41)

Cowper, who had been involved in the practice of law, left the asylum to stay with acquaintances. He eventually improved significantly but struggled repeatedly with very serious depressions throughout the rest of his life. Cowper's account of his treatment of insanity in *Ariel* and his thoughts on the relation of his own spirituality to his melancholia reflect the complexity of thought among evangelicals in eighteenth-century England regarding the nature and treatment of mental disorders.

RELIGION AND ASYLUM REFORM

The emergence of asylum reform in the eighteenth and nineteenth centuries was a complex phenomenon to which has been devoted a considerable body of historical literature. Among the many factors influencing reformers in England and the United States was the religious impulses of a variety of individuals, particularly of the Quakers who patterned their approach to the mentally ill after William and Samuel Tuke at the York Retreat. The importance of the religious impulse is not surprising, considering that religious themes are so common among psychiatric patients. Those who are depressed often feel that they are damned. Patients not uncommonly hear an audible voice of God telling them to do nonsensical things. Patients also frequently have impressions that they are on a grand religious mission or have special powers or abilities granted to them by God but unrecognized by others. Given the many ways in which psychiatric disorders overlap with religious themes, it would be unusual if these themes had been neglected by the very physicians attempting to treat the disorders involved.

Though histories of psychiatry often focus on institutional developments, sociological problems, or the evolution of a particular concept within psychiatry, psychiatric writers have sometimes attempted to sort out the manner in which a religious, spiritual, experiential, and biological forces shape the presentations of mental disorders. In the late eighteenth and early nineteenth centuries many medical writers wrote works on psychiatric topics. The late eighteenth century was also a time of reform in the care of the mentally ill. In France these reforms took place under the secular guidance of Philippe Pinel, who viewed religion as a negative force. Pinel wrote that it was very difficult to treat religious "enthusiasm." He believed that those who were religiously preoccupied should be separated from other patients, that every object relating to religion should be removed from these patients, that certain hours of the day should be devoted to philosophical readings, and that every opportunity should be taken to make adverse comparisons between "the distinguished acts of humanity and patriotism of the ancient, and the pious nullity and delirious extravagances of saints and anchorites" (Pinel, 1806/1962, p. 78).

Although convents and monasteries had historically offered comfort and care for the sick, hospitals gradually came under increasing secular control from the sixteenth century onward (Rosen, 1968). Bethlem Hospital in London offered care for the insane from 1247 onward, but it was not until the eighteenth century that madhouses and asylums became a significant source of care for the insane. Many factors contributed to the emergence of the asylum and private madhouses. These institutions, for all their shortcomings, provided some degree of care for the mad, but by the late eighteenth century, asylums and madhouses became the subject of reform. Some reformers acted out of secular motives and some reformers apparently sought personal recognition and gain, but some were motivated by religious commitment and moral indignation.

In many ways, the most fascinating of these people were the Tukes, the Quaker family instrumental in establishing the Retreat at York. William Tuke (1732–1822), a Quaker merchant, came to the conclusion that an institution for the care of insane Quakers should be established in their home town when a Quaker woman died in the York County asylum after apparent abuse. With the assistance of his son Henry, Quakers opened the Retreat, an institution that housed 30 patients, in 1796. Though the York Retreat was certainly not the first institution to incorporate humane treatment of the insane, the Tukes' particular style of treatment gained wide notoriety. William Tuke's grandson, Samuel Tuke (1784–1857), wrote *A Description of the Retreat at York* (1813), and this book in particular, which described the means of management of the insane at the York Retreat, received wide praise.

In contrast to Pinel's radically secular perspective, the retreat was permeated by the religious perspective of the Society of Friends. William, Henry, and Samuel Tuke believed that the insane should be treated with dignity and compassion because they were beings created in the image of God but deprived of the use of reason. In the Retreat's early days, the Bible was the principal source of reading matter (Digby, 1985, p. 45). The Tukes saw their work as a religious vocation and attempted to staff the retreat with Quakers or, if Quakers were not available, religiously committed individuals. The Retreat emphasized kindness, religious training, and the importance of spiritual factors in the restoration of sanity. It also stressed the importance of industriousness and orderliness in the treatment of mad patients (*Dictionary of National Biography,* 1885–1901; Digby, 1985).

BENJAMIN RUSH

This same complexity of thought is evident in the writings of Benjamin Rush (1746–1813), often referred to as the father of American psychiatry and undoubtedly the most influential American physician writing on the mind during the early nineteenth century. Rush's mother had taken him as a child to the second Presbyterian Church of Philadelphia, where Gilbert Tennent, an evangelist of the Great Awakening and associate of George Whitefield, had preached (D'Elia, 1974). He was also deeply influenced in his early years by the spirituality of his uncle, Samuel Finley, a "New Light" Presbyterian preacher of the Great Awakening, from whom he received his early formal education (D'Elia, 1974, pp. 9–20). On the other hand, Rush's exposure to the Scottish Enlightenment during his medical education in Edinburgh from 1766 to 1769 produced in him an intellectual commitment to the value of reason and natural philosophy. Consequently, Rush's philosophical approach was a fusion of evangelical pietism and Enlightenment philosophy that seems to have been particularly congenial to American physicians during the early years of the nineteenth century who often viewed him as a medical hero while eschewing most of his medical theories (Shryock, 1971).

In his influential book, *Medical Inquiries and Observations upon Diseases of the Mind* (1813/1962), Rush explained his view that the mind contained a "believing faculty" that could be diseased. Citing the New Testament as evidence for this view, Rush wrote that it was with this faculty that a person was able to believe in history, geography, public events, and family history. If the faculty were diseased, a person might believe things uncritically. On the other hand, if the faculty were affected in a different way, the sufferer might find that there was "an inability to believe things that are supported by all the evidence that usually enforces belief" (p. 273). This, for example, was what caused people to deny belief in the utility of medicine and to accept the medicine of quacks as well as the condition that caused a person to fail to accept the "truths of the Christian religion" while "believing in all the events of profane history" (p. 274). Reasoning and eloquent oration might help to alleviate this condition.

There were others who pursued a spiritual approach to psychiatry in the nineteenth century. Most notable was the German alienist Johann Christian Heinroth (1773–1843) of Leipzig whose *Lehrbuch der Störungen des Seelenlebens* (1818/1975) described the nature of mental disorder as being a result of spiritual disease and disorder. Heinroth devoted a significant part of this lengthy erudite book to a discussion of how disturbances of the soul could be prevented by a resolution of the soul's conflict (p. 428). Also, American asylum superintendents of the early nineteenth century, though not theoretically similar to Heinroth, often incorporated religious and spiritual elements into their treatment approach.

Historian Teresa Hill (1991) described the attitude toward religion in asylums in New England in the early nineteenth century. In 1838, Samuel B. Woodward (1787–1850) invited Thomas Hopkins Gallaudet (1787–1851) to become a regular chaplain to the Hartford Retreat (later the Institute of Living). At the McLean Asylum, superintendent Rufus Wyman (1778–1842), a Unitarian, and his successor Thomas G. Lee offered religious services to the patients of the McLean Asylum. Religion in the American asylums was generally of a variety that was noncontroversial and would not stir up religious delusions. Indeed, Isaac Ray (1807–1881), superintendent of the Butler Asylum and a pioneer of forensic psychiatry, thought religious services were of marginal benefit to patients.

Amariah Brigham (1798–1849), superintendent of the Utica Asylum and first editor of the *American Journal of Insanity,* believed that religious enthusiasm was a danger to mental health. However, most American superintendents of the first half of the nineteenth century seem to have viewed religion, rightly regarded, as having a beneficial effect on mental life. They also found that religion was a two-edged sword, and that a proper understanding of religion was important for patients. Indeed, many of the patients coming for care suffered from religious delusions and treatment of this condition was a major concern for the superintendents.

Psychiatry in the latter part of the nineteenth century focused on hereditarianism and the biological basis of madness. Pessimism about the prospects for improvement of the mad grew, and by the end of the century, psychiatry, like the rest of medicine, focused increasingly on physical pathology and, to a somewhat lesser extent, biological therapeutics. The latter part of the nineteenth century was the period in the United States when graduate schools emerged, professionalism in science took shape, and psychology separated from philosophy as an academic discipline (Ben-David, 1971).

Despite the radical secularism of psychoanalysis, early attempts were made by various clergy to incorporate psychoanalytic thought, viewed then as "scientific," into pastoral care. Freud's friend and admirer, Oskar Pfister (1873–1956), provided the earliest significant interchange between those of a religious point of view and early psychoanalytic thought. Pfister, a Swiss Lutheran pastor, developed an interest in psychoanalysis after he came across the work of Freud in 1908. He subsequently became a practicing lay psychoanalyst and developed a personal friendship with Freud that is reflected in their correspondence from 1909 until the time of Freud's death in 1939. Although Pfister remained a lifelong devotee of psychoanalysis, he objected to Freud's characterization of religion as an illusion or a delusion, and indeed, Freud, on one occasion, declared to Pfister (Meng & Freud, 1963, p. 17) that

> In itself psycho-analysis is neither religious nor non-religious, but an impartial tool which both priest and layman can use in the service of the sufferer. I am very much struck by the fact that it never occurred to me how extraordinarily helpful the psycho-analytic method might be in pastoral work, but that is surely accounted for by the remoteness from me, as a wicked pagan, of the whole system of ideas.

About the same time, liberal Protestant clergy in the United States developed an interest in psychology as a tool in pastoral care. The earliest notable manifestation of this interest was the Emmanuel movement, founded in 1905 by Elwood Worcester and Samuel McComb at Emmanuel Church, an Episcopalian church in Boston. Worcester, who had grown up in Rochester, New York, experienced a dramatic call to the ministry at age 16 and after attending Columbia College graduated from General Theological Seminary and, eventually, the University of Leipzig. At Leipzig, Worcester had come under the influence of two pioneers of modern experimental psychology, Wilhelm Wundt and Gustav Theodor Fechner. In 1904 Worcester was called to "Emmanuel Church" in Boston, where he subsequently combined forces with several prominent physicians to offer the insights of psychology to the Christian community. In 1905 Worcester was joined by Samuel McComb, a church historian born in Ireland who later taught at Queen's University at Kingston, Ontario.

The psychology of the Emmanuel movement was essentially a pre-Freudian form of psychotherapy that used suggestion, relaxation, and soothing talk to elicit relief of mental distress. Though the movement initially included prominent physicians such as James Jackson Putnam and Richard Cabot, these men eventually left because of concerns about the direction of the movement. Though the name Emmanuel movement was dropped when Worcester resigned from his parish in 1929, Worcester continued to treat troubled people until the time of his death in 1940.

Freud did not like the Emmanuel movement, with its religious overtones and therapeutic suggestion, and condemned it when he visited the United States in 1909. Although not harsh toward Freud, Worcester and McComb found psychoanalysis too rigid and dogmatic when they wrote of it in their book *Body, Mind and Spirit* (1931). Nonetheless, the Emmanuel movement led to an acceptance by Protestant churches of psychotherapeutic techniques and was an early forerunner of the modern pastoral care movement.

In certain circles in psychiatry and psychology in the twentieth century, religious ideas have sometimes been pathologized. In the nineteenth century, hospital superintendents noted that many of their patients suffered from religious delusions and sometimes referred to "religious insanity." Religious insanity had rarely been used as a formal diagnosis. Also, its disappearance from psychiatric discourse was at least in part related to the disappearance of the old diagnostic categories in the latter part of the century. Instead of classifying insanity under the broad categories such as mania, melancholia, and dementia, more sophisticated systems that took into account course and, where possible, pathophysiology came into use. As a result, interest in "exciting causes" and the various precipitants of mental disorder waned, and with it waned the interest in separating religious insanity from insanity caused by disappointment in romance, excessive study, sedentary life, or the loss of a loved one. Wilhelm Griesinger (1817–1868), in an influential textbook of psychiatry, largely ignored the topic of religion, though he did observe that religion seemed to have beneficial effects on mental health (Griesinger, 1867/1882, p. 347). A chapter on the delusions of the insane written in 1883 by E. C. Spitzka (1883, p. 28) noted that "systematized delusions of a religious character are usually rooted in an early developing devotional tendency, and brought to full bloom by incidental circumstances," but his discussion of religion forms a major part of a large work in insanity, and he viewed religious delusions as one of several forms of delusions that preoccupied an insane person.

During the early years of the twentieth century, psychiatry in the United States and Europe underwent a number of changes, most notable of which was an increasing emphasis on social progress and the general welfare of society. Several forces shaped the psychiatric stance toward things religious, most notably psychoanalysis but also an evolving body of literature on the psychology of religion, new religious movements such as New Thought, Christian Science, Theosophy, and spiritualism, as well as the growing social marginalization of fundamentalism, particularly after the Scopes Trial.

Furthermore, in terms of diagnosis, psychiatry was tending away from classifications based on the course and prognosis of disease so that psychiatrists such as Adolph Meyer came increasingly to view designations such as religious insanity or religious mania, which were based on the content of a delusion, as irrelevant to classification and treatment (Burnham, 1967, p. 67; Grob, 1983, pp. 112–118).

PROTESTANT LIBERALS AND PSYCHOANALYSIS IN THE UNITED STATES

Though the idea of religious insanity faded with the coming of twentieth-century psychiatry, it lived on in some form in the ideas of Sigmund Freud. Freud usually avoided viewing religion in terms of individual psychopathology. Rather, in several of his writings, most notably the *Future of an Illusion* (1927), he portrayed religion as something of a failed social phenomenon, a pathology of culture that had failed for thousands of years to cure the insecurities and unhappinesses of the human race. Despite Freud's antagonism toward religion, religionists found much to be admired in psychoanalysis and often sought rapprochement with it, particularly the liberal Protestants of the early twentieth century. As a result, even though

Freud viewed God as a projection of infantile wishes, psychoanalysis became one of the bases for the development of the clinical pastoral education movement of the early and mid portions of the twentieth century.

REINTEGRATION OF RELIGION INTO MENTAL HEALTH THINKING?

The report of the Group for the Advancement of Psychiatry on "The Psychic Function of Religion in Mental Illness and Health" (1968) took note of the fact that religious themes often surfaced during psychoanalysis, and that religion could be used in both psychically healthy and unhealthy ways. Just as the Menningers had sought to explore the relationship of religion and mental disorders in the early part of the nineteenth century, interest in religion continued in American psychiatry in the latter part of the twentieth century, despite the general abandonment of psychoanalytic thought and the ascendancy of a new interest in the neurosciences.

During the past 20 years, American psychiatry has undergone another transformation as the explosion of knowledge in the neurosciences and psychopharmacology has made the assumptions of classical psychoanalysis increasingly tangential to the concerns of psychiatry and has produced more physiologically based diagnoses and more effective pharmacological means for treating mental disorders.

The attempts of some to use psychiatric terms to legitimize the social stigmatization of cults and new religious movements have generally failed, though efforts to "deprogram" cult members using the rationale that cult leaders are using mind control or other mental means of authority have been used by some mental health professionals. The American Psychiatric Association has taken the position that it is not ethical for a psychiatrist to make a diagnosis of mental illness solely because the individual has joined a new religion or cult (Group for the Advancement of Psychiatry, 1968). In 1990 the American Psychiatric Association issued a position statement on possible conflict between a psychiatrist's religions commitments and psychiatric practice in which it condemned the use of psychiatry to promote a particular religious or political system of values (Ungerleider & Wellisch, 1989, p. 244).

One residue of the nineteenth-century interest in religious insanity could be found in the glossary of the third edition of the *Diagnostic and Statistical Manual of the American Psychiatric Association (DSM)*. Despite the absence of any terms that implied a religious origin of some mental illnesses, the glossary frequently used examples of psychopathology that had religious content, tacitly suggesting that religious themes often characterize mental illness. Several researchers criticized the *DSM* for its promotion of an unsubstantiated bias against religion and a new revision of the manual in 1995 exhibits a great sensitivity to religious belief and omits any potentially offensive references to religious belief (American Psychiatric Association, 1990). In addition, *DSM-IV* also included a diagnostic code, "Religious or Spiritual Problem," that can be used when individuals come to clinical attention who are experiencing distress as a result of conversion, a loss of faith, or a questioning of spiritual values (American Psychiatric Association, 1994). In this way, *DSM-IV* sought to recognize the importance of religion in the lives of people and to avoid a materialistic/reductionistic bias in psychiatric diagnosis.

Physicians who have treated mental disorders, and the sufferers of mental disorders, have inevitably had to face the problem of how the spiritual and religious dimensions of human existence relate to madness in all its various manifestations. Perhaps more than other conditions that are treated by physicians, disorders of the mind raise questions about the meaning of life, the presence of evil in the world, and the possibility that forces beyond our senses are influencing our lives. Since the earliest days of the practice of Western medicine, physicians working within the scientific tradition have recognized that religion and spirituality can affect the mind for both good and ill. Physicians, theologians, and philosophers have understood the nature and extent of this influence in a variety of ways. Though a comprehensive accounting of the historical relationship between religion and mental disorders may not soon (or ever) be possible, given the many religious perspectives of mankind and the manner in which mental disorders are culturally shaped, the scholarship available to date indicates that the relationship is a manifestly complex one. Perhaps a fuller understanding of this historical relationship will help us more accurately formulate our current notions of how faith and mental health are intertwined.

REFERENCES

American Psychiatric Association. (1990). Guidelines regarding possible conflict between psychiatrists' religious commitments and psychiatric practice (official actions). *American Journal of Psychiatry, 147,* 542.

American Psychiatric Association. (1994). *Diagnostic and statistical manual of mental disorders* (4th ed.). Washington, DC: Author.

Bartholomeus Anglicus. (1975). *Bartholomeus Anglicus on the Properties of Things: John Trevista's translation of Bartholomeus Anglicus De Proprietas Rerum. A critical text* (M. C. Seymour, Ed., 2 vols.). Oxford, UK: Clarendon. (Original work probably written mid-thirteenth century, translated by John Travista into English in 1398, and published in English in 1495)

Ben-David, J. (1971). *The scientist's role in society: A comparative study.* Englewood Cliffs, NJ: Prentice-Hall.

Boorde, A. (1552). *The Breviary of Healthe, for all manner of sicknesses and diseases the which may be in man or woman, doth folowe. Expressyng the obscure termes of Greke, Araby, Latyn, and Barbary, in Englishe concernyng Physicke and Chierurgerie, compyled by Andrew Boorde, of Physicke Doctour, an Englishe man.* London: W. Powell.

Burnham, J. C. (1967). *Psychoanalysis and American medicine, 1894–1918: Medicine, science, and culture.* New York: International Universities Press.

Burton, R. (1994). *The anatomy of melancholy.* (T. C. Faulkner, N. K. Kiessling, and R. L. Blair, Eds., 3 vols.). Oxford: Clarendon Press.

Caelius Aurelianus. (1950). *On acute and chronic diseases* (I. E. Drabkin, Ed. and Trans.). Chicago: University of Chicago Press. (This is Caelius Aurelianus's Latin translation of two lost works by the Greek physician Soranus of Ephesus [ca. 100 AD]. Original Latin translation was composed ca. fifth century AD)

Celsus. (1933). De medicina. Vol. 1. Loeb Classical Library. Celsus, De Medicina. Loeb Classical Library, Vol. 1.

Cheyne, G. (1991). *The English malady* (R. Porter, Ed.). London: Travestock/Routledge. (Original work published 1733)

Chrysostom, J. (1994). On the statues. In P. Schaff (Ed.), *Nicene and Post Nicene Fathers. Chrysostom: On the priesthood, ascetic treatises, select homilies and letters, homilies on the statues* (Ser. 1, Vol. 9). Peabody, MA: Hendrickson. (Chrosostom wrote ca. 400 AD; this translation originally published 1889)

Cowper, W. (1979). Adelphi: An account of the conversion of W. C. Esquire. In J. King & C. Ryskamp (Eds.), *The letters and prose writings of William Cowper* (Vol. 1). Oxford, UK: Oxford University Press. (Original work published 1772)

D'Elia, D. J. (1974). *Benjamin Rush: philosopher of the American revolution* (N.S. 64, Part 5, pp. 1–113). American Philosophical Society.

Dictionary of National Biography. (1885–1901). s.v. "Tuke, William" and "Tuke, Samuel." London: Smith, Elder.

Digby, A. (1985). *Madness, morality and medicine: A study of the York Retreat, 1796–1914.* Cambridge, UK: Cambridge University Press.

Dols, M. W. (1992). *Majnūn: The madman in medieval Islamic society.* Oxford: Clarendon Press.

Edelstein, L. (1967). *Ancient medicine: Selected papers of Ludwig Edelstein* (O. Temkin & C. L. Temkin, Eds.). Baltimore: Johns Hopkins University Press.

Edelstein, E. J. L., & Edelstein, L. (1945). *Asclepius: A collection and interpretation of the testimonies* (2 Vol.). Baltimore: Johns Hopkins Press.

Falshar, H. (1966). *Melancholie und Melancholiker in den medeizinischen Theorien der Antike* [Melancholy and the melancholic in the medical theories of antiquity.] Berlin: Weidemann.

Gregory of Nyssa. (1994). On the making of man. In P. Schaff & H. Wace (Eds.), *Nicene and post-Nicene fathers. Gregory of Nyssa: Dogmatic treatises, etc.* (Ser. 2, Vol. 5). Peabody, MA: Hendrickson. (Originally written mid-fourth century; this translation originally published 1893).

Griesinger, W. (1882). *Mental pathology and therapeutics* (C. L. Robertson & J. Rutherford, Trans., 2nd ed.). New York: William Wood. (Original work published as Die Pathologie und Therapie der psychischen Krankheiten in 1845, 2nd ed. 1867).

Grob, G. N. (1983). *Mental illness and American society, 1875–1940.* Princeton, NJ: Princeton University Press.

Group for the Advancement of Psychiatry, Committee on Psychiatry and Religion. (1968, January). The psychic function of religion in mental health and illness (No. 67). *Reports and Symposiums, 6,* 642–725.

Heinroth, J. C. (1975). *Textbook of disturbances of mental life: Or disturbances of the soul and their treatment* (Introduction by George Mora, 2 Vols.). Baltimore: Johns Hopkins University Press. (Original work published 1818)

Hill, T. L. (1991). *Religion, madness, and the asylum: A study of medicine and culture in New England, 1820–1840.* Unpublished doctoral dissertation, Brown University, Providence, RI.

Hunter, R., & McAlpine, I. (Eds.). (1963). *Three hundred years of psychiatry, 1535–1860.* London: Oxford University Press.

Jackson, S. (1986). *Melancholia and depression from Hippocratic times to modern times.* New Haven, CT: Yale University Press.

Jerome. (1994). Letters. In P. Schaff & H. Wace (Eds.), *Nicene and post-Nicene fathers. Jerome: Letters and select works* (Ser. 2, Vol. 6). Peabody,, MA: Hendrickson. (Jerome wrote ca. 400 AD; this translation first published 1894)

John of the Cross. (1962). *Ascent of Mount Carmel* (E. A. Peers, Trans.). Garden City, NY: Image Books. (Original work written 1578 and afterward)

Kroll, J., & Bachrach, B. (1984). Sin and mental illness in the Middle Ages. *Psychological Medicine, 14,* 507–514.

Lain Entralgo, P. (1970). *The therapy of the word in classical antiquity* (L. J. Rather & J. M. Sharp, Ed. and Trans.). New Haven, CT: Yale University Press. (Original work published 1958)

Larson, D. B., Thielman, S. B., et al. (1993). Religious content in the DSM-III-R "Glossary of Technical Terms." *American Journal of Psychiatry, 150,* 1884–1885.

McDonald, M. (1981). *Mystical bedlam: Madness, anxiety, and healing in seventeenth-century England.* Cambridge, UK: Cambridge University Press.

Meng, H., & Freud, E. L. (Eds.). (1963). *Psychoanalysis and faith: The letters of Sigmund Freud and Oskar Pfister.* New York: Basic Books.

Nemesius of Emesa. (1955). A treatise on the nature of man. In W. Telfer (Ed.), *Cyril of Jerusalem and Nemesius of Emesa.* Philadelphia: Westminster Press. (Original work probably written in the fourth century)

Pinel, P. (1962). *A treatise on insanity* (D. D. Davis, Trans.). New York: Hafner. (Davis's translation of Pinel's 1801 work. *Traité médico–philosophique sur l'aliénation mentale ou la manie,* originally published 1806)

Plato. (1977). *Timeaus and Critas* (L. Desmond, Trans.). New York: Penguin. (Original work written in fourth century BC)

Porter, R. (1987). *Mind forg'd manacles: A history of madness in England from the Restoration to the Regency.* Cambridge, MA: Harvard University Press.

Post, S. G. (1992). DSM-III-R and religion. *Social Science and Medicine, 35,* 81–90.

Rosen, G. (1968). *Madness in society: Chapters in the historical sociology of mental illness.* Chicago: University of Chicago Press.

Rush, B. (1962). *Medical inquires and observations upon diseases the mind.* New York: Hafner. (Original work published 1813)

Screech, M. A. (1980). *Ecstasy and the praise of folly.* London: Duckworth.

Shryock, R. H. (1971). The medical reputation of Benjamin Rush: Contrasts over two centuries. *Bulletin of the History of Medicine, 45,* 507–552.

Simon, B. (1978). *Mind and madness in ancient Greece.* Ithaca, NY: Cornell University Press.

Spitzka, E. C. (1883). *Insanity: Its classification, diagnosis and treatment: A manual for students and practitioners of medicine.* New York: Bermigham.

Temkin, O. (1971). *The falling sickness* (2nd ed.). Baltimore: Johns Hopkins University Press.

Temkin, O. (1991). *Hippocrates in a world of pagans and Christians.* Baltimore: Johns Hopkins University Press.

Thielman, S. B., & Thielman, F. S. (1997; April). *Constructing religious melancholy: Despair, melancholia, and spirituality in the writings of the church fathers of late antiquity.* Paper presented at the annual meeting of the American Association of the History of Medicine, Williamsburg, VA.

Ungerleider, J. T., & Wellisch, D. K. (1989). Deprogramming (involuntary departure), coercion, and cults. In M. Galanter (Ed.), *Cults and new religious movements: A report of the American Psychiatric Association.* Washington, DC: American Psychiatric Association.

Walton, F. R. (1970). Asclepius. In N. G. L. Hammond & H. H. Scullard (Eds.), Oxford classical dictionary (2nd ed.). Oxford, UK: Clarendon.

2

ETHICS, RELIGION, AND
MENTAL HEALTH

STEPHEN G. POST

Center for Biomedical Ethics
School of Medicine
Case Western Reserve University
Cleveland, Ohio 44106

Spirituality has to do with a sense of connectedness to nature, humanity, and the Transcendent. Although it need not be the case, spirituality often is contextualized within a religious tradition, i.e., a specific system of belief, worship, and conduct. Mounting empirical studies demonstrate that for many Americans, spirituality and/or religion are a very important means of coping with major illness. In recovery from illness, illness prevention and health enhancement, suicide prevention, substance abuse prevention, preventing heart disease and high blood pressure, negotiating with pain, and good dying, the clinical evidence for the impact of religious beliefs is increasingly strong (Larson & Milano, 1995). In a *Time/CNN* telephone poll of 1004 adult Americans, in response to the question "Doctors should join their patients in prayer if the patients request it?," 64% answered yes, 27% answered no, and the remainder were uncertain (*Time* 1996, June 24, p. 62).

Every Patient's Bill of Rights should include a statement that the patient has a right to practice his or her spirituality and religion in a respectful and supportive clinical environment. On the one hand, even the most skeptical clinician can be creatively concerned with the power of spirituality and religion rather than with their truth. Spirituality should not be disrespected in any clinical encounters. On the other hand, healthcare professionals with religious beliefs should not force religion on patients, but they should respond to the religious patient seeking some acknowledgment of his or her spirituality and religiousness and not have to worry about losing licensure for allowing a moment of silence or prayer.

Clinicians in modern industrialized cultures have placed a Jeffersonian wall of separation between the spheres of allopathic practice and religion and spirituality. Referral to pastoral care departments is the result, and this distinction in professional roles has probably served patients well in some respects, i.e., in preventing clinicians from using their power to impose a particular religion on the vulnerable patient (it is still possible that pastoral caregivers may impose their beliefs on the patient, but it is hoped that their training precludes this). However, the wall of separation has also blinded some clinicians to the importance of spiritual and religious concerns in the patient. Thus, there is now a movement afoot to replace the wall with a fence, since fences "make good neighbors" by allowing conversation as well as distinction.

This chapter constructively surveys a small number of the many areas of clinical care in which mental health professionals cannot fully succeed in establishing therapeutic empathy and efficacy without respecting and allowing a place for spirituality and religion.

SUFFERING AND DYING

Psychiatrists very often consult with patients who are dying and in discomfort. Psychiatrist F. Scott Peck, MD, argues that Americans cannot fully grapple with the issue of a good dying until discussion of spirituality is elevated to equal seating in the debate. There is an alternative to the overtreatment of the dying (with tubes in every orifice, natural and unnatural) and to assisted suicide (usually in the form of a physician prescribing lethal drugs) or voluntary euthanasia (physically unable to end their lives, patients request that this be done for them, usually by lethal injection). Specifically, the hospice tradition of a good dying, in which comfort, excellent pain relief, psychological and relational well-being, and pastoral–spiritual care combine to often tame the fear of death.

Often those who are dying face the problem of physical pain. Here Peck rebuffs his colleagues for their torturous ignorance of pain medication and its application. He points out "the bugaboo about addiction," for surely when a patient is fatally ill and in dire need of opiates, addiction is not even an issue. Physicians are not trained in palliative care so that the average patient in a hospital has no assurance of being kept comfortable. This is a point that no one familiar with the modern American hospital could question. Even with the best palliative care, a person with pain will generally ask why he or she undergoes such an ordeal, a question which invites discussion of the spirituality of meaning.

We seem to have forgotten the power of spirituality in dying. Physician priests in Tibet, for example, have long used and prescribed meditative techniques in the context of painful terminal illness. Meditation has caught on in many hospice settings and among thanatologists as a method to enhance terminal care. In the Western tradition, meditation and prayer were an integral part of the vast *ars moriendi* ("art of dying") literature that was among the most popular in the late Middle Ages. Peck argues that we need to regain the confidence of our forbears in the continuing love and presence of God in our experiences of dying.

Whether one wishes to accept Peck's faith stance or not, the psychiatrist should always harness the power of (in contrast to "the truth of") spirituality and religion by merely honoring it in the experiences of the dying (Post, 1993). Immanuel Jakobovits (1975), Chief Rabbi of the British Commonwealth of Nations, in his classic *Jewish Medical Ethics,* wrote that "disease forges an especially close link between God and man; the Divine Presence Itself, as it were, 'rests on the head of the sickbed'" (p. 2). Human beings wish to protect themselves through the security of daily routines that provide order and control over existence. When pain and dying break in, the routine is lost. As it turns out, the routine is not real because human beings are fragile and subject to contingencies over which they hold no ultimate control. At this point, many (but not all) people with a terminal diagnosis call out to some higher being in the universe who, according to their beliefs, does have control. One need not be a believer to recognize the historic interrelationship of medicine and spirituality–religion. All religious traditions provide the self with interpretations and coping strategies to navigate this fragility (Post, 1995b).

The literature on pain, suffering, and spiritual well-being is impressive. Pain is a complex, multidimensional perception with affective and sensory features; suffering refers to the self-perception of threat to the integrity of the self and the exhaustion of psychosocial and personal resources for coping (Chapman & Gavrin, 1993). Spirituality and religion are so much a part of these personal resources that any lack of appreciation for them in this context must be considered poor medical practice, if not malpractice.

THE PHENOMENON OF HOPE

Whether a terminal or a chronic diagnosis is revealed to the patient, hope is utterly important and falls within the concerns of any worthy psychiatrist. Hope is a multidimensional dynamic attribute of an individual that concerns dimensions of possibility and confidence in future outcome (Frankl, 1993). Hope can address secular matters, such as future plans and relationships, or religious matters of ultimate destiny. Hope is an aspect of spiritual well-being (Carson, Soeken, & Grimm, 1988). It has been studied in cancer patients (Brandt, 1987; Dufault, 1981; Herth, 1989; Kodish & Post, 1995; Nowotny, 1989; Owen, 1989) and in patients with AIDS (Carson, Soeken, Shanty, & Terry, 1990).

Preservation of hope can maximize a patient's psychological adjustment to a severe diagnosis. The cerebral neurobiology of hope and hopelessness has been carefully studied by a team of psychiatric researchers drawing on positron emission tomography (Gottschalk, Fronczek, & Buchsbaum, 1993). The importance of a spirituality of hope in the lives of people with disability has been summarized at the Conference on "The Roles of Religiousness and Spirituality in Rehabilitation and the Lives of those with Disability," held at the National Institutes of Health in May 1995 (Underwood-Gordon, 1995). Hope need not exist within the context of a world religion, although it often does.

A 1993 survey conducted in an inpatient rehabilitation unit indicated that 74% of patients hold their religious and spiritual beliefs to be important, 54% desire pastoral counseling, and 45% think not enough attention is given to spiritual and religious beliefs. The authors concluded that rehabilitation personnel should be aware of the diversity of religious beliefs held by patients and should address these when necessary with respect (Anderson, Anderson, & Felsenthal, 1993).

Hope is the subjective sense of having a meaningful future despite obstacles. In times of severe disabling injury, hope may be mediated through ritual, meditation, prayer, and traditional sacred narratives. The experience of many such patients is a spiritual–religious construct.

Much more active pastoral care in the clinical context of diagnosis could allow people to retain hope with diagnostic disclosure. Questions such as the following can be brought into the clinical context:

Do you believe there is a reason or purpose for your illness? If yes, what do you think that reason or purpose is?

Do you think that your religious beliefs and community can contribute to your well-being in these circumstances?

The spiritual history of patients can be very useful in understanding their sources of well-being and in helping them to identify spiritual resources in the community (Maugans, 1996). Psychiatrists should acknowledge the importance of spirituality and religion in maintaining hope in diagnosed individuals, refer to clergy, but also respond (if willing) to the patient's requests for spirituality in the physician–patient relationship.

SPIRITUALITY AND QUALITY OF LIFE IN CHRONIC ILLNESS

One of the finest autobiographical accounts of living with the diagnosis and initial decline of probably Alzheimer's disease (AD) is Rev. Robert Davis' *My Journey into Alzheimer's Disease* (1989). He writes as follows:

> One night in Wyoming, as I lay in a motel crying out to my Lord, my long desperate prayers were suddenly answered. As I lay there in the blackness silently shrieking out my often repreated prayer, there was suddenly a light that seemed to fill my very soul. The sweet, holy presence of Christ came to me. He spoke to my spirit and said, "Take my peace. Stop your struggling. It is all right. This is all in keeping with my will for your life. . . . Lie back in your Shepherd's arms, and take my peace. (p. 55)

As Rev. Davis (1989) "mourned the loss of old abilities," he nevertheless could draw on his Christianity: "I choose to take things moment by moment, thankful for everything that I have, instead of raging wildly at the things that I have lost" (p. 57). However, as he struggled to find a degree of peace amidst decline, he was also keenly aware of people who "simply cannot handle being around someone who is mentally and emotionally impaired" (p. 115). In his church community, and through the love of his wife, the journey was at least more navigable.

People with a diagnosis of AD often pray, for they are thrown back onto whatever faith they have in the meaningful and beneficent purposes underlying the universe. They pray because the routine and the control has been taken from their lives, and probably because they fear the future. They are shaken existentially and must begin a final phase of their journey in remarkable trust. The person with a diagnosis of AD will often desire to pray with family members, to pray in religious communities, and to pray alone. The word prayer comes from the Latin *precari*, "to entreat," or ask earnestly. It comes from the same root as the word precarious, and it is in the precariousness of emerging forgetfulness that often drives the person with dementia to prayer. Prayer is one way of enhancing hope in the future despite dementia.

To present the picture of people with dementia as meaning seeking, I borrow from an autobiographical account in my book, *The Moral Challenge of Alzheimer Disease* (Post, 1995a). The following story—only lightly edited—was told by a woman in her mid-40s with dementia, etiology unknown. She is conversant, although there are some days when she is too mentally confused to engage in much dialogue. She has more difficulty responding to open-ended questions but does very well if her conversation partner cues her by mentioning several alternative words from which she might choose, at which point she can be quite articulate:

> It was just about this time three years ago that I recall laughing with my sister while in dance class at my turning the big 40. "Don't worry, life begins at forty," she exclaimed and then sweetly advised her younger sister of all the wonders in life still to be found. Little did either of us realize what a cruel twist life was proceeding to take. It was a fate neither she nor I ever imagined someone in our age group could encounter.
>
> Things began to happen that I just couldn't understand. There were times I addressed friends by the wrong name. Comprehending conversations seemed almost impossible. My attention span became quite short. Notes were needed to remind me of things to be done and how to do them. I would slur my speech, use inappropriate words, or simply eliminate one from a sentence. This caused not only frustration for me but also a great deal of embarrassment. Then came the times I honestly could not remember how to plan a meal or shop for groceries.
>
> One day, while out for a walk on my usual path in a city in which I had resided for 11 years, nothing looked familiar. It was as if I was lost in a foreign land, yet I had the sense to ask for directions home.
>
> There were more days than not when I was perfectly fine; but to me, they did not make up for the ones that weren't. I knew there was something terribly wrong and after 18 months of undergoing a tremendous amount of tests and countless visits to various doctors, I was proven right.
>
> Dementia is the disease, they say, cause unknown. At this point it no longer mattered to me just what that cause was because the tests eliminated the reversible ones, my hospital coverage was gone, and my spirit was too worn to even care about the name of something irreversible.
>
> I was angry. I was broken and this was something I could not fix, nor to date can anyone fix it for me. How was I to live without myself? I wanted her back!

She was a strong and independent woman. She always tried so hard to be a loving wife, a good mother, a caring friend and a dedicated employee. She had self-confidence and enjoyed life. She never imagined that by the age of 41 she would be forced into retirement. She had not yet observed even one of her sons graduate from college, nor known the pleasures of a daughter-in-law, or held a grandchild in her arms.

> Needless to say, the future did not look bright. The leader must now learn to follow. Adversities in life were once looked upon as a challenge; now they're just confusing situations that someone else must handle. Control of *my life* will slowly be relinquished to others. I must learn to trust—completely.
>
> An intense fear enveloped my entire being as I mourned the loss of what was and the hopes and dreams that might never be. How could this be happening to me? What exactly will become of me? These questions occupied much of my time for far too many days.
>
> Then one day as I fumbled around the kitchen to prepare a pot of coffee, something caught my eye through the window. It had snowed and I had truly forgotten what a beautiful sight a soft, gentle snowfall could be. I eagerly but so slowly dressed and went outside to join my son, who was shoveling our driveway. As I bent down to gather a mass of those radiantly white flakes on my shovel, it seemed as though I could do nothing but marvel at their beauty. Needless to say, he did not share in my enthusiasm; to him it was a job, but to me it was an experience.
>
> Later I realized that for a short period of time, God granted me the ability to see a snowfall through the same innocent eyes of the child I once was, so many years ago. I am still here, I thought, and there will be wonders to be held in each new day; they are just different now.
>
> Quality of life is different to me now from the way it was before. I am very loved, in the early stages, and now my husband and my sons give back in love what I gave them. I am blessed because I am loved. That woman who killed herself, you know, with that suicide doctor. She didn't have to wind up that way. Not that I condemn her, but our lives can't really be that bad. Her choice is understandable if she wasn't loved or cared for. Now my quality of life is feeding the dogs, looking at the flowers. My husband says I am more content now than ever before! Love and dignity, those are the keys. This brings you back down to the basics in life, a smile makes you happy.

The most remarkable theology of dementia is David Keck's *Forgetting Whose We Are: Alzheimer's Disease and the Love of God* (1996). Keck describes the experience of his mother, who has suffered with AD for more than a decade. He asserts that asthetic experience is still open to his mother, who seems enchanted by the beauty of a wooded path; he believes that she thrives in church, stimulated by hymns, the sense of community, and well-known litanies. While her purposeful means–ends reasoning is seriously diminished, she still seems to appreciate the glory of God's creation. Keck suggests that his mother may in some respects be closer to this appreciation of creation than the routines of our busy lives usually permit.

SPIRITUALITY IN THE LIVES OF CAREGIVERS

Caregivers often pray for loved ones with dementia. There is no need to follow Sir Francis Galton, who in 1883 proposed that prayer is ineffective because clergy, who purportedly pray more than lawyers or physicians, nevertheless live slightly shorter lives based on mortality rates between 1758 and 1843 in England. The results of recent prayer studies can best be described as inconsistent. After all, in the Hebrew Bible Abraham prayed for the recovery of Abimelech, and God healed him (Gen. 20:17); but when David prayed for the recovery of his son, his son died (II Sam. 12:16). According to most rabbinic opinion, the claim that God must answer a prayer is presumptuous and represents a transgression. In the words of Rosnor (1986), the Hebrew Bible and the Talmud indicate that prayer is thought to be efficacious if offered by the proper person at the proper time with the proper intent and under the proper circumstances (pp. 355–362).

The fact remains that the vast majority of humankind prays for the sick. This is clearly the case with family members caring for loved ones with AD. In a recent study of religiosity variables in relation to perceived caregiver rewards, African American women caring for elderly persons with major deficits in activities of daily living perceived greater benefits through caring based on a spiritual–religious reframing of their situation. Religiosity indicators (i.e., "prayer, comfort from religion, self-rated religiosity, attendence at religious services") are especially significant as coping resources in African American women caregivers (Picot, Debanne, Namazi, & Wykle, 1997). Religiosity is a clear stress deterrent and therefore also impacts depression rates, which are extraordinarily high in AD caregivers. These authors suggest that "if religiosity indicators are shown to enhance a caregiver's perceived rewards, health care professionals could encourage caregivers to use their religiosity to reduce the negative consequences and increase the rewards of caregiving" (p. 89). This seems self-evident.

From a purely economic perspective, the spirituality of caregivers can sustain their abilities to care and thus keep people with AD out of nursing homes longer. While this is not an unambiguous goal, the fact is that nursing home care costs families and the medicaid system a great deal of money.

PSYCHIATRY: CAREER, PROFESSION, AND VOCATION

For those concerned about the moral drift of psychiatry downward toward pure self-interested careerism, spirituality may have much to offer the professional. The other-regarding solicitude in professional life may be facilitated by a better understanding of the ways in which a highly altruistic religious notion of vocation classically shaped and formed the ethos of Western medical professional life. The idea of "professionalism" implies that there is something rather unique to be "professed," namely, that care for the ill is at the motivational center of the physician's life.

With specific attention to the Roman Catholic tradition, and to a "Christocentric ethics" informed by the ministry of Jesus of Nazareth to the ill of mind and body, Pellegrino and Thomasma (1997) assert a well-established principle of Christian love and justice—the principle of care for the most vulnerable (or "the least") among us. Thus, the professional whose endeavors are seasoned by vocational idealism (the sense of a higher divine meaning and purpose that calls the professional to elevated heights of altruism) will want to direct attention to the socially marginal (e.g., the mentally ill, the demented, AIDS patients, and the poor).

There was a time when "Medicine as a means of livelihood, prestige, power, and preferments—as a career—was secondary to medicine as a calling" (Pellegrino and Thomasma, 1997, p. 87). Regardless of one's religious commitments, Pellegrino and Thomasma define one of the critical moral questions for all those concerned with professions and their decline: Can we anymore rise above greed and self-interest to rediscover the meaning and purpose of genuine service? If not, then the idea of the professional will be lost to the idea of the careerist, and perhaps the only moral idealism left will be discerned in those whose medical practice is elevated by the spirituality of vocational giving and self-denial. Professions are meant to be the most noble of callings, and yet they do seem to have lost some of their more elevating qualities. A good deal of moral idealism ("do unto others as you would have them do unto you") has been grounded in our spiritual–religious traditions, and these traditions may still contribute to the moral fiber of the psychiatric profession, as they did in the nineteenth century.

REFERENCES

Anderson, J. M., Anderson, L. J., & Felsenthal, G. (1993). Pastoral needs for support within an inpatient rehabilitation unit. *Archives of Physical Medicine and Rehabilitation, 74,* 574–578.

Brandt, B. T. (1987). The relationship between hopelessness and selected variables in women receiving chemotherapy for breast cancer. *Oncology Nursing Forum, 14,*(2), 35–39.

Carson, V., Soeken, K. L., & Grimm, P. M. (1988). Hope and its relationship to spiritual well-being. *Journal of Psychology and Theology, 16,* 159–167.

Carson, V., Soeken, K. L., Shanty, J., & Terry, L. (1990). Hope and spiritual well-being: Essentials for living with AIDS. *Perspectives in Psychiatric Care, 26*(2), 28–34.

Chapman, C. R., & Gavrin, J. (1993). Suffering and its relationship to pain. *Journal of Palliative Care, 9*(2), 5–13.

Davis, R. (with help from his wife Betty). (1989). *My journey into Alzheimer's disease: Helpful insights for family and friends.* Wheaton, IL: Tyndale House.

Dufault, K. J. (1981). Hope of elderly persons with cancer (Doctoral dissertation, Case Western Reserve University). *Dissertation Abstracts International, 42,* 1820-B.

Frankl, V. (1963). *Man's search for meaning.* Boston: Beacon.

Gottschalk, L. A., Fronczek, J., & Buchsbaum, M. S. (1993). The cerebral neurobiology of hope and hopelessness. *Psychiatry, 58,* 270–281.

Herth, K. A. (1989). The relationship between level of hope and level of coping response and other variables in patients with cancer. *Oncology Nursing Forum, 16*(1), 67–72.

Jakobovits, I. (1975). *Jewish medical ethics.* New York: Block.

Keck, D. (1996). *Forgetting whose we are: Alzheimer's disease and the love of God.* Nashville, TN: Abington.

Kodish, E., & Post, S. G. (1995). Oncology and hope. *Journal of Clinical Oncology, 13,* 1817–1822.

Larson, D. B., & Milano, M. A. (1995). Are religion and spirituality clinically relevant in health care? *Mind/Body Medicine, 1,* 147–157.

Maugans, T. A. (1996). The SPIRITual history. *Archives of Family Medicine, 5,* 11–16.

Nowotny, M. L. (1989). Assessment of hope in patients with cancer: Development of an instrument. *Oncology Nursing Forum, 16*(1), 57–61.

Owen, D. C. (1989). Nurses perspectives on the meaning of hope in patients with cancer: A qualitative study. *Oncology Nursing Forum, 16*(1), 75–79.

Peck, F. S. (1997). *Denial of the soul: Spiritual and medical perspectives on euthanasia and mortality.* New York: Harmony.

Pellegrino, E. D., & Thomasma, D. C. (1997). *Helping and healing: Religious commitment in health care.* Washington, DC: Georgetown University Press.

Picot, S. J., Dehanne, S. M., Namazi, K. H., & Wykle, M. L. (1997). Religiosity and perceived rewards of black and white caregivers. *The Gerontologist, 37*(1), 89–101.

Post, S. G. (1993). *Inquiries in bioethics.* Washington, DC: Georgetown University Press.

Post, S. G. (1995a). *The moral challenge of Alzheimer disease.* Baltimore: Johns Hopkins University Press.

Post, S. G. (1995b). Medicine and religion. In J. Z. Smith & W. S. Green (Eds.), *The HarperCollins dictionary of religion* (with the American Academy of Religion) (pp. 690–691). New York: HarperCollins.

Richard, W. C., & Kornfield, H. S. (1995). *Life to death: Harmonizing the transition.* Rochester, VT: Inner Traditions.

Rosnor, F. (1986). *Modern medicine and Jewish ethics.* New York: Yeshiva University Press.

Underwood-Gordon, L. (1995). A working model of health: Spirituality and religiousness as resources: Applications to persons with disability (unpublished). Bethesda, MD: National Institutes of Health.

A New Research Frontier

3

RESEARCH ON RELIGION AND MENTAL HEALTH: AN OVERVIEW OF EMPIRICAL FINDINGS AND THEORETICAL ISSUES

JEFFREY S. LEVIN

National Institute for Healthcare Research
Rockville, Maryland 20852

LINDA M. CHATTERS

Department of Health Behavior and Health Education
School of Public Health
University of Michigan
Ann Arbor, Michigan 48109

One of the central issues concerning the role of religion in human affairs has been its relationship to constructs such as mental health, emotional well-being, and adjustment. While debate concerning the positive versus negative contributions of religion to mental health and related concepts is long-standing, it is only recently that theory and research have addressed these issues in a systematic and rigorous manner. A considerable amount of work has been conducted on this topic, particularly in the fields of gerontology and geriatrics. Over the past decade, researchers in the areas of clinical practice, epidemiology, and the social sciences have contributed to the development and growth of a new field of religion, aging, and mental health.

This chapter provides an overview of research on the influence of religious involvement on psychiatric and mental health outcomes by summarizing existing empirical findings and recent theoretical developments in the field. First, empirical findings from studies of religious effects on mental health outcomes are briefly reviewed. This section includes summaries both of clinical and epidemiologic studies and of social and gerontological research. Second, several salutogenic mechanisms or pathways are proposed as possible explanations for religious effects on mental health, including health-related behavior, social support, positive emotions, health beliefs or personality styles, and optimism and hope. Third, midrange theoretical models are proposed as ways to understand the interrelation of these potential mediating factors with religion and mental and physical health. This discussion focuses on five distinct specifications, termed suppressor, distress-deterrent, prevention, moderator, and health effects models. Finally, implications of these findings and theories for researchers and clinicians are discussed.

EMPIRICAL RESEARCH ON RELIGION AND MENTAL HEALTH

For the past century, numerous epidemiologic and clinical studies have documented the influence of religious affiliation and religious involvement on physical and mental health outcomes. While remaining a generally obscure area of research, over 200 published studies have investigated religious differences in a wide range of health outcomes and have examined the effects of dimensions of religiosity on health status indicators and measures of disease states (Levin & Schiller, 1987). Nearly every major disease entity and cancer site has been studied with regard to religion. Especially large bodies of published data exist for cardiovascular disease (Levin & Schiller, 1987), hypertension and stroke (Levin & Vanderpool, 1989), cancer (Troyer, 1988), and overall and cause-specific mortality (Jarvis & Northcutt, 1987). This literature is not widely known perhaps because few of these studies were designed specifically to study the effects of religion on health. Rather, these investigations of atherosclerosis, cervical cancer, respiratory disease, life expectancy, colitis, and other outcomes collected data on a range of social, psychological, and biological variables, among which were one or more religious indicators. Subsequent statistical findings bearing on the impact of these religious variables on the respective health outcome or disease being studied often ended up buried in a table and then not discussed further, mentioned in the abstract, or indexed as a key word.

In large part, results from these studies have been consistent in indicating a salutary relationship between religious involvement and health status. However, since most of the studies in this literature were not designed solely and explicitly to investigate this issue, coupled with a paucity of true experimental evidence, no one study is ideally designed to "prove" that religion exerts a positive influence on health. Across this literature, however, the consistency of findings despite the diversity of samples, designs, methodologies, religious measures, health outcomes, and population characteristics actually serves to strengthen the inference of a positive association between religion and health. This finding has been observed in

studies of old, middle-aged, and young respondents; in men and women; in subjects from the United States, Europe, Africa, and Asia; in research conducted in
the 1930s and into the 1990s; in case-control, prospective cohort, cross-sectional,
and panel studies; in Protestants, Catholics, Jews, Muslims, Buddhists, Parsis, and
Zulus; in studies operationalizing religiosity as any of over a dozen variables (religious attendance, prayer, Bible reading, church membership, subjective religiousness, Yeshiva education, etc.); in research limited to *t* tests and bivariate correlations and in research testing structural–equation models with LISREL; and in
U.S. studies, among Anglo-whites, Hispanics, Asian Americans, and African
Americans (Levin, 1994a). The volume and consistency of findings have led to
calls for more systematic study of the "epidemiology of religion" (Levin & Vanderpool, 1987).

The influence of religious involvement on specifically mental health outcomes
has been a focus of considerable research for many years. However, this work, too,
is not widely known within the fields of psychiatry or mental health research. Literature reviews have identified hundreds of published studies reporting associations between religious variables and mental health outcomes (Bergin, 1983; Gartner, Larson, & Allen, 1991), generally pointing to a salutary religious effect
(Larson et al., 1992).

CLINICAL AND EPIDEMIOLOGIC RESEARCH

Over 10 years ago, *The American Journal of Psychiatry* published a systematic review critiquing research on religion published in psychiatry journals (Larson,
Pattison, Blazer, Omran, & Kaplan, 1986). The authors suggested that "the clinical practice of psychiatry is ill-served by the current inadequacies in the psychiatric literature" which serve to discourage "a sophisticated appreciation of the conceptual and empirical knowledge linking both psychiatry and religion" (p. 333). A
1992 follow-up review also published in *The American Journal of Psychiatry* (Larson et al., 1992) noted the persistence of earlier, paradoxical trends: Between 1978
and 1989, an impressive 139 quantified religious commitment measures appeared
in articles published in either *The American Journal of Psychiatry* or *Archives of
General Psychiatry*. However, for 78% of these measures no hypothesis was tested and for 64% of these no association with a mental health outcome was actually tested. Psychiatric researchers in considerable numbers apparently agree that religious involvement is worth studying as a potential protective or risk factor, yet
they are reluctant to pursue these questions or are unsure of how to proceed in the
absence of widespread dissemination of prior findings and theoretical work. Another significant factor may be the perception that consideration of "the *R* word"
(Larson, Sherrill, & Lyons, 1994) represents an "anti-tenure factor" (Sherrill &
Larson, 1994) for academic psychiatrists. According to Peck (1993), in an address
to the American Psychiatric Association in 1992, "Psychiatry has not only neglected but actively ignored the issue of spirituality" (p. 233), a situation he termed
"psychiatry's predicament" (p. 232).

For several decades, empirical research findings and literature reviews cumulating such findings have reported strong, positive associations between measures of religious involvement and mental health outcomes. Over 35 years ago, investigators from the seminal Midtown Manhattan Study (Srole & Langner, 1962) compared the prevalence of mental illness among active and currently "unchurched" Catholics, Protestants, and Jews. They found higher ratios of impaired to well respondents among currently nonaffiliated from all three religious groups, in comparison with such ratios among respondents still active in their religion of origin. About 10 years later, several new studies supported these findings. Longitudinal data from New Haven found an inverse, "dose–response" relationship between degree of psychological impairment and indicators of religious affiliation and frequent religious attendance (Lindenthal, Myers, Pepper, & Stern, 1970). Stark (1971) reviewed data from a case-control study of religious commitment among mental health clinic outpatients in California. He found that individuals diagnosed as mentally ill were less likely to be religiously affiliated, more likely to report that religion was not important to them, less likely to belong to a church or synagogue, and more likely never to attend services. Wilson (1972) studied a sample of Protestants from North Carolina who had undergone a "born-again" salvation experience. Respondents subsequently reported less depression, fear, confusion, anger, and pain.

Such findings are typical of early work from the 1960s and 1970s. A meta-analysis of 24 studies of religion and mental health published during this time period (Bergin, 1983) affirmed that religiousness maintains moderate but positive associations with psychological outcomes. A subsequent systematic review of this same literature through the 1980s (Gartner et al., 1991), uncovered over 200 studies, about half of which indicated a positive association and less than a quarter of which pointed to negative effects of religion. A salutary impact of religious involvement was observed for outcomes such as suicide, drug use, alcohol abuse, delinquent behavior, marital satisfaction, psychological distress, certain functional psychiatric diagnoses, and depression.

Much of this research is epidemiologic. That is, it involves studying well populations and comparing current rates (prevalence) or subsequent rates (incidence) of psychiatric morbidity or psychological dysfunction across certain categories of religious indicators. Recent work has begun to follow clinical populations forward in time in hopes of identifying religious factors that impede or promote recovery from illness. Koenig and associates (1992) conducted a prospective follow-up study of hospitalized, medically ill males from North Carolina. Upon readmission an average of 6 months later, religious coping was the only predictor of fewer depressive symptoms according to scores on a self-rated depression scales (Geriatric Depression Scale and Brief Carroll Depression Scale). Koenig has also reported similar findings with respect to cognitive symptoms of depression (Koenig, Cohen, Blazer, & Krishnan, 1995). Taken together, the studies reviewed here suggest that religious involvement exhibits both preventive and therapeutic effects on mental health outcomes.

SOCIAL AND GERONTOLOGICAL RESEARCH

Within social gerontology, religious research has never been mainstream, but, unlike in psychiatry, published studies have given considerable if sporadic and unsystematic attention to mental health and psychological well-being (Levin, 1989). The original *Handbook of Social Gerontology* (Tibbitts, 1960), forerunner of the definitive Academic Press handbook series in aging, included an extensive summary chapter on religion (Maves, 1960). From the 1950s through the early 1970s, the establishment and growth of research on religious factors in mental health was principally due to the pioneering work of gerontologist Moberg (1953, 1965, 1971). The further emergence of this field is documented in the first edition of *The Encyclopedia of Aging* (Markides, 1987). The years since have seen the publication of key literature reviews (Levin, 1989; Witter, Stock, Okun, & Haring, 1985), chapters (Moberg, 1990), and books (Koenig, 1994a, 1997; Koenig, Smiley, & Gonzales, 1988; Levin, 1994b; Thomas & Eisenhandler, 1994); several annotated bibliographies (Fecher, 1982; Koenig, 1995b; Levin, 1997); inclusion of a section on religion in the fourth edition of the authoritative *Handbook of the Psychology of Aging* (McFadden, 1996); and publication of *Aging, Spirituality, and Religion: A Handbook* (Kimble, McFadden, Ellor, & Seeber, 1995), which includes chapters on psychological well-being (Levin & Tobin, 1995) and health (Koenig, 1995a).

Researchers have identified effects of religious involvement on many mental and physical health outcomes in older adults. Statistically significant and mostly salutary effects have been found in relation to subjective health (Levin & Markides, 1986), functional disability (Idler, 1987; Idler & Kasl, 1992), mortality (Bryant & Rakowski, 1992), physical symptomatology (Hannay, 1990), hypertension prevalence (Larson et al., 1989), cancer prevalence (Koenig, Moberg, & Kvale, 1988), smoking and drinking behavior (Koenig et al., 1988), coping (Pargament et al., 1990), self-esteem and mastery (Krause & Tran, 1989), and dimensions of mental health and illness such as life satisfaction (Anson, Antonovsky, & Sagy, 1990; Levin, Chatters, & Taylor, 1995), depressive symptoms (Idler, 1987; Koenig et al., 1988), chronic anxiety (Koenig et al., 1988), dementia (Koenig et al., 1988), loneliness (Johnson & Mullins, 1989), happiness (Poloma & Pendleton, 1990), and emotional adjustment (Blazer & Palmore, 1976). Positive findings have emerged regardless of the specific measures used to assess mental health or psychological distress. Among studies of religion and mental health, most well-known mental health scales and indices have been used, including the ABS, CES-D, GWB, LSIA, LSIZ, Langner, Zung, Beck, Hamilton, MAS, GDS, MMPI, Cavan, Cantril, Gurin, Flanagan, and Diener measures (Levin & Tobin, 1995).

Over the past decade, religious research in social gerontology has become methodologically more sophisticated. No doubt this has helped the field to shed its perceived marginality and to enter into the mainstream of gerontology. One advance has been the examination of complex multifactorial models incorporating religious constructs and measures of psychological well-being. Krause and Tran

(1989) used a covariance-structure modeling (or LISREL) approach to test a model of the interrelationships among two dimensions of religiousness, stress, and self-esteem and mastery using data from the National Survey of Black Americans (NSBA). This outstanding and important study found that religion tends to bolster positive self-feelings independent of the current amount of life stress. Levin et al. (1995) also used NSBA data to show that a composite measure of organizational religious involvement (including frequency of religious attendance) is as strong or stronger a correlate of life satisfaction as is physical health status, a finding that persists even after controlling for effects of other religious dimensions, sociodemographic correlates of health and religiosity, and health status itself.

A second methodological advance has been the investigation of religious effects on well-being through longitudinal analyses. Williams, Larson, Buckler, Heckmann, and Pyle (1991), using data from the New Haven sample noted earlier, found that frequent religious attendance buffers the deleterious effects of stressful life events and physical health problems on subsequent symptoms of psychological distress (according to the Gurin checklist). Levin, Markides, and Ray (1996), in a panel study of three generations of Mexican Americans, found that frequent religious attendance in the youngest generation predicted less depression (according to the depressed affect subscale of the CES-D). These results withstood controlling for the effects of baseline depression, subsequent religious attendance, and a host of sociodemographic factors, as well as self-rated health. Finally, Anson et al. (1990) combined both methodological advances in a single study. In a two-wave LISREL model of retired Israelis, the authors found that the longitudinal effects of self-rated religiosity on subsequent psychological distress were ambiguous, with some evidence that this association is complicated by the possibility that poor well-being leads to increased religiosity. Overall, these longitudinal findings provide additional support for a preventive and therapeutic role of religious involvement in mental health.

SALUTOGENIC MECHANISMS
FOR RELIGIOUS EFFECTS

Given the extent of existing findings, a next logical step for research on religion and mental health would be to explore possible explanations for this mostly salutary religious effect. In other words, research should begin to address the "why" question by identifying or postulating the possible characteristics, functions, expressions, or manifestations of being religious or practicing religion that are known or believed to be salient for mental health (Levin, 1996). This involves describing salutogenic mechanisms whose effects may mediate or moderate in some way the impact of religious constructs on particular mental health outcomes.

For research on determinants of mental health or illness, or of morbidity in general, it is not typical to focus on identification of mechanisms or pathways which promote salutogenesis. The basic medical sciences, as well as epidemiology, tend to emphasize pathogenesis, the process or processes by which healthy individuals or populations become diseased. According to the concept of the natural history of disease, however, pathogenesis is only one portion of the "career" of disease in individuals and populations. According to classical formulations (Leavell & Clark, 1965), a given disease, as manifested in a human population, is expressed over a natural history that includes several sequential stages. In prepathogenesis, factors related to agent, host, and/or environment interact to produce present but not yet symptomatic pathology in healthy people. Pathogenesis is next, in which the clinical horizon has been crossed, symptoms are thus present, and clinical (i.e., diseased) status is joined by the personal perception of illness experience and, likely, the social role of sickness. In order to learn more about how disease originates and progresses, most basic science research and chronic disease epidemiology (including psychiatric epidemiology) are largely oriented toward identifying etiologic factors, pathogenic mechanisms, and risk factors for pathological states.

In epidemiology, the "flipside" of a risk factor is known as a protective factor. For a respective exposure (i.e., independent) variable, one category may denote a presumed risk-enhancing effect (e.g., type A behavior) and the opposite category or categories may designate the presumed protective or preventive effect (e.g., type B behavior). According to Levin (1996),

> The typical way to describe the effects of a protective factor are to state that it protects against or prevents morbidity. This implies that the force of this effect is somehow to "hold back" the tide of pathogenesis. Another way to conceive of this same effect is an active agent that reverses the course of the pathogenic process and moves an individual or population "back" to the prepathogenic state of normal health. The natural history of disease, viewed in this way, could be characterized as a natural history of health. This would require a framework to conceptualize the pathways and mechanisms by which a protective factor enhances the likelihood or probability of health, much as etiologic hypotheses exist for how risk factors initiate and shepherd pathogenesis. (p. 857)

Such a framework exists in Antonovsky's (1987) concept of salutogenesis, which "is not just the other side of the coin from the pathogenic orientation" (p. 2) but a dynamic, multifactorial process based on several assumptions, including defining health and disease as falling along a continuum as opposed to a dichotomy; recognizing that salutogenic factors may not just be the "opposite" categories of risk factors for pathogenesis but rather different constructs altogether; and affirming that epidemiologic research should emphasize factors that promote adaptation and coping instead of just diagnosable etiologic factors. Antonovsky believed that focusing on salutogenesis, in contrast to pathogenesis, would direct scientists to begin identifying mechanisms or pathways leading in the direction of health. In terms of the natural history of disease, such potentially salutogenic factors encompass both those preventing morbidity and those promoting health, the latter including both the elevation of healthy populations to a state of wellness and of clinical populations to a state of recovery.

In the context of the psychiatric epidemiology of religion, a salutogenic focus requires the identification of potential mediating factors or constructs which may help explain why dimensions of religiousness salutarily influence mental health. A variety of possible factors have already been identified in relation to the association between religious involvement and physical health status. Sociological explanations have been offered by Idler (1987), who proposed that religious belief and/or practice may influence health by way of providing or promoting social cohesiveness (i.e., socially supportive resources which buffer the impact of stress), theodicy (i.e., a context of meaning for coping with suffering), coherence (i.e., cognitive perceptions, such as optimism, which serve to reduce uncertainty), and health-related behavior (i.e., discouragement of known behavioral risk factors, such as smoking and drinking). Psychological explanations have been offered by McIntosh and Spilka (1990), who suggested that salutary effects of religiousness may be due to the impact of internal locus of control beliefs (i.e., such as characteristic of some religious believers and which motivate responsible health-related behavior) and faith in God (i.e., a perception that such beliefs and behaviors will be rewarded).

These perspectives and others were integrated in a comprehensive model of hypothesized social, psychological, behavioral, and biological explanations formulated in reference to the epidemiologic literature on religious factors in hypertension (Levin & Vanderpool, 1989). These possible explanations, however, can readily be adapted to the relationship between religion and mental health. These factors are best conceived of as a set of alternative hypotheses or competing explanations, and their underlying biobehavioral and psychosocial mechanisms and effects have since been elaborated (Levin, 1996). In this model, respective religious dimensions are linked to better mental health outcomes via several mediating pathways, each operationalized as one or more factors which, independent of religion, are known or believed to influence mental health through respective, established salutogenic mechanisms.

Religious commitment (e.g., subjective religious attitudes) may influence mental health through encouraging health-related behavior; that is, "lifestyle" or protective behaviors such as avoidance of smoking, alcohol consumption, drug use, poor diet, and physical health risks in general. Health-related behavior is important for well-being because it serves to lower disease risk and enhance physical health (Hamburg, Elliott, & Parron, 1982).

Religious involvement and fellowship (e.g., church or synagogue attendance or other forms of organizational religiosity) may influence well-being by providing social support, such as involvement in meaningful social relationships (in terms of quantity and quality) and integration into supportive networks (providing both tangible and emotional support). Social support is believed to be important for mental health because it serves to buffer the deleterious impact of stress, provide coping resources, help hosts adapt to stressful environments and pathogenic agents, and protect against morbidity and mortality (House, Landis, & Umberson, 1988).

Religious worship (e.g., prayer or other ritual activities) may influence mental health psychodynamically through the effects of positive emotions (such as hope, forgiveness, empowerment, self-esteem, contentment, and love). Positive emotions may be important for mental health due to their impact on health and physiology through possible psychoneuroimmunologic and psychophysiological mechanisms (Rossi, 1993).

Particular religious beliefs or worldviews characteristic of particular individuals or of specific religions or denominations (e.g., free will and the "Protestant ethic") may influence mental health through engendering salutary health beliefs or personality styles (e.g., internal locus of control and type A). Health beliefs and personality styles are important for mental health because of evidence linking them to preventive behavior and to health status in general (Jenkins, 1985), and because of the apparent consonance of respective religious and health-related cognitions or orientations (e.g., free will theology and internal locus of control; the Protestant ethic and type A) (Spector, 1979, pp. 114–123).

Religious faith (as reflected in the presence and intensity of particular beliefs or experiences) may influence mental health through generating optimism and hopeful expectations that God will reward expressions of piety or devotion with better health and well-being. Optimism is believed to be important for mental health because of the health-promoting qualities of positive mental attitudes (as in learned optimism or the placebo effect) (Taylor, 1989).

A final competing hypothesis is a multifactorial explanation—a "some or all of the above" explanation. Whenever possible, empirical investigators should attempt to include measures of as many of these constructs as is possible in given studies in order to examine the interrelationships and interactions among these potential mediating or moderating (i.e., effect-modifying) factors within particular analytical models.

THEORETICAL MODELS OF RELIGION AND MENTAL HEALTH

As studies continue to appear, efforts have been made to make sense of and interpret published findings in order to help understand how and why religion influences mental health. This includes work which (a) reviews theoretical perspectives underlying research on religion and mental health; (b) outlines theoretical frameworks from sociology, psychiatry, and theology for understanding the impact of religious involvement on mental health; and (c) proposes theoretical models for investigating the impact of religion on mental health while accounting for possible mediating factors. All of this theoretical work contributes to our understanding of the possible ways in which religion serves to mitigate or buffer the deleterious impact of poor health or other stressors on mental health (Koenig & Futterman, 1995).

In a review of findings through the middle 1980s, Levin (1989) identified six alternative theoretical perspectives which, explicitly or implicitly, underlie research in this area: an eschatological perspective, a deterioration perspective, activity theory, disengagement theory, a social decrement or isolation perspective, and the multidimensional disengagement perspective of Mindel and Vaughan (1978). Each perspective hypothesizes certain patterns of religious involvement in older adults and changes in involvement over the life course as well as the nature of religion's impact on mental health over time. Existing data seemed to best support the multidimensional disengagement perspective. This model hypothesizes that while old age may be accompanied by a decline in organizational religious involvement due to increased disability, nonorganizational and subjective religiosity remain steady or increase somewhat in compensation. Furthermore, organizational involvement may not necessarily increase in its salience for mental health, whereas nonorganizational and subjective religiosity may emerge as important inverse (and possibly spurious) predictors of mental health. This possible artifact may in part reflect increases in private, noninstitutional forms of religious expression in compensation for declines in organizational religiosity due to poor physical health. Such confounding between organizational religiosity and functional health status is often observed in samples of older adults (Levin & Vanderpool, 1987) and is considerable incentive for using longitudinal research designs, such as prospective cohort studies and multiwave panel studies, in clinical research on religion (Koenig et al., 1992).

Several researchers have attempted to interpret existing findings by developing theoretical frameworks and explanations for a salutary religious effect on the mental health of older adults. Ellison (1994), a sociologist, suggests that religious involvement may influence mental health by (a) reducing the risk of chronic and acute stressors, such as due to marital problems or consequences of deviant behavior; (b) offering cognitive or institutional frameworks, such as a sense of coherence, order, or meaning, that serve to buffer the deleterious impact of stress and facilitate coping; (c) providing concrete social resources, such as religious fellowship and congregational networks; and (d) enhancing internal psychological resources such as feelings of self-esteem and worthiness. Tobin (1991), writing from psychodynamic and developmental perspectives, observes that religion provides continuity across life-course stages by emphasizing the intrinsic and enduring meaning of life, fostering a sense of feeling blessed by God, and, similar to Ellison's (1994) view, providing both personal and community resources which enhance coping with age-related losses. Koenig (1994b), a geriatric psychiatrist, outlines the various ways that religious faith promotes the mental health of older adults suffering physical challenges. Foremost among these is that religious faith provides hope for change and healing as well as a paradigm and role models for understanding human suffering. Furthermore, the focus on interpersonal relationships, seeking forgiveness of oneself and others, a sense of control and self-determination, the provision of a supportive community, and promises of an afterlife and ready accessibility reflect positive cognitive perspectives and emotional states that are conducive to individual adjustment.

The formulation of theoretical models of the interrelationships among religion, mental health, and the possible mediating factors identified earlier is derived from similar models formulated to guide research on other sociomedical topics. Espe-

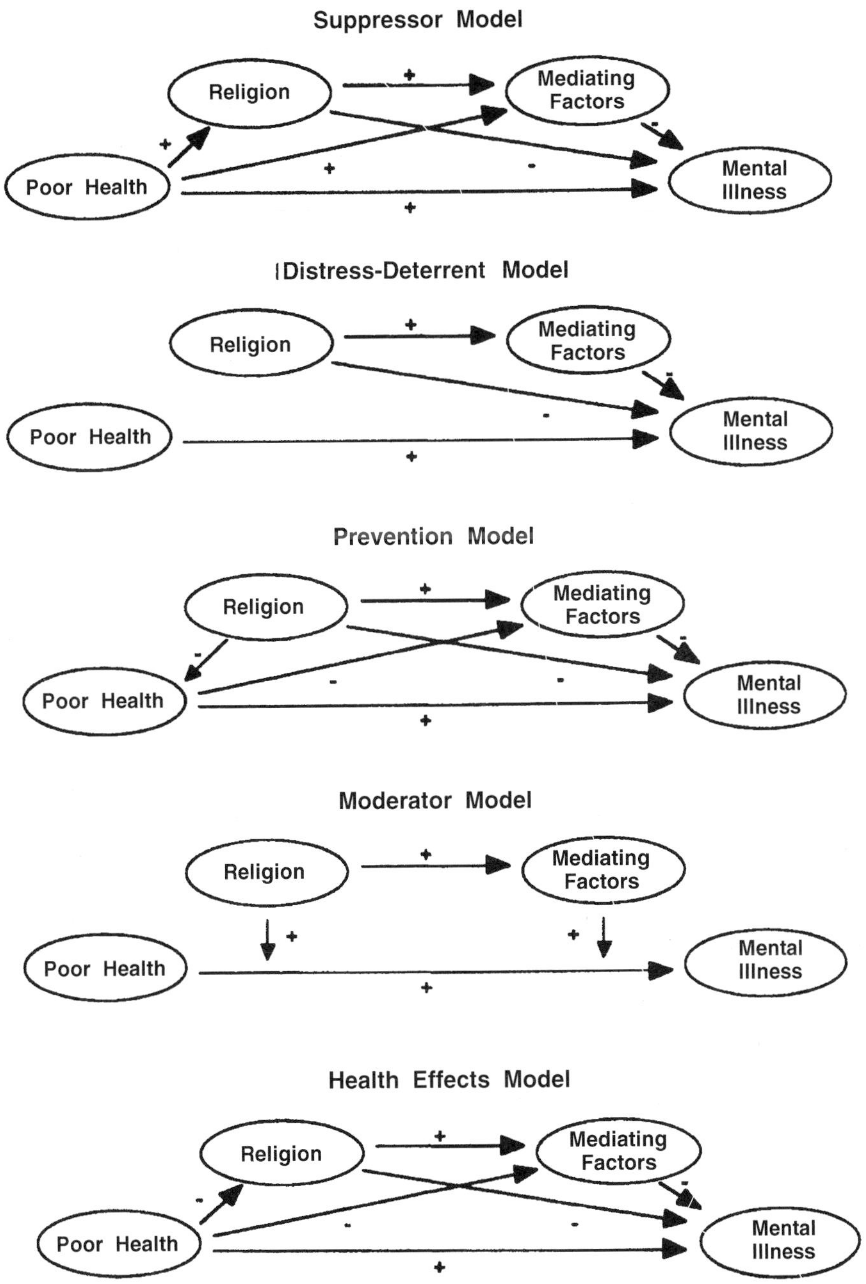

FIGURE 3.1 Alternative theoretical models of religion and mental health.

cially applicable are multifactorial theoretical models proposed for the stress-buffering functions of coping resources for health (Wheaton, 1985); the role of religion as a coping resource that enhances self-esteem and mastery (Krause & Tran, 1989); the impact of religious, social, and psychological resources in mediating the effects of stressful life events on health and life satisfaction (Levin et al., 1995); and the role of religion in buffering the impact of stress on health (Koenig & Futterman, 1995). Based on this work, five alternative theoretical models can be posited for how mediating factors, along with health status, impact the effects of religion on mental health (Fig. 3.1).

In the suppressor model, the overall relationship is, in sociological terms, fully recursive and, in epidemiologic terms, an indirect effects association. Poor health, or a stressor in general, leads to an increase in religious activity and other social, psychological, and behavioral coping responses, themselves also engendered by religion, which serve to reduce or suppress deleterious effects on mental health. This class of model is consistent with qualitative findings in the religious coping literature (Koenig & Futterman, 1995).

In the distress-deterrent model, the overall relationship, in epidemiologic terms, defines an independent effects association. Poor health (or stress in general) and religion have independent and opposite effects on mental health, and poor health does not engender either greater religiosity or a psychosocial coping response. This class of model, also known as a "counterbalancing model," is consistent with findings on stressful life events and self-esteem in older African Americans (Krause & Tran, 1989).

In the prevention model, religion exerts, in epidemiologic terms, both direct and indirect protective effects on mental health. Religious involvement, as well as psychosocial mediating factors, benefits mental health indirectly by preventing physical morbidity, which itself is a risk factor for psychological distress. This class of model is consistent with the epidemiologic literature on the primary preventive effects of religion for physical health (Levin, 1996; Levin & Schiller, 1987; Levin & Vanderpool, 1992) and is best tested with prospective or longitudinal data.

In the moderator model, the overall relationship is, in sociological terms, interactive and, in epidemiologic terms, an effect-modifying association. Poor health (or stress in general) interacts with religion and mediating factors such that its deleterious effect on mental health varies by degree of religious involvement. This class of model is consistent with findings from health-related studies in clinical populations (e.g., Idler, 1987; Koenig & Futterman, 1995) whose respondents are symptomatic or at more advanced stages of the natural history of disease. Such a model can be tested by cross-product terms in mathematical models (as done by sociologists) or by stratified analyses of risk or odds (as done by epidemiologists).

In the health effects model, the overall relationship is similar to that of the suppressor model, but the direction of effects is just the opposite. Poor health (typically age-related declines, on average, in functional activity) suppresses or prevents certain types of religious activity (e.g., organizational involvement) and may exert negative psychosocial effects in terms of the competing mediating factors identified previously (i.e., lead to harmful health-related behavior, increase social isolation, create negative emotions, promote pessimism, etc.). This class of model is consistent with findings in the gerontological literature on religious factors in health and well-being (Levin, 1989).

IMPLICATIONS

This overview of empirical findings and theoretical issues in research on religion and mental health suggests several important implications for mental health research and practice. First, the extant body of work in this area, while substantial, is somewhat uneven in quality. This results from a number of different circumstances, including a lack of theoretical clarity in defining distinct religious dimensions and specifying appropriate analytical relationships, methodological flaws in the measurement of religious involvement, and interpretive error when assessing empirical relationships. Although these shortcomings have been described previously (Levin & Vanderpool, 1987), it bears emphasizing that deficiencies in any one of these areas compromises the validity of an investigation. Researchers who are unfamiliar with the variety of issues attendant to the conceptualization and measurement of religious involvement may be particularly susceptible to difficulties in this area and are encouraged to consult with experts in empirical religious research.

Coupled with these concerns is a need to recognize the inherent complexity of constructs such as religious involvement, mental health, and the factors that have been proposed as mediators of religion–mental health associations. As the discussion of theoretical models illustrated, there are several alternative ways that religious involvement, mediating factors, and mental health are potentially related. The complexity and meaning of these constructs and their relationships are not trivial matters (Idler, 1995) and must be fully appreciated in order to arrive at a thorough understanding of the varied connections between religion and mental health.

Above and beyond these purely conceptual and empirical issues, this work suggests a number of theoretical and ideological implications for mental health research and practice. It is important first to recognize that psychiatry and the mental health field continue to embody an active prejudice (of long-standing) against issues of a religious nature. The modern origins of this antagonism date primarily from the writings of Freud (1961a, 1961b), but the roots of the conflict can be traced back to fundamental controversies between science and religion. Furthermore, antagonisms are sometimes mutual because strong adherents to religious worldviews may mistrust and disparage psychiatry and the field of mental health. Thankfully, this has been mitigated both by continued growth of the field of pastoral counseling and psychology and by exposure to psychological theories and concepts and human services practice models in the training of clergy at graduate divinity schools.

Notwithstanding the age-old conflicts between religion and science, it is easy to appreciate the current sources of (in)difference and distrust. Modern psychiatry and psychology purport to have effectively supplanted a number of religious concepts that are central to understanding human nature. For example, the concepts of a human soul and sin have been replaced with notions of human consciousness and psychological and social pathologies. Deficiencies in individual morality are viewed not as personal shortcomings to be ameliorated through a process of confession and redemption but as products of inadequacies in the processes by which people are socialized. These examples illustrate that while religion and modern psychiatry and psychology may be concerned with identical issues of human adjustment and well-being, many differences exist between them with respect to fundamental worldviews and the concepts and vocabularies used to describe, explain, and understand human motivation and behavior.

As a consequence, there is mutual reluctance to engage the "other" perspective. Among mental health researchers and practitioners, there are still pockets of resistance to examining the influence of religious issues in relation to mental health issues. For those willing to consider the relationships between religious involvement and mental health, there is frequently a basic naivete as to the conceptual and methodological complexities of such an undertaking. In addition, there are dissimilarities involving the basic characteristics of what constitutes an emotionally healthy individual as well as the types of behaviors that are regarded as normal and adaptive. For example, research on individual coping often emphasizes those efforts that involve adopting an active stance in the face of threatening events (i.e., problem-solving or active coping) as opposed to palliative forms of coping that are directed toward changing the meaning of the event (i.e., threat appraisal) and/or managing one's emotional response to it (Folkman & Lazarus, 1988). Religious coping (e.g., prayer) is typically categorized as a palliative coping strategy that is effective in altering threat perceptions and in managing associated emotions. In contrast, mobilization of social resources within a religious context would constitute a form of problem-solving coping. While largely ignored in mental health research, these particular aspects of religious coping (i.e., threat appraisal and emotional management) may actually function epidemiologically as protective factors against psychiatric disorders, thus contributing to positive mental health (Ellison, 1994).

Finally, the research findings and theoretical issues reviewed in this chapter underscore the importance of appreciating the conceptual diversity both of religious expression and of what constitutes mental health. Given that current perspectives on religious involvement in the mental health field are so severely limited, there is a tendency to view religious behaviors, attitudes, and beliefs in a fairly stereotypical (and prejudicially negative) manner. However, religious expression and meaning, and the adaptive function and efficacy of religion, vary widely within particular faith traditions and even within respective denominations, adding further to the complexity of conducting research in this area. Even straightforwardly "simple" variables such as frequency of prayer or frequency of religious attendance may mask profound variation in norms and meanings across even related religious groups, rendering hazardous any interpretation of their effects (Levin & Taylor, 1997; Levin & Vanderpool, 1987). While it is crucial to recognize and account for this diversity when interpreting findings bearing on relationships between religion and mental health, this is easier said than done, as evidenced by pervasive underappreciation of potential problems in religious measurement.

Frequency of attendance at religious services, for example, is widely known to vary across different faiths. Weekly attendance may be normative for observant Catholics and mainstream Protestants, whereas among Pentecostal groups more frequent attendance (two or three times weekly) may be expected. Interpretation of group differences in religious attendance is rarely informed, however, by an understanding of existing expectations and norms. Likewise, the varying effects of religious attendance on mental health outcomes across religions and religious denominations are more typically described than explained. Similarly, the manifestation of religious involvement, in general, as a representative human phenomenon is subject to the influence of social patterning. Considerable research documents the ways that factors such as age, gender, ethnicity, marital status, residence, and socioeconomic status function to shape various forms of religious expression (Levin, Taylor, & Chatters, 1994).

In conclusion, research and theory addressing the interrelationships among religion, potential mediating factors, and mental health outcomes have evidenced impressive growth and development in recent years. Current work demonstrates careful attention to issues of conceptualization and measurement as well as an appreciation for the value of prospective designs in studying the impact of religion. Research is just beginning to address whether the associations among religion, mediating factors, and mental health outcomes vary across diverse social groupings, such as religions or religious denominations. This work holds promise for helping to clarify the diverse functions of religious involvement for personal well-being and adjustment.

ACKNOWLEDGMENT

This work was supported by the National Institute on Aging under NIH Grant AG10135 (Dr. Robert Joseph Taylor, PI).

REFERENCES

Anson, O., Antonovsky, A., & Sagy, S. (1990). Religiosity and well-being among retirees: A question of causality. *Behavior, Health, and Aging, 1,* 85–97.

Antonovsky, A. (1987). *Unraveling the mystery of health: How people manage stress and stay well.* San Francisco: Jossey-Bass.

Bergin, A. E. (1983). Religiosity and mental health: A critical reevaluation and meta-analysis. *Professional Psychology: Research and Practice, 14,* 170–184.

Blazer, D., & Palmore, E. (1976). Religion and aging in a longitudinal panel. *The Gerontologist, 16,* 82–85.

Bryant, S., & Rakowski, W. (1992). Predictors of mortality among elderly African-Americans. *Research on Aging, 14,* 50–67.

Ellison, C. G. (1994). Religion, the life stress paradigm, and the study of depression. In J. S. Levin (Ed.), *Religion in aging and health: Theoretical foundations and methodological frontiers* (pp. 78–121). Thousand Oaks, CA: Sage.

Fecher, V. J. (1982). *Religion & aging: An annotated bibliography.* San Antonio, TX: Trinity University Press.

Folkman, S., & Lazarus, R. S. (1988). The relationship between coping and emotion: Implications for theory and research. *Social Science and Medicine, 26,* 309–317.

Freud, S. (1961a). *Civilization and its discontents.* New York: Norton. (Original work published 1930)

Freud, S. (1961b). *The future of an illusion.* New York: Norton. (Original work published 1927)

Gartner, J., Larson, D. B., & Allen, G. D. (1991). Religious commitment and mental health: A review of the empirical literature. *Journal of Psychology and Theology, 19,* 6–25.

Hamburg, D. A., Elliott, G. R., & Parron, D. L. (Eds.). (1982). *Health and behavior: Frontiers of research in the biobehavioral sciences.* Washington, DC: National Academy Press.

Hannay, D. R. (1990). Religion and health. *Social Science and Medicine, 14A,* 683–685.

House, J. S., Landis, K. R., & Umberson, D. (1988). Social relationships and health. *Science, 241,* 540–545.

Idler, E. L. (1987). Religious involvement and the health of the elderly: Some hypotheses and an initial test. *Social Forces, 66,* 226–238.

Idler, E. L. (1995). Religion, health, and nonphysical senses of self. *Social Forces, 74,* 683–704.

Idler, E. L., & Kasl, S. V. (1992). Religion, disability, depression, and the timing of death. *American Journal of Sociology, 97,* 1052–1079.

Jarvis, G. K., & Northcutt, H. C. (1987). Religion and differences in morbidity and mortality. *Social Science and Medicine, 25,* 813–824.

Johnson, D. P., & Mullins, L. C. (1989). Subjective and social dimensions of religiosity and loneliness among the well elderly. *Review of Religious Research, 31,* 3–15.

Kimble, M. A., McFadden, S. H., Ellor, J. W., & Seeber, J. J. (Eds.). (1995). *Aging, spirituality, and religion: A handbook.* Minneapolis, MN: Fortress Press.

Koenig, H. G. (1994a). *Aging and God: Spiritual pathways to mental health in midlife and later years.* New York: Haworth.

Koenig, H. G. (1994b). Religion and hope for the disabled elder. In J. S. Levin (Ed.), *Religion in aging and health: Theoretical foundations and methodological frontiers* (pp. 18–51). Thousand Oaks, CA: Sage.

Koenig, H. G. (1995a). Religion and health in later life. In M. A. Kimble, S. H. McFadden, J. W. Ellor, & J. J. Seeber (Eds.), *Aging, spirituality, and religion: A handbook* (pp. 9–29). Minneapolis, MN: Fortress Press.

Koenig, H. G. (1995b). *Research on religion and aging: An annotated bibliography.* Westport, CT: Greenwood.

Koenig, H. G. (1997). *Is religion good for your health?: The effects of religion on physical and mental health.* New York: Haworth Pastoral Press.

Koenig, H. G., Cohen, H. J., Blazer, D. G., & Krishnan, K. R. R. (1995). Religious coping and cognitive symptoms of depression in elderly medical patients. *Psychosomatics, 36,* 369–375.

Koenig, H. G., Cohen, H. J., Blazer, D. G., Pieper, C., Meador, K. G., Shelp, F., Goli, V., & DiPasquale, R. (1992). Religious coping and depression in elderly hospitalized medically ill men. *American Journal of Psychiatry, 149,* 1693–1700.

Koenig, H. G., & Futterman, A. (1995). *Religion and health outcomes: A review and synthesis of the literature.* Paper presented at Methodological Approaches to the Study of Religion, Aging, and Health, National Institute on Aging, Bethesda, MD, March 16–17.

Koenig, H. G., Moberg, D. O., & Kvale, J. N. (1988). Religious activities and attitudes of older adults in a geriatric assessment clinic. *Journal of the American Geriatrics Society, 36,* 362–374.

Koenig, H. G., Smiley, M., & Gonzales, J. A. P. (1988). *Religion, health, and aging: A review and theoretical integration.* New York: Greenwood.

Krause, N., & Tran, T. V. (1989). Stress and religious involvement among older blacks. *Journal of Gerontology: Social Sciences, 44,* S4–S13.

Larson, D. B., Koenig, H. G., Kaplan, B. H., Greenberg, R. F., Logue, E., & Tyroler, H. A. (1989). The impact of religion on blood pressure status in men. *Journal of Religion and Health, 28,* 265–278.

Larson, D. B., Pattison, E. M., Blazer, D. G., Omran, A. R., & Kaplan, B. H. (1986). Systematic analysis of research on religious variables in four major psychiatric journals, 1978–1982. *American Journal of Psychiatry, 143,* 329–334.

Larson, D. B., Sherrill, K. A., & Lyons, J. S. (1994). Neglect and misuse of the *r* word: Systematic reviews of religious measures in health, mental health, and aging. In J. S. Levin (Ed.), *Religion in aging and health: Theoretical foundations and methodological frontiers* (pp. 178–195). Thousand Oaks, CA: Sage.

Larson, D. B., Sherrill, K. A., Lyons, J. S., Craigie, F. C., Jr., Thielman, S. B., Greenwold, M. A., & Larson, S. S. (1992). Associations between dimensions of religious commitment and mental health reported in the *American Journal of Psychiatry* and *Archives of General Psychiatry:* 1978–1989. *American Journal of Psychiatry, 149,* 557–559.

Leavell, H. R., & Clark, E. G. (1965). Levels of application of preventive medicine. In *Preventive medicine for the doctor in his community* (3rd ed., pp. 14–38). New York: McGraw-Hill.

Levin, J. S. (1989). Religious factors in aging, adjustment, and health: A theoretical overview. In W. M. Clements (Ed.), *Religion, aging and health: A global perspective* (pp. 133–146). New York: Haworth. (Compiled by the World Health Organization)

Levin, J. S. (1994a). Religion and health: Is there an association, is it valid, and is it causal? *Social Science and Medicine, 38,* 1475–1482.

Levin, J. S. (Ed.). (1994b). *Religion in aging and health: Theoretical foundations and methodological frontiers.* Thousand Oaks, CA: Sage.

Levin, J. S. (1996). How religion influences morbidity and health: Reflections on natural history, salutogenesis and host resistance. *Social Science and Medicine, 43,* 849–864.

Levin, J. S. (1997). Religious research in gerontology, 1980 –1994: A systematic review. *Journal of Religious Gerontology, 10*(3), 3–31.

Levin, J. S., Chatters, L. M., & Taylor, R. J. (1995). Religious effects on health status and life satisfaction among black Americans. *Journal of Gerontology: Social Sciences, 50B,* S154–S163.

Levin, J. S., & Markides, K. S. (1986). Religious attendance and subjective health. *Journal for the Scientific Study of Religion, 25,* 31–40.

Levin, J. S., Markides, K. S., & Ray, L. A. (1996). Religious attendance and psychological well-being in Mexican Americans: A panel analysis of three-generations data. *The Gerontologist, 36,* 454–463.

Levin, J. S., & Schiller, P. L. (1987). Is there a religious factor in health? *Journal of Religion and Health, 26,* 9–36.

Levin, J. S., & Taylor, R. J. (1997). Age differences in patterns and correlates of the frequency of prayer. *The Gerontologist, 37,* 75–88.

Levin, J. S., Taylor, R. J., & Chatters, L. M. (1994). Race and gender differences in religiosity among older adults: Findings from four national surveys. *Journal of Gerontology: Social Sciences, 49,* S137–S145.

Levin, J. S., & Tobin, S. S. (1995). Religion and psychological well-being. In M. A. Kimble, S. H. McFadden, J. W. Ellor, & J. J. Seeber (Eds.), *Aging, spirituality, and religion: A Handbook* (pp. 30–46). Minneapolis, MN: Fortress Press.

Levin, J. S., & Vanderpool, H. Y. (1987). Is frequent religious attendance *really* conducive to better health?: Toward an epidemiology of religion. *Social Science and Medicine, 24,* 589–600.

Levin, J. S., & Vanderpool, H. Y. (1989). Is religion therapeutically significant for hypertension? *Social Science and Medicine, 29,* 69–78.

Levin, J. S., & Vanderpool, H. Y. (1992). Religious factors in physical health and the prevention of illness. In K. I. Pargament, K. I. Maton, & R. E. Hess (Eds.), *Religion and prevention in mental health: Research, vision, and action* (pp. 83–103). New York: Haworth.

Lindenthal, J. J., Myers, J. K., Pepper, M. P., & Stern, M. S. (1970). Mental status and religious behavior. *Journal for the Scientific Study of Religion, 9,* 143–149.

Markides, K. S. (1987). Religion. In G. L. Maddox (Ed.), *The encyclopedia of aging* (pp. 559–561). New York: Springer.

Maves, P. B. (1960). Aging, religion, and the church. In C. Tibbitts (Ed.), *Handbook of social gerontology: Societal aspects of aging* (pp. 698–749). Chicago: University of Chicago Press.

McFadden, S. H. (1996). Religion, spirituality, and aging. In J. E. Birren & K. W. Schaie (Eds.), *Handbook of the psychology of aging* (4th ed., pp. 162–177). San Diego: Academic Press.

McIntosh, D., & Spilka, B. (1990). Religion and physical health: The role of personal faith and control beliefs. *Research in the Social Scientific Study of Religion, 2,* 167–194.

Mindel, C. H., & Vaughan, C. E. (1978). A multidimensional approach to religiosity and disengagement. *Journal of Gerontology, 33,* 103–108.

Moberg, D. O. (1953). Church membership and personal adjustment in old age. *Journal of Gerontology, 8,* 207–211.

Moberg, D. O. (1965). Religiosity in old age. *The Gerontologist, 5*(2), 78–87.

Moberg, D. O. (Ed.). (1971). *Spiritual well-being: Background and issues.* Washington, DC: White House Conference on Aging.

Moberg, D. O. (1990). Religion and aging. In K. F. Ferraro (Ed.), *Gerontology: Perspectives and issues* (pp. 179–205). New York: Springer.

Pargament, K. I., Ensing, D. S., Falgout, K., Olsen, H., Reilly, B., Van Haitsma, K., & Warren, R. (1990). God help me: 1. Religious coping efforts as predictors of the outcomes of significant negative life events. *American Journal of Community Psychology, 18,* 793–824.

Peck, M. S. (1993). Psychiatry's predicament. In *Further along the road less traveled* [Epilogue] (pp. 232–255). New York: Simon & Schuster.

Poloma, M. M., & Pendleton, B. F. (1990). Religious domains and general well-being. *Social Indicators Research, 22,* 255–276.

Rossi, E. L. (1993). *The psychobiology of mind–body healing* (rev. ed.). New York: Norton.

Sherrill, K. A., & Larson, D. B. (1994). The anti-tenure factor in religious research in clinical epidemiology and aging. In J. S. Levin (Ed.), *Religion in aging and health: Theoretical foundations and methodological frontiers* (pp. 149–177). Thousand Oaks, CA: Sage.

Spector, R. E. (1979). *Cultural diversity in health and illness.* New York: Appleton-Century-Crofts.

Srole, L., & Langner, T. (1962). Religious origin. In L. Srole, T. S. Langner, S. T. Michael, M. K. Opler, & T. A. C. Rennie (Eds.), *Mental health in the metropolis: The Midtown Manhattan Study* (pp. 300–324). New York: McGraw-Hill.

Stark, R. (1971). Psychopathology and religious commitment. *Review of Religious Research, 12,* 165–176.

Taylor, S. E. (1989). *Positive illusions: Creative self-deception and the healthy mind.* New York: Basic Books.

Thomas, L. E., & Eisenhandler, S. A. (Ed.). (1994). *Aging and the religious dimension.* Westport, CT: Auburn House.

Tibbitts, C. (Ed.). (1960). *Handbook of social gerontology: Societal aspects of aging.* Chicago: University of Chicago Press.

Tobin, S. S. (1991). Preserving the self through religion. In *Personhood in advanced old age: Implications for practice* (pp. 119–133). New York: Springer.

Troyer, H. (1988). Review of cancer among 4 religious sects: Evidence that life-styles are distinctive sets of risk factors. *Social Science and Medicine, 26,* 1007–1017.

Wheaton, B. (1985). Models of the stress-buffering functions of coping resources. *Journal of Health and Social Behavior, 26,* 352–364.

Williams, D. R., Larson, D. R., Buckler, R. E., Heckmann, R. C., & Pyle, C. M. (1991). Religion and psychological distress in a community sample. *Social Science and Medicine, 11,* 1257–1262.

Wilson, W. P. (1972). Mental health benefits of religious salvation. *Diseases of the Nervous System, 33,* 382–386.

Witter, R. A., Stock, W. A., Okun, M. A., & Haring, M. J. (1985). Religion and subjective well-being in adulthood: A quantitative synthesis. *Review of Religious Research, 26,* 332–342.

4

WHAT SOCIOLOGY CAN HELP US UNDERSTAND ABOUT RELIGION AND MENTAL HEALTH

ELLEN L. IDLER

Department of Sociology and Institute for Health Care Policy and Aging Research
Rutgers University
New Brunswick, New Jersey 08903

LINDA K. GEORGE

Department of Sociology and Center for the Study of Aging and Human Development
Duke University
Durham, North Carolina 27710

To some readers, it may seem as if the sociological perspective on mental health and on religion is a quite distant one—marginally relevant at best. In our culture, for lay people and mental health professionals alike, mental illness is viewed as a condition of disordered individuals. Such illness is rooted in the personality, or the brain, of individuals and expressed in symptoms and behaviors that seem to come from somewhere inaccessibly deep within the isolated person. Just as the causes and symptoms of mental illness are located within the individual, so too are the culturally favored treatments of medication and psychotherapy.

Religion, too, may be thought of as something for which the social aspects are merely superficial. However, the earliest sociologists relied heavily on religion to help them formulate their thoughts about the very nature of society: Emile Durkheim and Max Weber both viewed religion as critical to the sociohistorical changes taking place in Europe in the nineteenth and twentieth centuries that were shaping the modern world. More important for the topic of this chapter, they also saw religion as critical in explaining the behaviors, motives, and well-being of individuals. Religious groups are social organizations with their own structures, beliefs, and patterns of interaction. Durkheim and Weber viewed the structures and beliefs of religious groups as exemplars of parallel structures in other social institutions. They chose to study religion because it illuminated all of society. The perspective of this chapter is that sociology has a great deal to offer us in understanding the complicated relationship between religion and mental health. The sociological perspective directs our attention to the social conditions which provide the background to mental health problems and to the social responses such disorders evoke. While there is no single sociological explanation of mental illness, there are a variety of approaches which can illuminate a phenomenon which many would not consider to be in the social domain at all.

THE ETIOLOGY OF MENTAL ILLNESS:
FROM THE ORIGINS OF THE DISCIPLINE

The sociology of religion, going back to its origins, supplies us with an overarching theoretical framework for thinking about religion and mental health. The French sociologist Emile Durkheim's original work (1897/1951) was about how and why religions protect believers from suicide; his later work (Durkheim, 1912/1995) revealed the importance of ritual and the recognition of the sacred. The German sociologist Max Weber (1904/1958) took the teachings of the Protestant church and showed how they created uncertainty for individuals, which resulted in changes in behavior that transformed the economic system of Europe. Together, these founders of the discipline mark out for us a complex set of structures and processes that are influencing research to this day.

Durkheim's work in *Suicide* (1897/1951) showed that religious groups provide rules for many areas of life, and that these rules have a preservative function for individuals. Religious groups, notably Catholicism more than Protestantism, Durkheim argued, regulate the behavior of individuals; they constrain individuals from following their own selfish desires and force them to consider the interests of the group ahead of their own self-interest. Social groups, and religious groups especially, provide structures which protect individuals from anomie, or "normlessness," a state in which individuals have insufficient guides for their behavior. Normless, rudderless, individuals, in Durkheim's work, were more prone to committing suicide than those with a strong sense of attachment to the collective conscience.

Religious groups, in Durkheim's view, have another important function in addition to providing rules: they provide support and integration. Durkheim argued that individuals who were isolated from social life, who were not active participants in families, religious groups, or other community organizations, were more prone to suicide as well. These individuals lack a sense of social solidarity and risk what Durkheim called egoistic suicide. While Durkheim's *Suicide* has frequently been subjected to criticism on methodological grounds, recent tests of the theory have elaborated it with contemporary social network theory and consistently provide support for it with suicide rates in the United States and abroad (Breault, 1986; Pescosolido & Georgianna, 1989; Stack & Wasserman, 1992). Durkheim's achievement is that he took what is at face value a highly individualistic act, most often contemplated and carried out in secrecy, and showed that it had profound social influences bearing on it. In fact, he established that rates of suicide must be thought of as characteristics of societies themselves, not simply as the sum total of the acts of isolated individuals. Like suicide, mental illness is a phenomenon we see in individual cases but which cannot be fully understood at that level.

It is easy to see the relevance of both the regulative and integrative functions of religion to mental health. Many religious groups have very specific rules proscribing the use of alcohol and drugs, for example, which could lower the rates of substance abuse and dependence among members. A recent review of the literature on substance abuse (Gorsuch, 1995) found a consistent inverse relationship: Highly religious people are less likely to abuse drugs and alcohol than less religious people (Cochran, Beeghley, & Bock, 1992; Koenig, Moberg, & Kvale, 1988). Many of these studies have been conducted in adolescent and college-age populations, in which the findings are especially significant given the vulnerability of these populations and the importance of lowering lifetime risk (Amoateng & Bahr, 1986; Benson & Donahue, 1989). It is important to note that not all religions have specific beliefs regarding alcohol or drug use, but as Kenneth Vaux (1976) argues, "purity of life" is a "generic religious value," and most religions have beliefs about the dangers of contamination and the maintenance of the purity of the mind, body, and soul. In the larger sense, these beliefs about purity are beliefs about molding the individual in the image of the social group, in conformity with its ideas about what is pure and what is impure.

It is also easy to see how Durkheim's ideas about religious groups as supportive, integrative communities are relevant to mental health. Just as individuals are prone to suicide when they are without sufficient constraint from the community, so are they vulnerable when they are lonely and isolated. Religious groups can be thought of as social network structures to which only members have access. Membership in a religious congregation then potentially expands the number of social ties individuals have available to them. From a functional perspective, religious groups provide support and nurturance for their members; compassion and care for others is a primary teaching of all of the major world religions. In the secular world, social support is often conceptualized as either instrumental or emotional in nature, and religious congregations are potential providers of both tangible assistance and spiritual support. Recent empirical studies have demonstrated support for these theories: Religious individuals in one study, especially those who believed in a "helpful" (as opposed to "wrathful") God, were less likely to be lonely (Schwab & Petersen, 1990). In a study from North Carolina, frequent attenders at religious services had larger social networks, more contacts with them, and more social support from them than infrequent attenders or nonattenders (Ellison & George, 1994); these findings were subsequently replicated with a U.S. national sample (Bradley, 1995).

Max Weber [1958(1904)], whose work forms the other theoretical pillar of the discipline, studied the effect of newly emergent Protestant belief systems on social and economic behavior. Religious groups offer members a complex set of beliefs about God, ethics, human relationships, life, and death, and many of them are directly relevant to health. In Weber's words, religion offers "coherent meaning" for "both social and cosmic events"; sociologist of religion Peter Berger (1967) calls religious belief systems "symbolic universes" in which the events of life and death take on spiritual significance. Individuals can call on the stories and beliefs of their faith to put their own lives into a much larger context, to learn lessons from others who have faced similar troubles, or to gain hope for the future. Recent research shows that this cognitive level of religion's influence is critically important: Ellison's (1991) analysis of U.S. national data shows that the beneficial effects of attendance at religious services and private devotional practices, such as prayer and Bible reading, on subjective well-being are primarily due to their role in strengthening religious belief systems. Individuals who describe themselves as having a strong religious faith report themselves to be happier and to be more satisfied with their lives (Ellison, 1991). Likewise, older adults with the highest levels of religious commitment also tend to have the highest feelings of self-worth (Krause, 1995). As Koenig, Smiley, and Gonzales (1988, p. 36) write, "The Judeo-Christian scriptures are full of references to the power of the thought life in affecting both emotional and spiritual states . . . [they] encourage positive thinking . . . and often direct thoughts toward helping others in worse situations."

This brief account of the intellectual contributions of the founders of the discipline of sociology is a modest attempt to demonstrate how critical religion was in their thinking about human behavior and human consciousness. The earliest contribution of the discipline to recent studies of mental health could be said to be primarily along etiological lines. That is, the contributions of Durkheim and Weber direct our attention to the social conditions which give rise to mental illness. They help us formulate research questions about which types of individuals are likely to develop symptoms or make predictions about rates of mental illness in different communities or cultures. In addition, this rich theoretical background provides a wealth of clues about the mechanisms through which the relationship between religion and mental health is worked out. The question for sociologists appraising the relationship between religion and mental health is not so much, "Is there a relationship?," but "What are the social and cognitive processes that are set in motion by religion which can help us understand it?"

THE SOCIAL RESPONSE TO MENTAL ILLNESS: LATER CONTRIBUTIONS OF THE DISCIPLINE

Sociologists studying mental illness have also focused on the ways individuals in society respond to mental illness in their community. This approach shifts attention to the nonmentally ill and their attitudes and responses to those who suffer symptoms. These approaches have asked, "When do social institutions label behavior 'mental illness' instead of calling it some other type of deviant behavior?" or "How do social factors in the community or the characteristics of individuals affect the type of treatment mentally ill individuals are likely to get?" These questions are relevant to religion in many ways. As a way of eliciting some of these questions, examine the following passage from the book of Mark in the New Testament which raises many of the issues we still face today:

> A man in the crowd spoke up: "Teacher, I brought my son for you to cure. He is possessed by a spirit that makes him dumb. Whenever it attacks him, it flings him to the ground, and he foams at the mouth, grinds his teeth, and goes rigid. I asked your disciples to drive it out, but they could not." Jesus answered: "What an unbelieving generation! How long shall I be with you? How long must I endure you? Bring him to me." So they brought the boy to him; and as soon as the spirit saw him it threw the boy into convulsions, and he fell on the ground and rolled about foaming at the mouth. Jesus asked his father, "How long has be been like this?" "From childhood," he replied; "it has often tried to destroy him by throwing him into the fire or into water. But if it is at all possible for you, take pity on us and help us." "If it is possible!" said Jesus. "Everything is possible to one who believes." At once the boy's father cried: "I believe; help my unbelief." When Jesus saw that the crowd was closing in on them, he spoke sternly to the unclean spirit. "Deaf and dumb spirit," he said, "I command you, come out of him and never go back!" It shrieked aloud and threw the boy into repeated convulsions, and then came out, leaving him looking like a corpse; in fact, many said, "He is dead." But Jesus took hold of his hand and raised him to his feet, and he stood up.
> Mark 9:17–27

This fascinating account from the Gospel of Mark uses some language that is unfamiliar to us, but it also contains many elements present in contemporary accounts of mental illness. The healing of both physical and mental illness through religious practices was a key element of early Christianity, thus this account is one of many that are similar. There are approximately 72 accounts of healings in the Gospels (with repetitions), and it is clear that the "casting out of unclean spirits" represents a significant proportion of Jesus' healing activity. The Gospel of Matthew (8:17) links these acts to the words of the Hebrew prophet Isaiah: "He took our illnesses from us and carried away our diseases." These healings, which often drew large crowds, were a primary way in which Jesus' ministry became known to the population. If the virtually instant, dramatic healing of the mentally ill with a few simple words seems strange to us, other parts of the story, representing persistent features of the effect of mental illness on social groups and the response they have to it, sound very familiar (Sheehan, 1983). We use the story to illustrate areas in which contemporary sociological research has already provided us with insights into the relationship between religion and health and also to suggest areas in which more work could fruitfully be done.

Mental illness has a big impact on families of the ill, and these families respond in different ways depending on their social location, particularly their religious affiliation and practices. Empirical research on mental illness done in the United States during the 1950s and 1960s revealed great complexity in the ways families deal with mental symptoms in their members. Mental symptoms are first noticed, interpreted, and responded to by those closest to the victim, and this is usually the family. The father in the previous passage reflects both this long knowledge of the condition and his reaction to it as he recounts the symptoms that have recurred over many years, and he pleads, "Take pity on us and help us." Early social scientific studies of mental illness showed how families grappled with new and developing symptoms, often finding ways of interpreting and "normalizing" them that would minimize the disruption to family life (Clausen & Yarrow, 1955). Most religious groups place a high value on preserving and supporting family life; research shows positive relationships between religious commitment and marital adjustment and strong families (D'Antonio and Aldous, 1983; Maton & Wells, 1995). The support of a religious congregation may provide very real assistance to the families of the mentally ill: One study of caregiving for ill (including mentally ill), handicapped, or older family members found that care-providing women who were religiously involved had better self-esteem and less depression than women who were providing care without the support of the religious group (Moen, Robison, & Dempster-McClain, 1995). Religious support for family caregivers for the mentally ill may even help explain one provocative finding in the literature: Researchers have noted, but not satisfactorily explained, ethnic differences in the caregiving duties of black and white family members (Horwitz, 1993). In one study, while black and white parents showed similar levels of caregiving duties, white parents reported significantly more feelings of burden; moreover, black siblings of the mentally ill reported simultaneously more caregiving duties and less caregiver burden than white siblings (Horwitz & Reinhard, 1995). The well-known higher levels of religious involvement among African Americans (Lincoln & Mamiya, 1990; Taylor & Chatters, 1991) may provide researchers with some hypotheses for future research in this area. In short, the impact of religion on the families of the mentally ill is an understudied area, but one which is likely to increase as care for the mentally ill devolves more to families and the community and away from psychiatric institutions.

Religious groups are especially effective at providing support during times of crisis. Chronic mental illness may be described as a series of crises, as in the life of the young boy in the Scripture passage. Mental illness, especially in the form of depression, may also be a response to a life crisis which is left unresolved. Religion, which can provide both social and cognitive support in times of crisis, recurringly appears in studies as a significant factor that predicts better outcomes. Studies of people in adverse, stressful situations are increasingly identifying religion as a coping resource (Ellison, 1994; Maton, 1989). Studies of the broad range of coping resources have shown religious coping to be especially effective in situations of loss or illness (Mattlin, Wethington, & Kessler, 1990). For example, one study of hospitalized veterans found that religious coping was the only significant predictor of lower depression scores over a 6-month period (Koenig et al., 1992); another study of elderly women with hip fractures showed that higher levels of religious belief were associated both with lower levels of depression and with better recovery from the fracture (Pressman, Lyons, Larson, & Strain, 1990; and a third found that, among men with severe disabilities, those who found strength and comfort in their religious beliefs had lower levels of depression (Idler & Kasl, 1992). Other studies have shown that the depression accompanying grieving is also moderated by religion for elderly men (Siegel & Kuykendall, 1990) and parents who have lost a child (McIntosh, Silver, & Wortman, 1993). Religious congregations may reach out to their members with considerable support during such crises, providing spiritual assistance in the material form of food, transportation, child care, or even financial aid. Perhaps even more important, religious faith provides cognitive resources for understanding tragic or stressful events; these religious meanings may have the power to bring individuals to a state of peace or acceptance of a situation which cannot be altered and give them the strength to live with it. As in the passage, the climax of a crisis situation may come with the turn away from earthly sources of help and the casting of the situation in religious terms.

Situations of illness, particularly mental illness, can be given religious interpretations, for which religious healing is a necessary and desired solution. The father of the little boy in the passage from Mark had defined his son's illness as a possession by spirits, an interpretation which he expected to be, and which was, shared by Jesus and his disciples. Ill individuals and their families come to terms with the symptoms of mental illness in many ways, which are to a large extent shaped by the symbolic and cultural repertoires they have at hand (Kleinman, 1980). Individuals and their families perceive symptoms, label and evaluate the disease, make social role adjustments for the disabled member, decide what to do about the symptoms, try remedies, and evaluate their success. In all of these activities, they use the beliefs and values that are available to them, and for many families in our culture, the interpretation of mental illness involves spiritual dimensions. Contemporary writing on religious healing commonly distinguishes between sickness of the body, sickness of the emotions, and sickness of the spirit, and while prayer is appropriate for the healing of all three, it is, by definition, the only way of resolving the latter (MacNutt, 1977; Stapleton, 1979).

In the religious sense, "healing" means "wholeness," or the restoration of a broken body, mind, or spirit. The cause of that brokenness, for many in the Judeo-Christian tradition, is sin, a break in the individual's relationship with God. The remedy for sin, of course, is forgiveness, a central feature of both the Jewish and Christian religions. Social scientists have only recently begun to explore the subject of forgiveness and its relevance to mental health. Enright and colleagues at the University of Wisconsin have for several years conducted a seminar on forgiveness as an aspect of moral development (Enright, Gassin, & Wu, 1992; see also Kaplan, Munroe-Blum, & Blazer, 1994). Clearly, the example of forgiveness does not begin to capture the range of religious interpretations available to individuals and their families. It is meant simply as an example of one way in which psychological distress could be given a religious interpretation. The question of sociological interest is, "How often are the relevant religious belief systems of patients elicited by physicians in treatment settings?" Would it improve care if they were? Writers suggesting this approach to physicians imply that the practice is relatively rare (Benson, 1996; Lynn, 1993). From a purely practical clinical standpoint, however, this is a sensible suggestion; as Favazza (1982, p. 734) points out, "[The psychiatrist] must understand and respect the patient's worldview and be willing to work within the patient's system, especially since complex and well-integrated belief systems tend to be stable and resistant to change."

The practice of religious healing frequently involves rituals. In the secular world, the term "ritual" very frequently connotes the empty repetition of meaningless acts, but to religious believers, rituals can be highly meaningful forms of religious practice. In the passage we have been exploring, Jesus employs a ritual form of language to cast out the evil spirits and then lays hands on the boy to bring him back to life. Prayer for healing and the laying on of hands were gifts given to the early Christians, and these remain important elements of Christian healing rituals today. In Durkheim's study of ritual in *Elementary Forms of Religious Life* (1912/1995), he shows the critical role ritual plays in renewing solidarity in social groups, strengthening social ties by reminding members of their origins and shared values. Performing rituals entails reenactment of ancient gestures, repeating of words that are heavily laden with symbolic meaning, and manipulating symbols that identify believers with one another and with the divine. Jerome Frank, in his classic work *Persuasion and Healing* (1961), observes that healing rituals "bring out the parallel between inner disorganization and disturbed relations with one's group, and indicate how patterned interaction of patient, healer, and group within the framework of a self-consistent assumptive world can promote healing" (p. 36). Thus, rituals link the internal, subjective world of the distressed individual with a culturally available scheme of shared meanings, bringing cognitions, emotions, and physical sensations into line.

Many forms of healing rituals are practiced today. McGuire's (1988) sociological study of religious healing in a New Jersey suburb found well-educated, middle-class Protestants, Catholics, and Jews engaged in a rich variety of symbolic and ritual healing practices, including meditation, speaking in tongues, anointing with oil, and the laying on of hands. Some of the insights of these traditional religious practices have been incorporated into secular healing practices which focus on relaxation and relief from stress (Benson, 1975, 1996). Conversely, other authors note the influence of psychoanalytic thinking on modern religious healing (Favazza, 1982).

The sociological contribution to our understanding of these practices and their importance for the mentally ill could be substantial. We need much more descriptive research on existing religious healing practices and their distribution in the community. With better descriptive information, the use of religious rituals as mental health resources could be adequately and accurately incorporated in psychiatric research.

People seek help for mental health problems from many diverse sources. Early studies of mental illness in the community indicated that a large proportion of persons with mental illness did not obtain any kind of treatment. Among those who sought help, a wide variety of sources were used, including mental health professionals, nonpsychiatric physicians, and the clergy (Hollingshead & Redlich, 1958;

Myers & Bean, 1968). Recent research suggests that as many as half of those suffering mental illness still receive no treatment (Regier et al., 1993). Moreover, many of those who seek help turn to clergy or religious professionals (20.8% of those who seek help) or simply to friends, family, and lay support groups (28.6%) (Narrow, Regier, Rae, Manderscheid, & Locke, 1993).

Although religious professionals have a long history of providing care to the mentally ill, we know little about the factors that lead to such therapeutic relationships or their effectiveness. Given the large numbers of persons who seek help for mental illness from religious sources, research on the effectiveness of clergy-based treatment is especially important. In addition, research on the proactive (e.g., identifying congregants with mental health problems and referring congregants who seek help to mental health professionals) and complementary (e.g., providing services to mentally ill persons or their families as an adjunct to treatment from mental health professionals) roles of religious professionals is of high priority.

METHODOLOGICAL CONTRIBUTIONS OF SOCIOLOGY TO THE STUDY OF RELIGION AND MENTAL HEALTH

This essay has been an attempt to suggest some of the many ways in which the sociological perspective can add to the substantive side of research on religion and mental health. Sociological research, since its inception, has been concerned with both religion and mental health, and sometimes even with the relationship between them. We know, for example, that a substantial minority of those seeking help for the symptoms of mental illness seek that help from clergy or other religious counselors, or that those in crisis situations of bereavement or serious illness do better if they have religious resources to call on. Many more research questions are suggested by the theoretical frameworks established by the sociological perspective, including the influence of religious beliefs on the interpretation of the symptoms of mental illness, the role of religious congregations in the support of family caregivers, and the effectiveness of religious rituals for the healing of mental illness.

The other contribution that the discipline of sociology has to make to this field of religion and mental health is a methodological one. The techniques and methods of social science, we believe, have two particular areas of expertise to offer to the field which come from the long history of field research and observational studies which have been conducted in health studies with a social scientific perspective.

MEASUREMENT OF THE CONCEPT OF RELIGIOUSNESS

Religiousness, as a characteristic of individuals, is a complex and multidimensional phenomenon. When it is included as a variable in mental health research, it is most often assessed with the single variable of religious affiliation, i.e., Protestant, Catholic, Jewish, or other membership (Larson, Pattison, Blazer, Omran, & Kaplan, 1986). This in itself, while useful, is only a crude indicator of the beliefs of the respondent that fails to differentiate between Protestant denominations or the large array of groups within the "other" category. The next most common indicator of the construct of religiousness is attendance at religious services, which is much more directly related to the extent of a respondent's religiousness but which still fails to capture any of the other important dimensions of religion, such as the private practices of prayer or the respondent's spiritual beliefs and feelings. Sociologists have been among the leaders in the field of the measurement of religiousness in identifying domains, developing instruments, and testing and refining them for use in systematic surveys. These ongoing efforts need to focus much more directly on the instruments needed for measurement in mental health research. They must be (a) brief and easily administered or self-administered in the survey or clinic situation, (b) multidimensional and inclusive of the many aspects of religiousness which might be relevant to mental health, and (c) inclusive in their language so that they are appropriate for use in religiously diverse populations.

DEVISING STUDY DESIGNS

Sociological research methods are extremely well suited to the types of observational studies that are needed to better understand the relationship between religion and mental health. We need longitudinal studies of representative populations with diverse religious group membership and good variation in religious involvement. We need to assess religious involvement at the initiation of the study and then follow respondents prospectively for changes in their mental health and/or their religious beliefs and practices. We also need to assess other competing risk factors, such as social networks and support, optimism, education, income, or stressful social conditions. Sociological data analysis methods will then allow us to examine and isolate the independent effects of these other important factors as well as to determine if they could help us explain any effect of religiousness. If people who attend religious services have more social contacts in the community, for example, this could explain why they are protected from depression during a period of unemployment. Sociological research methods provide us with the tools for adequately and sensitively measuring the concept of religiousness, for establishing time order in a prospective study design, and for evaluating competing and explanatory mechanisms.

In summary, sociological theories and methods have made important contributions to our understanding of mental illness and its consequences and have the potential to generate additional advances to the knowledge base in the future. An especially rich and fruitful direction for future research is combining sociological theories and methods with those from other disciplines.

REFERENCES

Amoateng, A. Y., & Bahr, S. J. (1986). Religion, family, and adolescent drug abuse. *Sociological Perspectives, 29,* 53–76.
Benson, H. (1975). *The relaxation response.* New York: William Morrow.

Benson, H. (1996). *Timeless healing.* New York: Simon & Schuster.

Benson, P. L., & Donahue, M. J. (1989). Ten-year trends in at-risk behaviors: A national study of black adolescents. *Journal of Adolescent Research, 4,* 125–139.

Berger, P. L. (1967). *The sacred canopy.* New York: Doubleday.

Bradley, D. E. (1995). Religious involvement and social resources: Evidence from the data set "Americans' Changing Lives." *Journal for the Scientific Study of Religion, 34,* 259–267.

Breault, K. D. (1986). Suicide in America: A test of Durkheim's theory of religious and family integration, 1933–1980. *American Journal of Sociology, 96,* 628–656.

Clausen, J. A., & Yarrow, M. R. (Eds.). (1955). The impact of mental illness on the family. *Journal of Social Issues, 11.*

Cochran, J. K., Beeghley, L., & Bock, E. W. (1992). The influence of religious stability and homogamy on the relationship between religiosity and alcohol use among Protestants. *Journal for the Scientific Study of Religion, 31,* 441–456.

D'Antonio, W. V., & Aldous, J. (Eds.). (1983). *Families and religions: Conflict and change in modern society.* Beverly Hills, CA: Sage.

Durkheim, E. (1951). *Suicide.* New York: Free Press. (Original work published 1897)

Durkheim, E. (1995). *The elementary forms of religious life.* New York: Free Press. (Original work published 1912)

Ellison, C. (1991). Religious involvement and subjective well-being. *Journal of Health and Social Behavior, 32,* 80–99.

Ellison, C. (1994). Religion, the life stress paradigm, and the study of depression. In J. Levin (Ed.), *Religion in aging and health: Theoretical foundations and methodological frontiers* (pp. 78–121). Thousand Oaks, CA: Sage.

Ellison, C., & George, L. (1994). Religious involvement, social ties and social support in a southeastern community. *Journal for the Scientific Study of Religion, 33,* 46–61.

Enright, R. D., Gassin, E. A., & Wu, G. R. (1992). Forgiveness: A developmental view. *Journal of Moral Education, 21,* 99–113.

Favazza, A. R. (1982). Modern Christian healing of mental illness. *American Journal of Psychiatry, 139,* 728–735.

Frank, J. (1961). *Persuasion and healing.* Baltimore: Johns Hopkins Press.

Gorsuch, R. L. (1995). Religious aspects of substance abuse and recovery. *Journal of Social Issues, 51,* 65–83.

Hollingshead, A. B., & Redlich, F. C. (1958). *Social class and mental illness: A community study.* New York: John Wiley.

Horwitz, A. V. (1993). Adult siblings as sources of social support for the seriously mentally ill: A test of the serial model. *Journal of Marriage and the Family, 55,* 623–632.

Horwitz, A. V., & Reinhard, S. C. (1995). Ethnic differences in caregiving duties and burdens among parents and siblings of persons with severe mental illnesses. *Journal of Health and Social Behavior, 36,* 138–150.

Idler, E. L., & Kasl, S. V. (1992). Religion, disability, depression, and the timing of death. *American Journal of Sociology, 97,* 1052–1079.

Kaplan, B., Munroe-Blum, H., & Blazer, D. G. (1994). Religion, health, and forgiveness: Traditions and challenges. In J. Levin (Ed.), *Religion in aging and health: Theoretical foundations and methodological frontiers* (pp. 52–77). Thousand Oaks, CA: Sage.

Kleinman, A. (1980). *Patients and healers in the context of culture: An exploration of the borderland between anthropology, medicine, and psychiatry.* Berkeley: University of California Press.

Koenig, H. G., Moberg, D. O., & Kvale, J. N. (1988). Religious activities and attitudes of older adults in a geriatric assessment clinic. *Journal of the American Geriatrics Society, 36,* 362–374.

Koenig, H. G., Smiley, M. & Gonzales, J. P. (1988). *Religion, health, and aging: A review and theoretical integration.* New York: Greenwood Press.

Krause, N. (1995). Religiosity and self-esteem among older adults. *Journal of Gerontology: Psychological Sciences, 50B,* P236–P246.

Larson, D. B., Pattison, E. M., Blazer, D. G., Omran, A. R., & Kaplan, B. H. (1986). Systematic analy-

sis of research on religious variables in four major psychiatric journals. *American Journal of Psychiatry, 143,* 329–334.

Lincoln, C. E., & Mamiya, L. (1990). *The black church in the African American experience.* Durham, NC: Duke Press.

Lynn, J. (1993). Travels in the valley of the shadow. In H. Spiro, M. McCrea Curnen, E. Peschel, & D. St. James (Eds.), *Empathy and the practice of medicine* (pp. 40–53). New Haven, CT: Yale University Press.

MacNutt, F. (1977). *The power to heal.* Notre Dame, IN: Ave Maria Press.

Maton, K. I. (1989). The stress-buffering role of spiritual support: Cross-sectional and prospective investigations. *Journal for the Scientific Study of Religion, 28,* 310–323.

Maton, K. I., & Wells, E. (1995). Religion as a community resource for well-being: Prevention, healing, and empowerment pathways. *Journal of Social Issues, 51,* 177–193.

Mattlin, J. A., Wethington, E., & Kessler, R. (1990). Situational determinants of coping and coping effectiveness. *Journal of Health and Social Behavior, 31,* 103–122.

McGuire, M. B. (1988). *Ritual healing in suburban America.* New Brunswick, NJ: Rutgers Press.

McIntosh, D. N., Silver, R. C., & Wortman, C. B. (1993). Religion's role in adjustment to a negative life event: Coping with the loss of a child. *Journal of Personality and Social Psychology, 65,* 812–821.

Moen, P., Robison, J. & Dempster-McClain, D. (1995). Caregiving and women's well-being: A life course approach. *Journal of Health and Social Behavior, 36,* 259–273.

Myers, J. K., & Bean, L. L. (1968). *A decade later: A follow-up of social class and mental illness.* New York: John Wiley.

Narrow, W. E., Regier, D. A., Rae, D. S., Manderscheid, R. W., & Locke, B. Z. (1993). Use of services by persons with mental and addictive disorders: Findings from the National Institute of Mental Health Epidemiologic Catchment Area Program. *Archives of General Psychiatry, 50,* 95–107.

Pescosolido, B. A., & Georgianna, S. (1989). Durkheim, suicide, and religion: Toward a network theory of suicide. *American Sociological Review, 54,* 33–48.

Pressman, P., Lyons, J. S., Larson, D. B., & Strain, J. J. (1990). Religious belief, depression, and ambulation status in elderly women with broken hips. *American Journal of Psychiatry, 147,* 758–760.

Regier, D. A., Narrow, W. E., Rae, D. S., Manderscheid, R. W., Locke, B. Z., & Goodwin, F. K. (1993). The de facto U.S. mental and addictive disorders service system: Epidemiologic Catchment Area prospective 1-year prevalence rates of disorders & services. *Archives of General Psychiatry, 50,* 85–94.

Schwab, R., & Petersen, K. U. (1990). Religiousness: Its relation to loneliness, neuroticism and subjective well-being. *Journal for the Scientific Study of Religion, 29,* 335–345.

Sheehan, S. (1983). *Is there no place on earth for me?* New York: Vintage.

Siegel, J. M. & Kuykendall, D. H. (1990). Loss, widowhood, and psychological distress among the elderly. *Journal of Consulting and Clinical Psychology, 58,* 519–524.

Stack, S., & Wasserman, I. (1992). The effect of religion on suicide ideology: An analysis of the networks perspective. *Journal for the Scientific Study of Religion, 31,* 457–466.

Stapleton, R. (1979). *The experience of inner healing.* Waco, TX: Word Books.

Taylor, R. J., & Chatters, L. (1991). Religious life of black Americans. In J. S. Jackson (Ed.), *Life in black America* (pp. 105–123). Newbury Park, CA: Sage.

Vaux, K. (1976). Religion and health. *Preventive Medicine, 5,* 522–536.

Weber, M. (1958). *The Protestant ethic and the spirit of capitalism.* New York: Scribner. (Original work published 1904)

5

RELIGION AND PERSONALITY

ROBERT A. EMMONS

Department of Psychology
University of California, Davis
Davis, California 95616

Thirty years ago, the psychology of religion and the psychology of personality appeared to be lifeless fields of inquiry. Destined to become archaic relics nostalgically and romantically associated with a more wistful time in psychology's past, researchers were discouraged from intellectual inquiry in what were perceived as terminal fields. In the opening sentence of a section titled "Religion and Personality Characteristics" in a chapter on religion in *The Handbook of Social Psychology,* Dittes (1968) stated, "It is a confession of the poverty and primitive state of this field to propose a section so grossly focused as the heading above indicates" (p. 636). The same year, Walter Mischel (1968) published his devastating critique of the field of personality, leaving academic personality psychology reeling for the next two decades.

Interestingly, 30 years later, both the psychology of religion and the psychology of personality are experiencing something of a renaissance, with vigorous empirical and conceptual work being carried out in both fields. A revival of personality psychology has been noted by several writers (Emmons, 1993; McAdams, 1996a; Singer & Salovey, 1993) and the psychology of religion is similarly alive and well (Paloutzian, 1996; Wulff, 1996). The field of personality emerged from the post-Mischellian age with renewed vigor over the past decade. To be sure, differences of opinion remain, but consensus has slowly emerged regarding the answers to fundamental issues in the field, such as the genetic and evolutionary basis of personality traits and the degree to which personality changes versus remains stable over time (Caprara, 1996; Loehlin, 1992).

Research into spiritual matters is burgeoning as well and has not been limited only to what is normally seen as the purview of "religious psychology." Various fields of psychology, in particular clinical and health psychology, are becoming increasingly aware of, and impressed by, the centrality of religious concerns in people's lives as well as the impact that these concerns have on mental, physical, and interpersonal outcomes (Bergin, 1991; Kimble, McFadden, Ellor, & Seeber, 1995; Paloutzian & Kirkpatrick, 1995; Pargament & Park, 1995; Schumaker, 1994; Shafranske, 1996). Once considered off limits for serious injury, there now appears to be considerable momentum and interest building in the study of the psycho-spiritual component of people's lives.

Despite progress in both these subdisciplines of psychology, advances at the interface of personality and religion have been unsystematic, scattered, and generally unintegrated within an overall organizational framework that could promote progress and stimulate theoretical and methodological advances. In comparison to its neighboring subdisciplines, contemporary academic personality psychology has lagged behind in acknowledging the spiritual reality of the person. This is a perplexing state of affairs for two reasons. First, early pioneers in the psychology of religion, such as Gordon Allport (1950) and Gardner Murphy (Murphy, 1990), were identified primarily as personality psychologists. Though it was often regarded with suspicion, disdain, outright hostility, or a mixture of these, religion received considerable attention in Freudian, neo-Freudian, and other classical personality theories. However, somewhere along the line, religion pulled a vanishing act from personality theory and from psychology more generally. Nearly half a century ago, Allport (1950) began his classic book on personality and religion by stating that,

> Among modern intellectuals—especially in the universities—the subject of religion seems to have gone into hiding. . . . The persistence of religion in the modern world appears as an embarrassment to the scholars of today. Even psychologists, to whom presumably nothing of human concern is alien, are likely to retire into themselves when the subject is broached. (p. 1)

Allport would therefore have been chagrined, but probably not surprised, to learn that a volume devoted to celebrating the 50th anniversary of his textbook (Craik & Hogan, 1993) made no mention of his extensive writings on the central role of religiosity within the structure of personality. In addition, two recent, comprehensive handbooks of personality (Hogan, Johnson, & Briggs, 1997; Pervin, 1990) fail to include religion as a topic of inquiry. A singular reference that appears in one book (Megargee, 1997) bemoans this very neglect of the topic.

The second surprising reason for the neglect of religion is that personality psychology has long claimed to be concerned with understanding the whole person. Spiritual or religious goals, beliefs, and practices are central to many people's lives and are powerful influences on cognition, affect, motivation, and behavior. Because spirituality and religiousness are profound aspects of people's lives, it would seem that in order to know a person (McAdams, 1995), personality psychologists must know about the religious side of that person's life. Because personality psychologists purport to study the whole person, I examine the links between personality and religion, both in terms of what the study of personality can contribute to the scientific study of religion and what possible insights into personality structure and functioning that an acknowledgment of the religious side of life can offer.

THE GOALS OF PERSONALITY PSYCHOLOGY

The primary question that personality psychologists are concerned with, at the broadest level is, What is a person like? Shoda and Mischel (1996) view the central mission of the field as the "understanding of individuals as deeply, completely, and precisely as possible" (p. 425). McAdams (1995) posed the question as follows: What do we know when we know a person? He suggests that of all the questions that can be posed about persons from a scientific point of view, there is none more fundamental. Other issues of central relevance to psychologists concerned with personality (e.g., issues of development, stability, and change) must remain in the personological queue until there is a description—an account of what a person is like. Personality deals with the whole person, the total functioning organism, and therefore requires knowledge of significant aspects of the interior life of persons. Also, because of its unique position within psychology, personality psychology may serve as a bridge between research on basic processes and clinical practice (Caprara, 1996).

A complete understanding of the role of personality in religious experience and in the expression of religious impulses requires an extended discussion of how personality is conceptualized by contemporary personality psychologists. It is only after this that the interplay between personality and religion, at the levels of both theory and method, can be effectively approached. The balance of this chapter will be devoted to a presentation of McAdams' (1995, 1996b) articulated framework for the understanding of human individuality and its' application to research on religious and spiritual constructs within personality.

LEVELS OF PERSONALITY: THREE TIERS

Recent advances in the development of comprehensive frameworks for understanding persons suggest the possibility of advances in understanding links between personality and religion. The history of personality psychology is synonymous with the search for appropriate units of analysis for studying the person. What units of analysis should be used to describe persons? A bewildering array of possibilities await the contemporary personologist. McAdams (1995, 1996a, 1996b) proposes that knowing a person requires being privy to information at three distinct levels or domains of personality description: (a) comparative dispositional traits, (b) contextualized personal concerns, and (c) integrative life stories. Each level contains different constructs and a different focus and is accessed through different assessment operations. The three levels are relatively orthogonal realms of functioning, unfolding independently of each other and differing in their accessibility to consciousness. They provide different vantage points or perspectives with which to view the scientific study of persons.

The first level, level I, is composed of relatively nonconditional, decontextualized, and comparative dimensions of personality called "traits." Characteristics at this level are essential in describing the most general and observable aspects of a person's typical behavioral patterns. Personality trait psychology has recently culminated in what many have argued is a consensus around the five-factor model of personality traits (Digman, 1990; McCrae & Costa, 1990). Five traits—openness to experience, conscientiousness, extraversion, agreeableness, and neuroticism (OCEAN)—offer a unifying frame of reference that seems to have been readily adopted by many inside and outside the field of personality psychology proper. OCEAN has proven to be a powerful framework for organizing existing trait questionnaire measures and for predicting important life outcomes, such as health, psychological well-being, and therapeutic outcomes. The five-factor model has also been bolstered by behavior genetic studies demonstrating substantial heritabilities of many personality traits (Loehlin, 1992).

Traits are valuable descriptive features of persons, owing to their normative and nonconditional properties. However, people are not identical with their traits. Ryan (1995) stated, "Life is not lived as a trait" (p. 416). The limitations of decontextualized trait units for understanding individuality have been discussed elsewhere (Block, 1995; McAdams, 1992; Pervin, 1994). Diener (1996) argued that traits are not enough for understanding the multiply determined phenonomena of subjective well-being. He demonstrates that trait constructs fail to offer a complete account of people's evaluative responses to their lives. McAdams (1992) argued that trait descriptions yield at best a "psychology of the stranger"; they are literally a first-stab attempt at describing a person.

Level II is composed of contextualized strategies, plans, and concerns which enable a person to solve various life tasks and achieve personally important life goals. In recent years, there has been increasing articulation of constructs at this level of analysis as personologists turn their attention to self-regulatory mechanisms and structures that guide behavior purposefully to achieve desired goals. Constructs at this level, which include personal objects (Little, Lecci, & Watkinson, 1992), life tasks (Cantor, 1990), and personal strivings (Emmons, 1986), are characterized by intentionality and goal-directedness, in comparison to the stylistic and habitual tendencies at level I. These units are sometimes noncomparative, frequently highly contingent, and contextualized in time and space. Little et al. (1992) referred to these units using the acronym "PAC" (personal action contructs) and explicitly contrasted them with broad dispositions. Constructs at this level tend to be motivational and developmental in nature because they focus explicitly on what a person is consciously trying to do during a particular period in his or her life. As McAdams (1992) and Pervin (1994) have forcefully argued, concepts at this level are fundamentally different from traits and cannot be reduced to traits. In a sense, level I speaks to what a person "has" (Cantor, 1990), whereas level II speaks to what a person "does."

The third level or domain is identity or the life narrative, which consists of the stories that people construct that provide them with a sense of overall meaning and purpose to their lives. It is the life story that renders the array of traits, strivings, and various other level I and II elements into a more or less coherent and constantly evolving integrative unity. Singer and Salovey (1993) stated, "The stories individuals tell about their own lives are the life blood of personality" (p. 70). As opposed to the having and doing sides of personality, which are encapsulated in levels I and II, respectively, level III is concerned with the "making" of the self (McAdams, 1996b).

The study of narrative, both as a methodology and as a theoretical construct, has increasingly impacted personality psychology in the past decade (e.g., Rosenwald & Ochberg, 1992). Narrative approaches have not been limited to the field of personality. Sarbin (1986) suggested that the organization of life experiences into a narrative can serve as a root metaphor for general psychology. Sarbin's thesis is that narrative modes of explanation provide for a more satisfactory account of human action than do formistic or mechanistic models. Since identity is a story, it must be understood in story terms. McAdams (1993, 1996b) outlines several component features of life stories: narrative emotional tone, symbolic and metaphoric use of imagery, motivational themes, ideological setting, nuclear episodes (e.g., turning points in life), imagoes (idealized characters), and the ending provided by the generativity script. An appraisal of these features enables life stories to be systematically quantified, classified, and analyzed much like any other data source for personologists.

APPLYING THE THREE LEVELS TO THE PSYCHOLOGY OF RELIGION

The three levels of personality structure can be used to organize current knowledge and to suggest future directions for research on religion and personality. How can this integrative three-level model of personality offer a helpful framework for guiding conceptual and empirical efforts on personality and religion? Various constructs that have been studied in the psychology of religion can be organized using this tri-level conceptual framework. Beginning with James' (1902) distinction between feelings, acts, and experiences, psychologists have historically partitioned religious experience into meaningful clusters of activity. The levels of personality framework offer an alternative to the conventional decomposition of religiousness into beliefs, practices, feelings, and knowledge (Glock, 1962), suggesting that the richest picture of the religious life of the person would require, at a minimum, collecting information at all three levels of analysis, covering dispositional traits, personal concerns, and integrative stories.

LEVEL I: DISPOSITIONAL TRAITS

The bulk of psychological research on religion has focused on level 1, dispositional traits. From this vantage point, religiosity is expressed in broad, decontextualized trans-situational tendencies such as the intrinsic/extrinsic orientation (Paloutzian, 1996). Researchers examining individual differences in religiousness have emphasized that people are not religious in the same ways. Allport (1950) was the first to systematically distinguish between religion as a means to an end (extrinsic) and religion as a way of life (intrinsic). Measures of the former generally show a very different pattern of correlation with criterion variables, such as church attendance, prejudice, and mental health, than measures of the latter (Ventis, 1995). Even a rudimentary distinction between intrinsic and extrinsic religiousness, however, fails to begin to capture the complexity inherent in the construct of religiosity or spirituality (Kirkpatrick & Hood, 1990).

Piedmont (1996) demonstrated the value of the five-factor model (FFM) for advancing religious research. He suggested that the FFM can provide an empirical reference point for evaluating the development of new measures of religiousness and for evaluating the meaning of existing measures, and it might also be profitably used in clergy selection and assessment. Ozer and Reise (1994) advise that researchers routinely correlate their particular measure with the FFM. Given the proliferation of measurement instruments in the psychology of religion, researchers would do well to heed this advice. However, as Piedmont points out, the FFM might not always be appropriate because the five factors are not religiously based. Instead, measures of intrinsic and extrinsic religiosity might be comparably employed as a defining marker to be correlated with new measures of spiritual constructs.

LEVEL II: PERSONAL CONCERNS

The limitations of focusing solely on the trait level in psychology of religion research while relying exclusively on the questionnaire measurement paradigm have been noted by Gorsuch (1984). Thus, an important agenda for future research is identifying and rigorously measuring contextualized and conditional units of analysis. Level II (contextualized personal concerns and goals) and level III (identity or the life narrative) constructs remain largely unexplored and have much to offer the psychologist interested in religious issues within personality.

Given the frequency of religious beliefs, at least in the United States (Paloutzian, 1996), it would be surprising if concerns over ultimate questions of meaning and existence did not find expression in one form or another through the personal concerns of people in their everyday lives. One of the functions of a religious belief system and a religious worldview is that it provides "an ultimate vision of what people should be striving for in their lives" (Pargament & Park, 1995, p. 15) and the strategies to reach those ends. Similarly, Apter (1985) views the religious state of mind as "telic," providing a guide to "the most serious and far-ranging goals there can possibly be" (p. 69). Spiritual personal concerns can be conceptualized as "ultimate concerns," a term used by the existential theologian Paul Tillich (1957) in his classic analysis of the affective and cognitive bases of faith. The essence of religion, in the broadest and most inclusive sense, is ultimate concern. An ultimate concern (a) is one in which maximal value is invested, (b) possesses the power to center one's life, and (c) demands "total surrender" (Tillich, 1957, p. 3). When ultimate concerns center on the transcendent (Pargament & Park, 1995) they are considered spiritual.

Personal concerns offer advantages for both conceptualizing and measuring spirituality. Constructs at this level of analysis offer a vantage point on spirituality that transcends measures of denominational affiliation, retrospective reports of church attendance or prayer or other spiritual activity, and general attitudes toward religion to encompass the diversity of daily goals, enduring strivings, and ultimate concerns of a spiritually oriented lifestyle under the same theoretical umbrella or "sacred canopy" (Berger, 1967). Measurement approaches to personal goals exploit the power of a combined idiographic/nomothetic assessment strategy. They reflect the idiosyncratic ways in which individuals strive to obtain or maintain a concern with the sacred in their everyday lives. At the same time, they allow for conclusions to be drawn about the relation between spiritual goals and well-being that generalize across persons.

Emmons, Dank, and Mongrain (1997) provide an example of how constructs at this level might lead to progress in understanding the effect of religiosity on subjective well-being. These researchers first developed a set of coding criteria to classify strivings as spiritual based on a categorical accounting of the target of the individual striving as directed toward transcendent concerns. Examples of spirituality in strivings include trying to "be aware of the spiritual meaningfulness of my life," "share my faith with others," and "be less self-centered." Spiritual strivings, elicited through both self-reports and spouse ratings, were found to be highly predictive of various indices of mental health, including individual life satisfaction and marital satisfaction, purpose in life, and reduced psychological distress.

Examining religion as personal concerns holds implications for therapeutic assessment and intervention. Clinically mindful investigators such as Karoly (1993) have described the potential benefits of incorporating a goal-based approach into the design of treatment programs. A goals or concerns assessment can pinpoint problematic goal appraisals within the person's hierarchy that might be associated with psychological, somatic, or interpersonal distress. For example, an identification of goals that are overvalued, undervalued, unrealistic, conflict producing, or self-defeating would be a first step in designing an appropriate, workable intervention that would enable an individual to experience greater self-efficacy and positive states of well-being.

LEVEL III: LIFE NARRATIVES

Level III concerns how persons make sense of who they are in the world, and how they create life stories that provide their lives with overall unity, meaning, and purpose. Religious considerations play a major role in this level of personality because people construct a life story often rooted in a religious ideology that gives a unique meaning to their life. Beit-Hallahmi (1989) argues that religion is an identity-maintenance system, providing a bridge between individualistic and collectivist identities. In several collections of life stories (Colby & Damon, 1992; Franz & Stewart, 1994; McAdams, 1993), spirituality as a guiding, integrating, and empowering force is a recurring theme, with religious narratives functioning as potent identity stories in the diverse lives of these men and women. Conversion narratives in the form of the personal testimony are a powerful means of consolidating and strengthening one's new religious identity (Beit-Hallahmi, 1989; Rambo, 1993; Stromberg, 1993). McAdams (1996b) notes that the use of metaphor is a defining feature of personal identity. The richness of metaphor that religious systems provide (e.g., viewing major life changes such as divorce and remarriage as involving the death and burial or an old life and a resurrection to a new one) may be a potent means of constructing identity (Atkinson, 1995; Rambo, 1993) and thus are ideally suited to story-based methodologies.

Because the problem of identity is the problem of constructing unity, purpose, and coherence in one's life, religion may offer a particularly attractive solution for many. Allport (1950) was impressed by the coherence and integration in personality that personal religion can foster:

> The religious sentiment . . . is the portion of personality that arises at the core and that has the longest range intentions, and for this reason is capable of conferring marked integration upon personality. . . . It is man's ultimate attempt to enlarge and to complete his own personality. (p. 142)

Religion or spirituality can provide a unifying philosophy of life and serve as an integrating and stabilizing force in the face of constant environmental and cultural pressures that push for fragmentation, particularly in postmodern cultures (McAdams, 1996b). Tillich (1957) stated that "the ultimate concern gives depth, direction, and unity to all other concerns, and with them, to the whole personality" (p. 105). This religion-as-integration hypothesis is a promising one that is amenable to empirical scrutiny. After all, the root of religion originates in the term *religare,* which means to bind things together or to bring them back together again. If there are inherent integrating tendencies within persons (Ryan, 1995), might not these be religious in nature?

Constructs at levels II and III might have utility in gauging cultural trends in spirituality. Personal concerns and life stories reflect broader societal concerns and shared cultural stories (Cantor, 1990; McAdams, 1996b; Singer & Salovey, 1993). Singer and Salovey lament the dearth of self-transcendent themes in self-defining memories generated by their college student samples. They ask, "Where are the memories of religious community . . . of an active pursuit of social justice . . . of responsibility to the elderly and appreciation of the knowledge they might have to share?" (p. 209). Instead, their memories reflect the dominant themes of contemporary Western culture: autonomous, individualistic pursuits and accomplishments—an indictment of the prevailing cultural ideology. If the present times are indeed a period of spiritual renewal as some historians and social commentators have suggested (Roof, 1993; Tickle, 1995), indications of this trend should appear in the nature of the data collected by personality psychologists—the personal concerns, self-defining memories, and life stories told by research participants.

CONCLUSIONS AND RECOMMENDATIONS

There is, of course, more to understanding the religious lives of persons than can be captured within the three-tiered framework described in this chapter. However, these three levels provide some conceptual tools and measurement guidelines for locating mapping religious variables onto a broader personological framework. In so doing, significant advances in understanding the role of religion in personality structure and functioning might be realized. Dealing as it does with daily life concerns and the affective, cognitive, and motivational functioning of persons, the field of personality might also succeed in making theology more relevant to the ups and downs of everyday life.

There is much to be gained by an increased dialogue between personality psychology and theology. Taking as its subject matter the development, functioning, and degree of transformation of the person over time, personality psychology is ideally situated to stimulate progress in understanding religious influences in persons' lives. Although this chapter has stressed the applicability of frameworks for understanding the person for research on spiritual phenomena, theological perspectives might also profitably inform personality theory and research. Personality psychology deals with fundamental questions of human nature; indeed, theologies are psychological theories as well (Ingram, 1996; Spilka & Bridges, 1989). Personality theory and theology should be natural allies; both are concerned, ultimately, with what it means to be a human being. Theological formulations offer a complementary perspective on human nature, one that transcends historical and cultural circumstances. Personality theory and research cannot take place in a theological black hole. To stay silent on theological matters is to take the position that they are unimportant for understanding individuality; there is ample evidence to argue against this position. Personality may have more to do with theology than most personality psychologists are comfortable admitting. Personality psychologists cannot afford to be parochial in outlook; the health and vitality of their discipline depends on interdisciplinary outreach (Baumeister & Tice, 1996).

At the same time, personality researchers must avoid the temptation to reduce theological principles to psychological concepts. Mixing a pinch of theism with a dash of psychologism is likely to result in a psychotheological soup that is distasteful for personologists and theologians alike. Psychological and theological accounts have different ranges of convenience and cannot be reduced to each other (Jeeves, 1997). To the degree that it incorporates religious constructs into its models of persons, personality theory needs to be guided by sophisticated theological doctrine; Donahue (1989) has aptly illustrated the pitfalls of disregarding theology in the scientific study of religion.

Fifty years ago, Gardner Murphy (1947) concluded his biosocial text on personality by boldly speculating,

> In a future psychology of personality there will surely be a place for directly grappling with the questions of man's response to the cosmos, his sense of unity with it, the nature of his aesthetic demands upon it, and his feelings of loneliness or of consummation in his contemplation of it. . . . They have felt incomplete as human beings except as they have endeavored to understand their filial relations to the cosmos. . . . Our study of man must include the study of his response to the cosmos of which he is a reflection. (p. 919)

The future personality psychology that Murphy envisioned may be right around the corner.

REFERENCES

Allport, G. W. (1950). *The individual and his religion.* New York: Macmillan.

Apter, M. J. (1985). Religious states of mind: A reversal theory interpretation. In L. B. Brown (Ed.), *Advances in the psychology of religion* (pp. 62–75). Oxford: Pergamon.

Atkinson, R. (1995). *The gift of stories.* Westport, CT: Bergin & Harvey.

Baumeister, R. F., & Tice, D. M. (1996). Rethinking and reclaiming the interdisciplinary role of personality psychology: The science of human nature should be the center of the social sciences and humanities. *Journal of Research in Personality, 30,* 363–373.

Beit-Hallahmi, B. (1989). *Prolegomena to the psychological study of religion.* Lewisburg, PA: Bucknell University Press.

Berger, P. L. (1967). *The sacred canopy: Elements of a sociological theory of religion.* Garden City, NY: Doubleday.

Bergin, A. E. (1991). Values and religious issues in psychotherapy and mental health. *American Psychologist, 46,* 394–403.

Block, J. (1995). A contrarian view of the five-factor approach to personality description. *Psychological Bulletin, 117,* 187–215.

Cantor, N. (1990). From thought to behavior: "Having" and "doing" in the study of personality and cognition. *American Psychologist, 45,* 735–750.

Caprara, G. V. (1996). Reflections on the scientific status and perspectives of personality psychology. In J. Georgas, M. Manthouli, E. Besevegis, & A. Kokkevi (Eds.), *Contemporary psychology in Europe* (pp. 103–117). Seattle: Hogrefe & Huber.

Colby, A., & Damon, W. (1992). *Some do care.* New York: Free Press.

Craik, K. H., & Hogan, R. (Eds.). (1993). *Fifty years of personality psychology.* New York: Plenum.

Diener, E. (1984). Subjective well-being. *Psychological Bulletin, 95,* 542–575.

Diener, E. (1996). Traits can be powerful, but are not enough: Lessons from subjective well-being. *Journal of Research in Personality, 30,* 389–399.

Digman, J. M. (1990). Personality structure: Emergence of the five-factor model. *Annual Review of Psychology, 41,* 417–440.

Dittes, J. (1968). Psychology of religion. In G. Lindzey & E. Aronson (Eds.), *The handbook of social psychology* (2nd ed., Vol. 5, pp. 602–659). Reading, MA: Addison-Wesley.

Donahue, M. J. (1989). Disregarding theology in the psychology of religion: Some examples. *Journal of Psychology and Theology, 17,* 329–335.

Emmons, R. A. (1986). Personal strivings: An approach to personality and subjective well-being. *Journal of Personality and Social Psychology, 51,* 1058–1068.

Emmons, R. A. (1993). Current status of the motive concept. In K. H. Craik, R. Hogan, & R. N. Wolfe (Eds.), *Fifty years of personality psychology* (pp. 187–196). New York: Plenum.

Emmons, R. A., Dank, M., & Mongrain, M. (1997). *Spirituality through personal strivings: Ultimate concerns and psychological well-being.* Manuscript submitted for publication, University of California, Davis.

Franz, C., & Stewart, A. J. (Eds.). (1994). *Women creating lives: Identities, resilience, and resistance.* Boulder, CO: Westview.

Glock, C. Y. (1962). On the study of religious commitment. *Religious Education, 57,* 98–109.

Gorsuch, R. L. (1984). Measurement: The boon and bane of investigating religion. *American Psychologist, 39,* 228–236.

Hogan, R., Johnson, J., & Briggs, S. (Eds.). (1997). *Handbook of personality psychology.* San Diego: Academic Press.

Ingram, J. A. (1996). Psychological aspects of the filling of the Holy Spirit: A preliminary model of post-redemptive personality functioning. *Journal of Psychology and Theology, 24,* 104–113.

James, W. (1902). *The varieties of religious experience.* White Plains, NY: Longmans.

Jeeves, M. A. (1997). *Human nature at the millenium.* Grand Rapids, MI: Baker Books.

Karoly, P. (1993). Goal systems: An organizational framework for clinical assessment and treatment planning. *Psychological Assessment, 3,* 273–280.

Kimble, M. A., McFadden, S. H., Ellor, J. W., & Seeber, J. J. (Eds.). (1995). *Aging, spirituality, and religion: A handbook.* Minneapolis, MN: Fortress Press.

Kirkpatrick, L., & Hood, R. W., Jr. (1990). Intrinsic–extrinsic religious orientation: The "boon" or "bane" of contemporary psychology of religion? *Journal for the Scientific Study of Religion, 29,* 442–462.

Little, B. R., Lecci, L., & Watkinson, B. (1992). Personality and personal projects: Linking Big Five and PAC units of analysis. *Journal of Personality, 60,* 501–525.

Loehlin, J. (1992). *Genes and environment in personality development.* New York: Guilford.

McAdams, D. P. (1992). The five-factor model in personality: A critical appraisal. *Journal of Personality, 60,* 329–361.

McAdams, D. P. (1993). *The stories we live by: Personal myths and the making of the self.* New York: Morrow.

McAdams, D. P. (1995). What do we know when we know a person? *Journal of Personality, 63,* 365–396.

McAdams, D. P. (1996a). Alternative futures for the study of human individuality. *Journal of Research in Personality, 30,* 374–388.

McAdams, D. P. (1996b). Personality, modernity, and the storied self: A contemporary framework for studying persons. *Psychological Inquiry, 7,* 295–321.

McCrae, R. R., & Costa, P. T., Jr. (1990). *Personality in adulthood.* New York: Guilford.

McDonald, M. (1994). The new spirituality: Mainstream North American is on a massive search for meaning in life. *Maclean's, 107,* 44–48.

Megargee, E. (1997). Internal inhibitions and controls. In R. Hogan, J. Johnson, & S. Briggs (Eds.), *Handbook of personality psychology* (pp. 581–614). San Diego: Academic Press.

Mischel, W. (1968). *Personality and assessment.* New York: John Wiley.

Murphy, G. (1947). *Personality: A biosocial approach to origins and structure.* New York: Harper & Row.

Murphy, L. B. (1990). *Gardner Murphy: Integrating, expanding, and humanizing psychology.* Jefferson, NC: McFarland.

Ozer, D. J., & Reise, S. P. (1994). Personality assessment. *Annual Review of Psychology, 45,* 357–388.

Paloutzian, R. F. (1996). *Invitation to the psychology of religion* (2nd ed.). Needham Heights, MA: Allyn & Bacon.

Paloutzian, R. F., & Kirkpatrick, L. A. (1995). Introduction: The scope of religious influences and personal and society well-being. *Journal of Social Issues, 51,* 1–12.

Pargament, K. I., & Park, C. L. (1995). Merely a defense? The variety of religious means and ends. *Journal of Social Issues, 51,* 13–32.

Pervin, L. A. (Ed.). (1990). *Handbook of personality: Theory and research.* New York: Guilford.

Pervin, L. A. (1994). A critical analysis of current trait theory. *Psychological Inquiry, 5,* 103–113.

Piedmont, R. L. (1996, August). *Strategies for using the five-factor model in religious research.* Paper presented at the annual convention of the American Psychological Association, Toronto, Canada.

Rambo, L. R. (1993). *Understanding religious conversion.* New Haven, CT: Yale University Press.

Roof, W. C. (1993). *A generation of seekers: The spiritual journeys of the baby boom generation.* San Francisco: Harper.

Rosenwald, G. C., & Ochberg, R. C. (Eds.). (1992). *Storied lives.* New Haven, CT: Yale University Press.

Ryan, R. M. (1995). Psychological needs and the facilitation of integrative processes. *Journal of Personality, 63,* 397–428.

Sarbin, T. (1986). *Narrative psychology: The storied nature of human conduct.* New York: Praeger.

Schumaker, J. F. (Ed.). (1994). *Religion and mental health.* New York: Oxford University Press.

Shafranske, E. (Ed.). (1996). *Religion and the clinical practice of psychology.* Washington, DC: American Psychological Association.

Shoda, Y., & Mischel, W. (1996). Toward a unified, intra-individual dynamic conception of personality. *Journal of Research in Personality, 30,* 414–428.

Singer, J. A., & Salovey, P. (1993). *The remembered self.* New York: Free Press.

Spilka, B., & Bridges, R. A. (1989). Theology and psychological theory: Psychological implications of some modern theologies. *Journal of Psychology and Theology, 17,* 343–351.

Stromberg, P. G. (1993). *Langauage and self-transformation: A study of the Christian conversion narrative.* New York: Cambridge University Press.

Tickle, P. A. (1995). *Re-discovering the sacred: Spirituality in America.* New York: Crossroads.

Tillich, P. (1957). *Dynamics of faith.* New York: Harper & Row.

Ventis, W. L. (1995). The relationships between religion and mental health. *Journal of Social Issues, 51,* 33–48.

Wulff, D. M. (1996). *Psychology of religion: Classic and contemporary* (2nd ed.). New York: John Wiley.

6

THE NEUROPSYCHOLOGY

OF SPIRITUAL EXPERIENCE

ANDREW B. NEWBERG*, †
AND EUGENE G. D'AQUILI†

*Division of Nuclear Medicine
†Department of Psychiatry
Hospital of the University of Pennsylvania
Philadelphia, Pennsylvania 19104

This chapter will consider the neuropsychology of religious and spiritual experience. An analysis of the neuropsychological basis of these experiences serves several important purposes: (a) to illuminate the biological roots of these experiences and provide new information regarding the function of the human brain, (b) to provide a new understanding of how and why these experiences have played such a significant role in human thought and history, and (c) to lead to an understanding of the relationship between these experiences and human health and psychological well-being.

Religious and spiritual experiences, such as meditation, prayer, and ritual, have been described in the biomedical, psychological, anthropological, and religious literature. Furthermore, there are a large number of studies which have already begun to examine the neuropsychological and physiological correlates of such experiences. It is likely that such experiences became possible with the evolution of various structures in the brain of early primates and eventually of *Homo sapiens*. The concatenation of "religiogenic" brain mechanisms in *H. sapiens* was accompanied historically by an explosion of religious traditions that have continued to permeate human societies since prehistoric times. In light of this evolutionary pattern, neurobiological and neuropsychological correlates of religious and spiritual experiences have begun to be identified. Furthermore, by considering other relevant studies in neurobiology, a more complex model of neurophysiological events during religious and spiritual experience can be developed. More specifically, brain function can be considered in relation to its interconnection with other body physiology that can be mediated by the autonomic nervous system as well as the neuroendocrine system. A consideration of this relation between cognitive processes in the brain and the autonomic nervous system may yield a more complete understanding of a variety of spiritual experiences ranging from "awe" to intense unitary states. Thus, from the current literature, a foundation for the development of a neuropsychological model can be considered in order to guide future studies in the neurobiology of religious and spiritual experiences. In addition, the use of state-of-the-art brain imaging techniques, as well as other measures of brain activity, has been and will continue to be applied to investigate brain function during experiences such as meditation, prayer, and ritual experiences.

THE NEUROEVOLUTION OF SPIRITUAL EXPERIENCE

Evolution has led to the development of the complex neuronal connections that exist within the brain's cerebral hemispheres. The higher centers in the brain are also connected to the more primitive structures such as the limbic system. For the most part, the brain evolved its complexity to provide human beings improved abilities to delineate order in the external environment and to solve cognitive problems necessary for survival. In addition to purely cognitive aspects, the evolution of the brain led to human socialization. The ability to form family units, communities, and societies had a tremendous evolutionary advantage. The question is, How did these evolutionary changes in the brain lead to the development of spiritual experience, religion, and ritual?

The brain can be divided functionally into several primary cognitive functions (d'Aquili, 1978, 1983, 1986). We have previously referred to these functions as cognitive operators. Cognitive operators simply refer to the neurophysiological mechanisms that underlie certain broad categories of cognitive function. Thus, these operators do not exist in the literal sense but can be useful when considering overall brain function. The cognitive operators include abstraction of generals from particulars, the perception of causality in external reality, the perception of spatial or temporal sequences in external reality, and the ordering of elements of reality into causal chains giving rise to explanatory models of the external world whether scientific or mythical. Space does not permit us to describe in detail the neurophysiological substrates and neuroanatomical networks of all these operators. However, several operators require consideration.

The causal operator accounts for the causal sequencing of elements of reality as abstracted from sense perceptions (d'Aquili, 1978). This causal operator derives its function from the inferior parietal lobule in the left hemisphere, the anterior convexity of the frontal lobes, primarily in the left hemisphere, and their reciprocal neural interconnections (Luria, 1966; Pribram, 1973). The causal operator has important relevance to the development of religious and spiritual experience (d'Aquili, 1978). This operator organizes any given strip of reality into what is subjectively perceived as causal sequences back to the initial terminus of that strip. In view of the apparently universal human trait of positing causes for any given strip of reality, we postulate that if the initial terminus is not given by sense data, the causal operator generates automatically an initial terminus. Western science refuses to postulate an initial terminus or first cause for any strip of reality unless it is observed or can be immediately inferred from observation. Under more usual (nonscientific) conditions the causal operator simply generates an initial terminus or first cause for a strip of reality. We are proposing that when no observational or "scientific" causal explanation is forthcoming for a strip of reality, gods, powers, spirits, or some other causative construct is automatically generated by the causal operator. Thus, the causal operator simply operates spontaneously on reality, positing an initial causal terminus when none is given.

If it is true that the causal operator necessarily analyzes reality, then human beings have no choice but to construct myths filled with personalized power sources to explain their world. The myths may be social in nature or they may be individual in terms of dreams, daydreams, or other fantasy aspects of the individual person. Nevertheless, as long as human beings are aware of the contingency of their existence in the face of what often appears to be a capricious universe, they must construct myths to orient themselves within that universe. Thus, they construct gods, spirits, demons, or other personalized power sources with whom they can deal contractually in order to gain control over a capricious environment.

A second operator that has particular significance regarding spiritual experience is the holistic operator. The holistic operator permits reality to be viewed as a whole or as a gestalt. This operator allows for the abstraction from particulars or individuals into a larger contextual framework. The holistic operator likely resides in the parietal lobe in the nondominant hemisphere, more specifically in the posterior superior parietal lobule and adjacent areas that have been found to be involved in generating gestalt understanding about both sensory input and various abstract concepts (Bogen, 1969; Gazzaniga & Hillyard, 1971; Levy-Agresti & Sperry, 1968; Nebes & Sperry, 1971; Sperry, Gazzaniga, & Bogen, 1969; Trevarthen, 1969). It is also interesting to note that this area sits adjacent to the area in the dominant hemisphere that provides the neuroanatomical substrate for logical–grammatical operations. Thus, the right parietal lobe is involved in a holistic approach to things and the left parietal lobe is involved in more reductionist processes. We will consider how the holistic operator, in addition to the causal operator, functions with regard to spiritual experience.

METHODS OF ATTAINING SPIRITUAL EXPERIENCES

In further considering a neuropsychological and neuroevolutionary approach to the study of religious and spiritual experiences, it is important to consider two major avenues toward attaining such experiences: group ritual and individual contemplation or meditation. A phenomenological analysis reveals that the two practices are similar in kind, if not in intensity, along two dimensions: (a) intermittent emotional discharges involving the subjective sensation of awe, peace, tranquillity, or ecstasy; and (b) varying degrees of unitary experience correlating with the emotional discharges just mentioned (d'Aquili & Newberg, 1993b). These unitary experiences consist of a decreased sense or awareness of the boundaries between the self and the external world (d'Aquili, 1986; d'Aquili & Newberg, 1993a, 1993b; Smart, 1958, 1967, 1969, 1978; Stace, 1961). The latter dimension can also lead to a sense of oneness between other perceived individuals, thereby generating a sense of community. At the extreme, unitary experiences can eventually lead to the abolition of all boundaries of discrete being, thus generating a state of what we have called absolute unitary being (AUB; d'Aquili & Newberg, 1993a, 1993b).

It should be noted that the experiences of group ritual and individual meditation have a certain degree of overlap such that each may play a role in the other. In fact, it may be that human ceremonial ritual actually provides the "average" person access to mystical experience (average in distinction to those regularly practicing intense contemplation such as highly religious monks). This by no means implies that the mystic or contemplative is impervious to the effects of ceremonial ritual. Precisely because of the intense unitary experiences arising from meditation, mystics are likely to be more affected by ceremonial ritual than the average person. Viewed dispassionately, one must conclude that ceremonial ritual, at its most effective, is an incredibly powerful technology whether for good or ill. Furthermore, because of its essentially communal aspects, it tends to have immeasurably greater social significance than meditation or contemplation. Although meditation and contemplation may produce more intense and more extended unitary states compared to the relatively brief flashes generated by group ritual, the former are almost always solitary experiences.

With regards to human ceremonial ritual, it is a morally neutral technology. Therefore, depending on the myth in which it is imbedded and which it expresses, ritual can either promote or minimize the structural aspects of a society and promote or minimize overall aggressive behavior. Utilizing Turner's concept of *communitas* (Turner, 1969) as the powerful unitary social experience usually arising out of ceremonial ritual, we can state that if a myth achieves its incarnation in a ritual that defines the unitary experience as applying only to the tribe, then the result is only the *communitas tribus*. It is certainly true that aggression within the tribe has been minimized or eliminated by the unifying experience generated by the ritual. However, this may only serve to emphasize the special cohesiveness of the tribe vis-à-vis other tribes. The result may be an increase in intertribal aggression even though intratribal aggression is diminished. The myth and its embodying ritual may, of course, apply to all members of a religion, a nation state, an ideology, all of humanity, and all of reality. Obviously, as one increases the scope of what is included in the unitary experience, the amount of overall aggressive behavior decreases. If indeed a ceremonial ritual were giving flesh to a myth of the unity of all being, then one would presumably experience brief senses of *communitas omnium*. Such a myth–ritual experience approaches meditative states such as Bucke's (1961) cosmic consciousness or even AUB (d'Aquili & Newberg, 1993a, 1993b). However, such grand scope is, unfortunately, unusual for group ritual in human ethnographic experiences.

A NEUROPHYSIOLOGICAL REVIEW

Any understanding of the neuropsychological basis of spiritual experience necessarily requires at least a basic understanding of neurobiology. Therefore, it is helpful to consider here the neurobiological concepts that are particularly relevant to spiritual experience. We will consider some of the major anatomical and functional components of human neurobiology. Furthermore, we will try to build this review using a "bottom-up" approach, considering the more primitive evolutionary aspects first and finishing with the cerebral cortex.

THE AUTONOMIC NERVOUS SYSTEM

The autonomic nervous system is responsible, in conjunction with the rest of the brain, for maintaining baseline bodily function. Thus, this system keeps us alive but also plays a crucial role in the overall activity of the brain as well as in the generation of fundamental emotions such as fear. The autonomic nervous system is traditionally understood to be composed of two subsystems, the sympathetic and parasympathetic systems (Joseph, 1990; Kandel & Schwartz, 1993). The sympathetic system subserves the so-called fight-or-flight response, the physiological basis of our adaptive strategies either to noxious stimuli or to highly desirable stimuli in the environment (Gellhorn, 1967; Gellhorn & Loofbourrow, 1963). The principal function of the sympathetic system is control of short-range adaptation to events in the environment. It initiates and carries out action directed either at acquiring or avoiding stimuli of survival interests to the animal. The sympathetic system mediates the expenditure of vital resources, increasing heart rate and blood pressure, increasing muscle efficiency, dilation of the pupils of the eye, erection of body hair, ejaculation, and increased respiration (Gellhorn, 1967; Gellhorn & Loofbourrow, 1963; Joseph, 1990; Kandel & Schwartz, 1993). Since all these functions are involved in the expenditure of the body's energy and metabolism, the total of the sympathetic system with its associated brain structures has been called the ergotropic system (Lex, 1979).

The parasympathetic system, on the other hand, is responsible for maintaining homeostasis (Gellhorn, 1967; Gellhorn & Loofbourrow, 1963; Kandel & Schwartz, 1993). It regulates physiological maintenance activities and vegetative functions, such as growth of cells, digestion, relaxation, and sleep. Parasympathetic functions include a storage of vital resources, decrease of heart rate and blood pressure, collection of waste products, penile erection, and slowing of respiration (Gellhorn, 1967; Gellhorn & Loofbourrow, 1963; Joseph, 1990; Kandel & Schwartz, 1993). Since all these functions are involved with the conservation of body energy and the maintenance of baseline metabolism, the total of the parasympathetic system with its associated brain structures has been called the trophotropic system (Lex, 1979).

The ergotropic and trophotropic systems have often been described as "antagonistic" to each other, but they can be complementary to each other under certain conditions. Normally, the increased activity of one tends to produce a decreased activity in the other. Thus, each system is designed to inhibit the functioning of the other in most circumstances. During normal waking consciousness, the specific balance between these two systems helps to characterize our baseline emotional state that we bring to the world, i.e., whether we are "uptight" or "laid-back." However, studies have shown that if either system is driven to its maximal capacity, one can induce "reversal" or "spillover" phenomena (Gellhorn & Keily, 1972). This spillover phenomenon occurs when continued stimulation of one system to maximal capacity begins to produce activation responses (rather than inhibitory) in the other system.

We have proposed, in a previous work (d"Aquili & Newberg, 1993b), four basic categories of ergotropic/trophotropic events and their sensorial concomitants which may occur during extraordinary phases of consciousness. The hypertrophotropic state, in which trophotropic activity is exceptionally high, may result in extraordinary states of quiescence. This activity can occur during normal sleep but may occur during deep meditation, prayer, or other related activities. In extreme form, a hypertrophotropic state may result in vivid, hyperlucid hallucinations via activation of the hippocampus. It is known that stimulation of the hippocampus, as well as the amygdala, can result in fully formed visual and auditory hallucinations (Halgren, Babb, & Crandel, 1978; Horowitz, Adams, & Rutkin, 1968). In addition, there may be an experience of oceanic tranquillity in which no thought or fantasy intrudes upon consciousness and no bodily sensations are felt. The hyperergotropic state occurs when ergotropic activity is exceptionally high. This results in an extraordinary stage of unblocked arousal and excitation and is associated with keen alertness and concentration in the absence of superfluous thought and fantasy (Czikszentmihalyi, 1975).

The next two autonomic states involve hyperactivation of one system with spillover into excitation of the other system. Thus, the hypertrophotropic state with ergotropic eruption is the state in which trophotropic activity is so extreme that spillover occurs and the ergotropic system becomes activated (Gellhorn & Keily, 1972). In the case of meditation, a person begins by activating the trophotropic system. As the hypertrophotropic state creates a sense of oceanic bliss, the ergotropic eruption results in the experience of a sense of a tremendous release of energy. The mediator may experience one of the so-called "active" blisses or energy rushes. The hyperergotropic state with trophotropic eruption occurs when ergotropic activity is so extreme that spillover occurs and the trophotropic system becomes activated. This may be associated with the experience of an orgasmic, rapturous, or ecstatic rush arising from a generalized sense of flow and resulting in a trance-like state. If the trophotropic breakthrough is intense enough, vivid, hyperlucid hallucinations also may occur (Laughlin, McManus, & d'Aquili, 1992).

A fifth and final state involves maximal discharge of both the ergotropic and trophotropic systems (d'Aquili & Newberg, 1993a, 1993b). This state is associated with the experience of the total breakdown of discrete boundaries between objects, an absence of a sense of time, and the elimination of the self–other dichotomy. In other words, this ergotropic/trophotropic state is associated with the most intense forms of mystical experience and may lie at the heart of compelling spiritual experiences, meditative states, near death experiences, and other types of human experiential phenomena (d'Aquili & Newberg, 1993a, 1993b; Newberg & d'Aquili, 1994).

BRAIN STRUCTURE AND FUNCTION

The brain itself is divided into a number of subdivisions. The first subdivision separates the brain into a left and right hemisphere. The cerebral hemispheres are generally regarded as the seat of higher level cognitive and emotional functions. It is the cerebral cortex that is believed to separate human beings from other animals and has led to the development of thought, language, religion, art, and culture. There are also subcortical structures which are involved in basic life support, hormone regulation, and primal emotions (Joseph, 1990; Kandel & Schwartz, 1993).

In addition to the cerebral cortex, there is a group of structures near the base of the brain that is called the limbic system. This system evolved initially from subcortical structures but has come to be incorporated into parts of the cerebral cortex in human beings and some other primates (Joseph, 1990; Kandel & Schwartz, 1993). The limbic system is associated with the more complex aspects of emotions and is involved with assigning emotional feelings to various objects and experiences and directing these emotions outward via behavior. The limbic system is also interconnected with the autonomic nervous system with its ergotropic and trophotropic components. The limbic system is the neuroanatomical substrate that subserves the generation and modulation of feelings and emotions (Joseph, 1990; Kandel & Schwartz, 1993). The limbic system has also been implicated as having a major role in religious and spiritual experiences (d'Aquili & Newberg, 1993a, 1993b; Saver & Rabin, 1997).

The hypothalamus is one of the most ancient structures in the brain from an evolutionary perspective. The medial hypothalamus is an extension of the trophotropic system into the brain, whereas the lateral hypothalamus seems to be an extension of the ergotropic system into the brain (Joseph, 1990). The amygdala is more recently developed evolutionarily than the hypothalamus and is preeminent in the control and modulation of all higher order emotional and motivational functions (Kling, Lloyd, & Perryman, 1987; Perryman, Kling, & Lloyd, 1987; Schutze, Knuepfer, Eismann, Stumpf, & Stock, 1987; Steklis & Kling, 1985). It has extensive interconnections with many parts of the brain through which it is able to monitor and determine which sensory stimuli are of motivational significance to the animal (Steklis & Kling, 1985). This includes the ability to discern and express even quite subtle social–emotional nuances such as love, affection, friendliness, fear, distrust, and anger. In addition to emotional and motivational functioning, the amygdala is also involved in attention, learning, and memory. Although the function of the amygdala is complex, it is becoming clear that the amygdala has primarily an ergotropic function, particularly in the lateral part (Chapman et al., 1954; Mark, Ervin, & Sweet, 1972; Ursin & Kaada, 1960). However, it does have some trophotropic functions as well.

The final structure of the limbic system that requires discussion is the hippocampus, which is shaped like a telephone receiver and is located slightly behind the amygdala. A number of investigators have assigned a major role to the hippocampus in information processing, including memory, new learning, cognitive mapping of the environment, attention, and some orienting reactions. The hippocampus is greatly influenced by the amygdala, which in turn monitors and responds to hippocampal activity (Joseph, 1990). The amygdala also acts to relay certain forms of information from the hippocampus to the hypothalamus. Thus, the hippocampus and amygdala complement each other and interact in regard to attention and generation of emotionally linked images as well as in regard to learning and memory. The hippocampus also partially regulates the activity in another structure that connects the autonomic nervous system to the cerebral cortex called the thalamus (Joseph, 1990). Since the thalamus is a major relay between a variety of brain structures, the hippocampus can sometimes block information input to various neocortical areas via the thalamus. It is important to note that while the amygdala may enhance information transfer between neocortical regions, the hippocampus usually tends to do the reverse. Through interconnections with the amygdala and the hypothalamus, in addition to other parts of the brain, the hippocampus can inhibit activity in these areas, thus preventing emotional extremes (Redding, 1967). This ability to inhibit the transfer of information from one region to another, in addition to its control over emotional responses, is very important in generating certain experiences such as mystical phenomena.

TERTIARY ASSOCIATION AREAS

Returning to the cerebral cortex, with its structures involved in higher cognitive, sensory, and emotional functioning, we note that there are four tertiary association areas that integrate neuronal activity from various other areas in the brain (Joseph, 1990; Kandel & Schwartz, 1993). These cortical regions are the inferior temporal lobe (ITL), the inferior parietal lobule (IPL), the posterior superior parietal lobule (PSPL), and the prefrontal cortex (PFC).

The PSPL is heavily involved in the analysis and integration of higher order visual, auditory, and somaesthetic information. Through the reception of auditory and visual input, the PSPL is also able to create a three-dimensional image of the body in space (Lynch, 1980). Some cells in the PSPL, exerting "command" functions (Montcastle, 1976; Montcastle, Motter, & Anderson, 1980), can direct visual attention, become excited when certain objects are within grasping distance, and can motivate and guide hand movements toward these objects. There is some difference in function between the PSPL on the right and the PSPL on the left. It has been observed that the right parietal lobe appears to play an important role in generalized localization and the sense of spatial coordinates per se, whereas the left PSPL exerts influences in regard to objects that may be directly grasped and manipulated (Joseph, 1990; Kandel & Schwartz, 1993). That some neurons in the left PSPL respond most to stimuli within grasping distance and other neurons respond most to stimuli just beyond arms reach led Joseph (1990) to postulate that the distinction between self and world may ultimately arise from the left PSPL's ability to judge these two categories of distances. Thus, it seems probable that the self–other dichotomy is a left PSPL function that evolved from its more primitive division of space into the graspable and the nongraspable.

The ITL neurons scan the entire visual field so as to alert the organism to objects of interest or motivational importance through its interconnections with the limbic nuclei (Herzog & Van Hoesen, 1976; Kling et al., 1987; Turner, Mishkin, & Knapp, 1980; Van Hoesen, Pandya, & Butters, 1972). When such objects are detected from the PSPL, the ITL's visual form recognition neurons are activated, and the neurons with wide nonspecific visual fields are inhibited. In this manner, objects of interest are detected and fixated upon. Brain imaging studies using position emission tomography (PET) have also shown that the ITL and PSPL are involved in the visual perception and learning of complex geometric patterns (Roland, 1995).

The IPL is located at the confluence of the temporal, parietal, and occipital lobes. The IPL is an association area of association areas and maintains rich interconnections with the visual, auditory, and somaesthetic association areas. This area is responsible for the generation of abstract concepts and relating them to words (Joseph, 1990). It is also involved in conceptual comparison, automatic ordering of conceptual opposites, the naming of objects and categories of objects, and, in general, higher order grammatical and logical operations (Bruce, Desimone, & Gross, 1986; Burton & Jones, 1976; Geschwind, 1965; Jones & Powell, 1970; Seltzer & Pandya, 1978; Zeki, Symonds, & Kaas, 1982).

DEAFFERENTATION

One other aspect of brain function that may play an important role in spiritual experience is the ability of certain brain structures to block input into other structures. This blocking of input into a brain structure is called deafferentation. There is much evidence of such phenomena arising from natural (i.e., stroke or neuronal degeneration) or induced lesions in various parts of the brain (Baron et al., 1986; Gilbert & Peterson, 1991; Jeltsch, et al., 1994; Kataoka, Hayakawa, Kuroda, Yuguchi, & Yamada, 1991). Deafferentation of a brain structure also can occur via the activity of inhibitory fibers from other nervous system structures. For example, Hoppe (1977) has shown that one hemisphere can be prevented from knowing what is occurring in the opposite hemisphere by suppressive actions of the frontal lobes. There is similar evidence that intrahemispheric information transmission can be partially or totally prevented by impulses originating in the prefrontal cortex and passing via the hippocampus (Green & Adey, 1956; Joseph, Forrest, Fiducis, Como, & Siegal, 1981; Nauta, 1958).

When a brain structure that ordinarily processes input has been deafferented to a significant degree, the structure is required to extract meaning from its own random neural activity. Such meaning takes the form of the intrinsic function of that structure (Joseph, 1990). Thus, a deafferented area of the brain that normally functions to analyze visual input will tend to interpret any neural activity as visual input resulting in a visual hallucination as occurs in patients with cortical blindness. Deafferentation via inhibitory mechanisms from other brain structures may ultimately give rise to various components of spiritual experiences.

A NEUROPHYSIOLOGICAL MODEL
FOR THE SPIRITUAL CONTINUUM

It appears that there are a variety of spiritual experiences which, although they seem to be fundamentally different, actually have a similar neuropsychological and neuroevolutionary origin and therefore lie along the same spiritual continuum. Frederick Streng (1978) notes,

> The term mysticism has been used to refer to a variety of phenomena including occult experience, trance, a vague sense of unaccountable uneasiness, sudden extraordinary visions and words of divine beings, or aesthetic sensitivity. For our purposes, we will narrow the definition to: an interior illumination of reality that results in ultimate freedom. Ninian Smart has correctly distinguished mysticism in this sense from "the experience of a dynamic external presence." (p. 142)

Smart (1958, 1967, 1969, 1978) has further argued that certain sects of Hinduism, Buddhism, and Taoism differ markedly from prophetic religions, such as Judaism and Islam, and from religions related to the prophetic-like Christianity in that the religious experience most characteristic of the former is "mystical," whereas that most characteristic of the latter is "numinous."

Somewhat similar to Smart's distinction between mystical and numinous experiences is that of W. B. Stace (1961), who distinguishes between what he calls extrovertive mystical experiences and introvertive mystical experiences. Stace characterizes these respectively as follows:

Extrovertive mystical experiences

1. The Unifying Vision—all things are one
2. The more concrete apprehension of the One as an inner subjectivity, or life, in all things

3. Sense of objectivity or reality
4. Blessedness, peace, etc.
5. Feeling of the holy, sacred, or divine
6. Paradoxicality
7. Alleged by mystics to be ineffable

Introvertive mystical experiences

1. The Unitary Consciousness; the One, the Void; pure consciousness
2. Nonspatial, nontemporal
3. Sense of objectivity or reality
4. Blessedness, peace, etc.
5. Feeling of the holy, sacred, or divine
6. Paradoxicality
7. Alleged by mystics to be ineffable

Stace then concludes that characteristics 3–7 are identical in the two lists and are therefore universal common characteristics of mystical experiences in all cultures, ages, religions, and civilizations of the world. However, it is characteristics 1 and 2 in which the distinction is made between extrovertive and introvertive mystical experiences in his typology. One can see the similarity between Stace's extrovertive mystical experience and Smart's numinous experience and between Stace's introvertive mystical experiences and Smart's mystical experience proper.

A neurobiological analysis of mysticism and other spiritual experiences might clarify some of the issues regarding mystical and spiritual experiences by allowing for a typology of such experiences based on the underlying brain functions. In terms of the effects of ceremonial ritual, we, along with other colleagues, have proposed that rhythmicity in the environment (i.e., visual, auditory, or tactile) drives either the ergotropic or trophotropic system to maximal capacity with the possibility of spillover and simultaneous activation of the other system creating unusual subjective states (d'Aquili, 1983; d'Aquili and Newberg, 1993a, 1993b). For the most part, this neurophysiological activity occurs as a result of the rhythmic driving of ceremonial ritual. This ultimately results in a progressive deafferentation of certain parts of the right PSPL (which, the reader will recall, is the neurobiological basis of the the holistic operator), creating an increasing sense of wholeness progressively more dominant over the sense of the multiplicity of baseline reality. Ceremonial ritual may be described as generating these spiritual experiences from a bottom-up approach since it is rhythmic sounds and behaviors of the ritual that eventually drive the ergotropic and trophotropic systems. It should also be mentioned that the particular system initially activated (ergotropic or trophotropic) depends on the type of ritual. Rituals themselves might therefore be divided into "slow" and "fast" rituals. Slow rituals might involve calm, peaceful music and soft chanting to generate a sense of quiescence via the trophotropic system (d'Aquili & Newberg, 1993b). Fast rituals might utilize rapid or frenzied dancing to generate a sense of heightened arousal via the ergotropic system (d'Aquili & Newberg, 1993b).

However, activation of the holistic operator (the right PSPL and adjacent structures) and the attainment of ecstatic and blissful unitary states can also be achieved via other mechanisms. For example, meditation approaches the situation from the opposite direction from ceremonial ritual and highly rhythmic behavior (d'Aquili & Newberg, 1993a, 1993b). Thus, meditation appears to utilize a top-down mechanism using cognitive/emotional activity to drive the ergotropic/trophotropic system to maximum activation. This appears to occur via a complex mechanism of neural interactions.

A detailed mechanism for the neurophysiological basis of meditative experiences has been previously described (d'Aquili & Newberg, 1993a, 1993b). However, it may be helpful to review some of the major components of that model in order to develop a better understanding of the spiritual continuum. One form of meditation begins with the subject willing or intending to focus either on a mental image or on an external physical object. In our model, impulses pass from the right PFC to the PSPL via the thalamus, which functions as a relay. These impulses are correlated with the person subjectively focusing their attention on a visual object. This object is presented by the ITL, which is subsequently spatially oriented by the PSPL.

We postulate that continuous fixation on the image presented by the right ITL begins to stimulate the right hippocampus, which in turn stimulates the right amygdala. The result is a stimulation of the lateral portions of the hypothalamus generating a mildly pleasant sensation. Impulses then pass back to the right amygdala and hippocampus, recruiting intensity as they go along. This then feeds back to the right PFC, reinforcing the whole system with progressively intense concentration upon the object. Thus, a reverberating loop is established.

In our model, the circuit continues to reverberate and to augment in intensity until the stimulation of the hypothalamic ergotropic centers (lateral part) reaches maximum, thus leading to a spillover such that maximal stimulation of the hypothalamic trophotropic centers (medial part) occurs. At this point, there would be maximal stimulation feedback through the limbic structures to both the left and right PFCs. This results in instantaneous maximal stimulation of the left PFC, with immediate total blocking of input into the left PSPL tending to obliterate the self–other dichotomy. In the right hemisphere, even though from the moment of spillover there should be likewise maximal limbic stimulation of the right PFC which should generate total deafferentation of the right PSPL, there is already an ongoing, powerful stimulation system from the right PFC to the right PSPL. This stimulation has been reinforced by a constant feedback loop going through the right ITL (the neurophysiological basis of "focusing on an object").

Therefore, the inhibitory ability of the right PFC, although at maximum, must fight against a preexistent and very strong facilitatory or stimulating system that is generated by fixating and focusing on the original object. Since the meditating subject is still intending to focus on the object of meditation, this system continues to be reinforced even in the presence of ecstatic feelings generated by the limbic system and the progressively stronger activity of the inhibitory system. Throughout the period of time when there is conflict in the right hemisphere between facilitatory and inhibitory mechanisms there has been total instantaneous blocking of input into the left PSPL. Thus, the self–other dichotomy has been obliterated during a period of time, perhaps fairly long, when the image still remains a focus of meditation. We suggest that this is the period of time when the subject feels absorbed into the object or describes a sense of becoming one with the object of meditation. Eventually, in the face of maximal ergotropic and trophotropic activity, either the meditator surrenders or, possibly even against his or her will, the inhibitory influences take over and total blocking of input into the right PSPL occurs. Since the left PSPL has already been totally blocked, the self–other dichotomy has been obliterated for some time. Thus, the endpoint of the meditation is maximal stimulation of the ergotropic and trophotropic systems with total blocking of input into both the right and left PSPL, creating the experience of AUB. The period of time from spillover to the final assertion of dominance of the inhibitory neurons of the right prefrontal cortex is the period of absorption of the meditator into the object of meditation.

Regarding a comparison of ceremonial ritual with meditation, the end result can be the same in both situations (d'Aquili and Newberg, 1993a, 1993b). In other words, both methods can result in simultaneous activation of the ergotropic and trophotropic systems with concomitant deafferentation of the left and right PSPL. This results in the experience of bliss and ecstasy as well as in profound unitary states. It should be noted that AUB is unlikely to occur in ceremonial ritual since it is very difficult to maintain the level of rhythmic activity necessary for the continued driving of the ergotropic system to result in simultaneous maximal activity of both the ergotropic and trophotropic systems. However, ceremonial ritual still can result in powerful unitary experiences.

In terms of a spiritual continuum, unitary states play a crucial role. While it is clearly difficult to define what makes a given experience spiritual, the sense of having a union with some higher power or fundamental state seems an important part of spiritual experiences. To that end, this union helps reduce existential anxiety as well as provides a sense of control over the environment (d'Aquili, 1978; Smart, 1967, 1969). The bottom line in understanding the phenomenology of subjective religious experience is to understand that every religious experience involves a sense of the unity of reality at least somewhat greater than the baseline perception of unity in day to day life (d'Aquili, 1986). This is another way of saying that a more intense application of the holistic operator to incoming stimuli, over and above its baseline function, coupled with the limbic or emotional stimulation that accompanies such increased functioning, results in experiences which are usually described as religious or spiritual. Whatever the mechanism for the increased functioning of the holistic operator may be, whether it is an external rhythmic driver, profound meditation, extreme fasting, or other physiological alterations, the bottom line is activation of the holistic operator with accompanying experiences of increased unity over multiplicity.

AUB is a state of ultimate unity and is described in the mystical literature of all the world's great religions. When a person is in this state he or she loses all sense of discrete being and even the difference between self and other is obliterated. There is no sense of the passing of time, and all that remains is a perfect timeless undifferentiated consciousness. However, it is important to realize that the limbic system is intimately involved in the perception of these experiences (Saver & Rabin, 1997). Thus, when such a state is suffused with positive affect there is a tendency to describe the experience, after the fact, as personal. Such experiences are often described as a perfect union with God (the *Unio mystica* of the Christian tradition) or else the perfect manifestation of God in the Hindu tradition. When such experiences are accompanied by neutral affect they tend to be described, after the fact, as impersonal. These states are described in concepts such as the abyss of Jacob Boeme, the void or nirvana of Buddhism, or the absolute of a number of philosophical/mystical traditions. There is no question that whether the experience is interpreted personally as God or impersonally as the absolute, it nevertheless possesses a quality of transcendent wholeness without any temporal or spatial division whatsoever.

We have postulated that these rare states of AUB are attained through the "absolute" functioning of the holistic operator (d'Aquili, 1982; d'Aquili and Newberg, 1993a, 1993b). As described in the previous model, the neurological substrate for the holistic operator involves the function of the right PSPL. However, during AUB, not only would there be absolute functioning of the holistic operator but also there would be an intense activity of structures in the left cerebral hemisphere associating with that wholeness the intense consciousness of the reflexive ego associated with normal left hemispheric functioning. Thus, the experience of AUB is not a vague sense of undifferentiated wholeness but one of intense consciousness.

We propose, however, that even in more ordinary perceptions, whenever the sense of wholeness exceeds the sense of multiplicity of parts or of discrete elements in the sensorium, there is an affective discharge via the right brain–limbic connections that Schwartz, Davidson, and Maer (1975) have shown to be of such importance. This tilting of the balance toward an increased perception of wholeness, depending on its intensity, can be experienced as beauty, romantic love, numinosity or the religious awe described by Smart, religious exaltation in the perception of unity in multiplicity (described by Stace as extrovertive mystical experience), and eventually various trance states culminating in AUB.

We propose that the spiritual continuum is based on the activation of the holistic operator with the subsequent experience of greater senses of unity within the sensorium. As there is an increasing sense of unity, there is the perception of ever greater approximations of a more fundamental reality (d'Aquili, 1986). Furthermore, the more the holistic operator functions in excess of a state of balance with the analytic functions of the left hemisphere, the stronger will be the associated emotional charge. Thus, in any perception, such as a piece of music, a painting, a sculpture, or a sunset, there is a sense of meaning and wholeness which transcends the constituent parts. In aesthetic perceptions such as those just described, this transcendence is slight to moderate. We would locate the overarching sense of unity between two persons in romantic love as the next stage in this spiritual continuum. The next stage is characterized as numinosity or religious awe and occurs when the holistic operator functions with a degree of intensity which generates a very marked sense of meaning and wholeness extending well beyond the parts perceived or well beyond the image generated but in a "wholly other" context. Both Otto (1970) and Smart (1969) have described this experience in detail. It is often considered (rather incorrectly we believe) to be the dominant Western mystical experience. It is experienced when an archetypal symbol is perceived or when certain archetypal elements are externally constellated in a myth. As we move from numinosity along the continuum—that is, as the function of the holistic operator increasingly overwhelms synthetic perception—we reach the state of religious exaltation which Bucke (1961) has called cosmic consciousness. This state is characterized by a sense of meaning and wholeness extending to all discrete being whether subjective or objective. The essential unity and purposefulness of the universe is perceived as a primary datum despite the perception and knowledge of evil in the world. During this state, there is nothing whatsoever that escapes the mantle of wholeness and purposefulness. However, this state does not obliterate discrete being, and it certainly exists within a temporal context. This roughly corresponds to Stace's extrovertive mystical experience.

PROOF OF THE MODEL

Clearly, one of the most important aspects of a study of spiritual experiences is to find careful, rigorous methods for empirically testing hypotheses. One such example of empirical evidence for the neurophysiological basis of the spiritual continuum described previously comes from a number of studies which have measured neurophysiological activity during states in which there is activation of the holistic operator. Meditative states comprise perhaps the most fertile testing ground because of the predictable, reproducible, and well-described nature of such experiences. Studies of meditation have evolved over the years to utilize the most advanced technologies for studying neurophysiology.

Originally, studies analyzed the relationship between electrical changes in the brain (measured by electroencephalography) and meditative states. Corby, Roth, Zarcone, and Kopell (1978) showed that during meditation, proficient practitioners had increased alpha and theta amplitudes compared to baseline. These changes were associated with increased autonomic activation. Banquet (1972) found an increased intensity of a frontal alpha pattern during the early stages of meditation. Later stages of meditation were characterized by bursts of theta waves on electroencephalography (EEG) associated with short shallow breathing and the disappearance of tonic electromyographic activity. Another study found hemispheric asymmetries in alpha and beta activity associated with meditation (Benson, Malhotra, Goldman, Jacobs, & Hopkins, 1990). Unfortunately, EEG is limited in its ability to distinguish particular regions of the brain that may have increased or decreased activity.

For this reason, recent studies of meditation have utilized brain imaging techniques such as single photon emission computed tomography (SPECT) and PET. Future studies may also use functional magnetic resonance imaging. There are limitations of each type of technique for the study of meditation. It is important to ensure that the technique is sensitive enough to measure the changes. Also, each of these techniques may interfere with the normal environment of meditation. For this reason, we have performed our initial studies with SPECT, which measures changes in cerebral blood flow.

Our initial data of highly proficient meditators (Newberg, Alavi, Baime, & d'Aquili, 1997a; Newberg, Alavi, Baime, Mozley, & d'Aquili, 1997b) showed significant increases in brain activity in the region comprising the PFC consistent with focusing attention during meditation. We have also observed significant decreases of activity in the area of the PSPL possibly consistent with deafferentation of the PSPL. Interestingly, there was also a strong inverse correlation between activity in the PFC and in the PSPL. This might indicate that the more active the PFC, the more the PSPL is deafferented. These results, although preliminary, are consistent with the model for the neurophysiological basis of meditative experiences presented in this chapter, a model that was developed prior to these imaging studies. Furthermore, our results corroborate an earlier PET study of meditation that showed an increased frontal:occipital ratio of cerebral glucose metabolism (Herzog et al., 1990/1991). However, more studies, using improved methods, will be necessary to further elucidate the neuropsychology of meditation and spiritual experiences. That the underlying neurophysiology of extreme meditative states can be considered at all allows for the conceptualization of many other spiritual experiences that lie along the spiritual continuum. Different spiritual experiences might be explained using the previously mentioned physiological mechanisms. They can be derived from either a top-down or bottom-up approach; either way, they eventually activate the holistic operator via the PSPL and ultimately generate their emotional value via activation of the limbic system and autonomic nervous system.

CONCLUSION: SPIRITUAL EXPERIENCE IN PSYCHOLOGICAL PRACTICE

In this section, using a neurophysiological analysis of spiritual experiences, we consider how these experiences impact clinical practice. Western society has historically emphasized the importance of causality, technological advances, and empiricism. It is from these values that Western medicine, psychiatry, and psychology have developed. We propose that regardless of the connotation of the concept of spirituality in Western society, mystical and meditative experiences are natural and probably measurable processes that are and can be experienced by a diversity of people of different races, religions, and cultures. Those having spiritual experiences can have a variety of neuropsychological constitutions.

In addition, it is important for clinicians to be sensitive and knowledgeable regarding spiritual and philosophical beliefs (Worthington, McCullough, & Sandage, 1996). Professionals need to be capable of distinguishing normal, healthy spiritual growth from psychopathology. It is hoped that some of the neurophysiological analysis described previously might allow for a distinction between normal spiritual experiences and pathological states. Such a distinction might depend on the ergotropic/trophotropic balance created by the experience or by the alterations in the functioning of the brain structures subserving the holistic or causal operators. However, the fact that spiritual experiences have an effect on autonomic function as well as other cortically mediated cognitive and emotional processes suggests that such experiences not only affect the human psyche but also may be utilized to assist in the therapy of various disorders.

Studies have demonstrated that prayer and meditation can improve both physical and psychological parameters (Carson, 1993; Kabat-Zinn, Lipworth, & Burney, 1985; Kaplan, Goldenberg, & Galvin-Nadeu, 1993; Worthington et al., 1996). The more the underlying neurophysiological correlates of spiritual experiences are understood, the more such experiences can be analyzed and utilized in clinical practice. Therefore spiritual experience can be very useful in clinical psychological and psychiatric practice. Furthermore, clinicians themselves can be instrumental in helping their patients with personal and spiritual growth by discussing various meditative and/or spiritual practices and encouraging patients to approach these practices in an unambiguous manner. According to Rowan (1983), a humanistic psychologist, "[the self] is the missing link between the psychological and the spiritual. And it offers a safe way into the difficult and apparently dangerous realms of mysticism" (p. 24). Therefore, it seems natural that spiritual experiences, such as those encountered in meditation and prayer, could become an adjunct to Western therapeutic practices and that developing oneself spiritually could become an important part of psychosocial development.

REFERENCES

Banquet, J. P. (1972). EEG and meditation. *Electroencephalography and Clinical Neurophysiology, 33,* 454.

Baron, J. C., D'Antona, R., Pantano, P., Serdaru, M., Samson, Y., & Bousser, M. G. (1986). Effects of thalamic stroke on energy metabolism of the cerebral cortex. A positron tomography study in man. *Brain, 109,* 1243–1259.

Benson, H., Malhotra, M. S., Goldman, R. F., Jacobs, G. D., & Hopkins, J. (1990). Three case reports of the metabolic and electroencephalographic changes during advanced Buddhist meditation techniques. *Behavioral Medicine, 16,* 90–95.

Bogen, J. E. (1969). The other side of the brain. II: An appositional mind. *Bulletin of Los Angeles Neurological Society, 34,* 135–162.

Bruce, C. J., Desimone, R., & Gross, C. G. (1986). Both striate and superior colliculus contribute to visual properties of neurons in superior temporal polysensory area of *Macaque* monkey. *Journal of Neurophysiology, 58,* 1057–1076.

Bucke, R. M. (1961). *Cosmic consciousness.* Secaucus, NJ: Citadel Press.

Burton, H., & Jones, E. G. (1976). The posterior thalamic region and its cortical projections in new world and old world monkeys. *Journal of Comparative Neurology, 168,* 249–302.

Carson, V. B. (1993). Prayer, meditation, exercise, special diets: Behaviors of the hardy person with HIV/AIDS. *Journal of the Association of Nurses in AIDS Care, 4,* 18–28.

Chapman, W. P., Schroeder, H. R., Geyer, G., Brazier, M. A. B., Fager, C., Poppen, T. L., Solomon, H. C., & Yakovlev, P. I. (1954). Physiological evidence concerning importance of the amygdaloid nuclear region in the integration of circulatory functioning and emotion in man. *Science, 177,* 949–951.

Corby, J. C., Roth, W. T., Zarcone, V. P., & Kopell, B. S. (1978). Psychophysiological correlates of the practice of tantric yoga meditation. *Archives of General Psychiatry, 35,* 571–577.

Czikszentmihalyi, M. (1975). *Beyond boredom and anxiety.* San Francisco: Jossey-Bass.

d'Aquili, E. G. (1978). The neurobiological bases of myth and concepts of deity. *Zygon, 13,* 257–275.

d'Aquili, E. G. (1982). Senses of reality in science and religion. *Zygon, 17*(4), 361–384.

d'Aquili, E. G. (1983). The myth–ritual complex: A biogenetic structural analysis. *Zygon, 18,* 247–269.

d'Aquili, E. G. (1986). Myth, ritual, and the archetypal hypothesis: Does the dance generate the word? *Zygon, 21,* 141–160.

d'Aquili, E. G., & Newberg, A. B. (1993a). Religious and mystical states: A neuropsychological substrate. *Zygon, 28,* 177–200.

d'Aquili, E. G., & Newberg, A. B. (1993b). Liminality, trance and unitary states in ritual and meditation. *Studia Liturgica, 23,* 2–34.

Gazzaniga, M. S., & Hillyard, S. A. (1971). Language and speech capacity of the right hemisphere. *Neuropsychologia, 9,* 273–280.

Gellhorn, E. (1967). *Principles of autonomic–somatic integration: Physiological basis and psychological and clinical implications.* Minneapolis: University of Minnesota Press.

Gellhorn, E., & Kiely, W. F. (1972). Mystical states of consciousness: Neurophysiological and clinical aspects. *Journal of Nervous and Mental Disease, 154,* 399–405.

Gellhorn, E., & Loofbourrow, G. N. (1963). *Emotions and emotional disorders: A neurophysiological study.* New York: Norton.

Geschwind, N. (1965). Disconnexion syndromes in animals and man. *Brain, 88,* 585–644.

Gilbert, M. E., & Peterson, G. M. (1991). Colchicine-induced deafferentation of the hippocampus selectively disrupts cholinergic rhythmical slow wave activity. *Brain Research, 564*(1), 117–126.

Green, J. D., & Adey, W. R. (1956). Electrophysiological studies of hippocampal connections and excitability. *Electroencephalography and Clinical Neurophysiology, 8,* 245–262.

Halgren, E., Babb, T. L., & Crandel, P. H. (1978). Activity of human hippocampal formation and amygdala neurons during memory tests. *Electroencephalography and Clinical Neurophysiology, 45,* 585–601.

Herzog, H., Lele, V. R., Kuwert, T., Langen, K.-J., Kops, E. R., & Feinendegen, L. E. (1990/1991). Changed pattern or regional glucose metabolism during yoga meditative relaxation. *Neuropsychobiology, 23,* 182–187.

Herzog, A. G., & Van Hoesen, G. W. (1976). Temporal neocortical afferent connections to the amygdala in the rhesus monkey. *Brain Research, 115,* 57–59.

Hoppe, K. D. (1977). Split brains and psychoanalysis. *Psychoanalytic Quarterly, 46,* 220–244.

Horowitz, M. J., Adams, J. E., & Rutkin, B. B. (1968). Visual imagery on brain stimulation. *Archives of General Psychiatry, 19,* 469–486.

Jeltsch, H., Cassel, J. C., Jackisch, R., Neufang, B., Greene, P. L., Kelche, C., Hertting, G., & Will, B. (1994). Lesions of supracallosal or infracallosal hippocampal pathways in the rat: Behavioral, neurochemical, and histochemical effects. *Behavioral and Neural Biology, 62*(2), 121–133.

Jones, E. G., & Powell, T. P. S. (1970). An anatomical study of converging sensory pathways within the cerebral cortex of the monkey. *Brain, 93,* 793–820.

Joseph, R. (1990). *Neuropsychology, neuropsychiatry, and behavioral neurology.* New York: Plenum.

Joseph, R., Forrest, N., Fiducis, D., Como, P., & Siegal, J. (1981). Behavioral and electrophysiological correlates of arousal. *Physiological Psychology, 9,* 90–95.

Kabat-Zinn, J., Lipworth, L., & Burney, R. (1985). The clinical use of mindfulness meditation for the self-regulation of chronic pain. *Journal of Behavioral Medicine, 8,* 163–190.

Kandel, E. R., & Schwartz, J. H. (1993). *Principles of neural science.* New York: Elsevier.

Kaplan, K. H., Goldenberg, D. L., & Galvin-Nadeu, M. (1993). The impact of a meditation-based stress reduction program on fibromyalgia. *General Hospital Psychiatry, 15,* 284–289.

Kataoka, K., Hayakawa, T., Kuroda, R., Yuguchi, T., Yamada, K. (1991). Cholinergic deafferentation after focal cerebral infarct in rats. *Stroke, 22*(10), 1291–1296.

Kling, A. S., Lloyd, R. L., & Perryman, K. M. (1987). Slow wave changes in amygdala to visual, auditory, and social stimuli following lesions of the inferior temporal cortex in the squirrel monkey. *Behavioral and Neural Biology, 47,* 54–72.

Laughlin, C. D., McManus, J., & d'Aquili, E. G. (1992). *Symbol & Experience: Toward A Neurophenomenology of Human Conciousness.* New York: Columbia University Press.

Levy-Agresti, J., & Sperry, R. W. (1968). Differential perceptual capacities in major and minor hemispheres. *Proceedings of the National Academy of Science, USA, 61,* 1151.

Lex, B. (1979). The neurobiology of ritual trance. In E. G. d'Aquili, C. D. Laughlin, Jr., & J. McManus (Eds.), *The spectrum of ritual: A biogenetic structural analysis* (pp. 117–151). New York: Columbia University Press.

Luria, A. R. (1966). *Higher cortical functions in man.* New York: Basic Books.

Lynch, J. C. (1980). The functional organization of posterior parietal association cortex. *Behavioral Brain Sciences, 3,* 485–499.

Mark, V. H., Ervin, F. R., & Sweet, W. H. (1972). Deep temporal lobe stimulation in man. In B. E. Eleftheriou (Ed.), *The neurobiology of the amygdala* (pp. 207–240). New York: Plenum.

Montcastle, V. B. (1976). The world around us: Neural command functions for selective attention. *Neurosciences Research Progress Bulletin, 14,* 1–47.

Montcastle, V. B., Motter, B. C., & Andersen, R. A. (1980). Some further observations on the functional properties of neurons in the parietal lobe of the waking monkey. *Brain Behavioral Sciences, 3,* 520–529.

Nauta, W. J. H. (1958). Hippocampal projections and related neural pathways to the midbrain in cat. *Brain, 81,* 319–340.

Nebes, R. D., & Sperry, R. W. (1971). Hemispheric disconnection syndrome with cerebral birth injury in the dominant arm area. *Neuropsychologia, 9,* 249–259.

Newberg, A., Alavi, A., Baime, M., & d'Aquili, E. (1997a). *Cerebral blood flow during intense meditation measured by HMPAO-SPECT: A preliminary study.* Paper presented at the American College of Nuclear Physicians Annual Meeting, February 1997, Palm Springs, CA.

Newberg, A., Alavi, A., Baime, M., Mozley, P., & d'Aquili, E. (1997b). The measurement of cerebral blood flow during the complex task of meditation using HMPAO-SPECT imaging. *Journal of Nuclear Medicine, 38,* 95P.

Newberg, A. B., & d'Aquili, E. G. (1994). The near death experience as archetype: A model for "prepared" neurocognitive processes. *Anthropology of Consciousness, 5,* 1–15.

Otto, R. (1970). *The idea of the holy.* New York: Oxford University Press.

Perryman, K. M., Kling, A. S., & Lloyd, R. L. (1987). Differential effects of inferior temporal cortex lesions upon visual and auditory-evoked potentials in the amygdala of the squirrel monkey. *Behavioral and Neural Biology, 47,* 73–79.

Pribram, K. H. (1973). The primate frontal cortex—Executive of the brain. In K. H. Pribram & A. R. Luria (Eds.), *Psychophysiology of the frontal lobes.* New York: Academic Press.

Redding, F. K. (1967). Modification of sensory cortical evoked potentials by hippocampal stimulation. *Electroencephalography and Clinical Neurophysiology, 22,* 74–83.

Roland, P. E., & Gulyas, B. (1995). Visual memory, Visual imagery, and visual recognition of large field patterns by the human brain: Functional anatomy by positron emission tomography. *Cerebral Cortex, 5,* 79–93.

Rowan, J. (1983). The real self and mystical experiences. *Journal of Humanistic Psychology, 23*(2), 9–27.

Saver, J. L., & Rabin, J. (1997). The neural substrates of religious experience. *Journal of Neuropsychiatry and Clinical Neurosciences, 9,* 498–510.

Schutze, I., Knuepfer, M. M., Eismann, A., Stumpf, H., & Stock, G. (1987). Sensory input to single neurons in the amygdala of the cat. *Experimental Neurology, 97,* 499–515.

Schwartz, G. E., Davidson, R. J., & Maer, F. (1975). Right hemisphere lateralization for emotion in the human brain: Interactions with cognitions. *Science, 190,* 286–288.

Seltzer, G., & Pandya, D. N. (1978). Afferent cortical connections and architectonics of the superior temporal sulcus and surround cortex in the rhesus monkey. *Brain Research, 149,* 1–24.

Smart, N. (1958). *Reasons and faiths: An investigation of religious discourse, Christian and non-Christian.* London: Routeledge Kegan Paul.

Smart, N. (1967). History of mysticism, In P. Edwards (Ed.), *Encyclopedia of philosophy.* London: Macmillan.

Smart, N. (1969). *The religious experience of mankind.* London: Macmillan.

Smart, N. (1978). Understanding religious experience. In S. Katz (Ed.), *Mysticism and philosophical analysis.* New York: Oxford University Press.

Sperry, R. W., Gazzaniga, M. S., & Bogen, J. E. (1969). Interhemispheric relationships: The neocortical commisures; Syndromes of hemisphere disconnection. In P. J. Vinken & C. W. Bruyn (Eds.), *Handbook of clinical neurology, Vol. 4.* Amsterdam: North Holland.

Stace, W. T. (1961). *Mysticism and philosophy.* London: Macmillan.

Steklis, H. D., & Kling, A. (1985). Neurobiology of affiliative behavior in nonhuman primates. In M. Reite & T. Field (Eds.), *The psychology of attachment and separation.* Orlando, FL: Academic Press.

Streng, F. (1978). Language and mystical awareness. In S. Katz (Ed.), *Mysticism and philosophical analysis.* New York: Oxford University Press.

Trevarthen, C. (1969). *Brain bisymmetry and the role of the corpus callosum in behavior and conscious experience.* Paper presented at the International Colloquium on Interhemispheric Relations, June, Czechoslovakia.

Turner, B. H., Mishkin, M., & Knapp, M. (1980). Organization of the amygdalopetal projections from modality-specific cortical association areas in the monkey. *Journal of Comparative Neurology, 191,* 515–543.

Turner, V. (1969). *The ritual process: Structure and anti-structure.* Ithaca, NY: Cornell University Press.

Ursin, H., & Kaada, B. R. (1960). Functional localization within the amygdaloid complex in the cat. *Electroencephalography and Clinical Neurophysiology, 12,* 1–20.

Van Hoesen, G. W., Pandya, D. N., & Butters, N. (1972). Cortical afferents to entorhinal cortex of the rhesus monkey. *Science, 175,* 1471–1473.

Worthington, E. L., McCullough, M. E., & Sandage, S. J. (1996). Empirical research on religion and psychotherapeutic processes and outcomes: A 10-year review and research prospectus. *Psychological Bulletin, 119,* 448–487.

Zeki, J. T., Symonds, L. L., & Kaas, J. H. (1982). Cortical and subcortical projections of the middle temporal area (MT) and adjacent cortex in galagos. *Journal of Comparative Neurology, 211,* 193–214.

7

FUTURE DIRECTIONS
IN RESEARCH

MICHAEL E. MCCULLOUGH

National Institute for Healthcare Research
Rockville, Maryland 20852

DAVID B. LARSON

Duke University Medical Center
Durham, North Carolina 27705
and
National Institute for Healthcare Research
Rockville, Maryland 20852

In the past 15 years, researchers in religion and mental health have been in-creasingly generative. Following Bergin's (1980, 1983) early investigations into the relationships between religion and mental health, other comprehensive reviews (Larson, Pattison, Blazer, Omran, & Kaplan, 1986; Worthington, 1986) also helped to usher in a period of intensified scientific interest in the relationship be-tween religion and mental health. Since the 1980s, the publication of several schol-arly books (Pargament, 1997; Schumaker, 1992; Shafranske, 1996) and several comprehensive field reviews (Gartner, Larson, & Allen, 1991; Gorsuch, 1995; Lar-son, et al., 1992; Worthington, Kurusu, McCullough, & Sandage, 1996) in impor-tant mental health journals has signaled that religion and mental health have ac-quired a degree of legitimacy as an area of scientific investigation; to some extent, it is now respectable (or at least permissible) for academic scholars in the mental health professions to study religion. Given this recently acquired degree of legitimacy, it might perhaps be time to assess the existing scientific landscape and set new goals for crossing the scientific frontiers in religion and mental health.

MOVING FROM CONSCIOUSNESS-RAISING
TO SCIENTIFIC PROGRESS

One of the major effects of the previous years of research on religion and mental health has been to raise scientific awareness about the potentially salutary effects of religion on mental health, despite the vocal minority (e.g., Ellis, 1992; Watters, 1992) who continue to insist that committed religiousness is conducive to mental disorder. Through the accretion of studies in the fields of psychiatry, family medicine, geriatrics, psychology, sociology, counseling, and social work, most informed scholars would probably now agree that religious factors are relevant to a comprehensive understanding of mental health.

Nevertheless, the field of religion and mental health has a long way to go before it yields a hard core of consensually validated scientific findings regarding the relationship between religion and mental health. To date, there are few replicated, well-demonstrated "facts" about the relationship between religion and mental health on which most experts would agree. While the accretion of such replicated, well-demonstrated facts is surely not the only goal of science, our perception is that this field would be helped immensely by the strategic development of a body of generally accepted knowledge about the relationship between religion and mental health. Such facts might help us to develop, for instance, an understanding of which elements of religious experience are relevant to the course of which mental health conditions for which groups of people.

If the field is far from a body of well-accepted, replicated facts, it is even further away from a hard core of research findings that could inform practitioners about how to influence mental health via the appropriate treatment of religion and spirituality. Knowledge is lacking that would allow clinical professions, on the basis of scientific knowledge, to draw clinically useful conclusions, such as "Given that this client is highly committed to religion X and has this set of psychological symptoms, I should be thinking about diagnosis Y", "Given that this client comes from this particular religious or spiritual background, his MMPI scale 2 score is going to be of limited validity in assessing depression. Therefore, I should use another tool for assessing depression as well", or "This patient is expressing spiritual distress that seems to be exacerbating her depressive symptoms. I should refer her to a chaplain for more thorough spiritual assessment."

There does not seem to be any *a priori* reason why the field of religion and mental health could not yield consensually validated and clinically useful findings such as these. However, the development of such a body of knowledge has not been the focal point for the field of research on religion and mental health. We believe that moving from a general recognition that religion is relevant to mental health to the strategic development of consensually validated and clinically useful knowledge is the next great frontier for this field.

TO BUILD A KNOWLEDGE BASE, RESEARCHERS SHOULD BEGIN TO SPECIALIZE

Currently, most of the researchers who are actively involved in conducting research on religion and mental health are generalists. As such, most have tried to keep up with trends in the measurement of religiousness, religion and depression, religion and anxiety, religion and coping, religion and substance use, and research on using religious approaches to the treatment of psychological disorders. While the generalist approach served the field well through early years of development (e.g., 1980–1997), being a generalist in religion and mental health is becoming increasingly difficult as the scope of the subject grows. Many scientific fields eventually outgrow the abilities of the generalist to monitor the existing literature and, as a result, specialties form.

LACK OF SPECIALIZATION LEADS TO BLAND GENERALIZATIONS

As early as 1983, the published research on religion and mental health portended the eventual need for greater specialization. In his meta-analysis of 24 published studies on religion and mental health, Bergin (1983) found that the overall relationship between measures of religiousness and measures of mental health was very small (mean $r = .09$) providing, in Bergin's words, "little positive information or incentive for further inquiry" (p. 176). Based on other relevant research in the social sciences, Bergin suggested that his bland meta-analytic results were probably the result of synthesizing many diverse measures of mental health that were likely to be influenced by religious involvement in different (and perhaps opposite) directions. Adding to the blandness, Bergin's meta-analytic effect size combined the results of studies that had used many diverse measures of religiousness. Finally, Bergin acknowledged that the studies included in his review included both clinical and nonclinical (e.g., captive undergraduate) samples. Given this aggregation across clinical measures, measures of religiousness, and samples, it is not surprising the Bergin found such meager evidence for a relationship between religion and mental health.

Building on Bergin's (1983) review, Gartner et al. (1991) used a different approach to reviewing the research on religion and mental health. By dividing the research according to clinical outcomes (e.g., depression and anxiety),Gartner et al. concluded that religious involvement appears to have a beneficial role on some indexes of mental health but an ambiguous or negative relationship on others. Gartner et al.'s review shows that monolithic statements about the relationship between religion and mental health are clearly unwarranted; religious commitment can influence various aspects of mental health in very different ways. In the following sections, we delineate several of the dimensions along which the research on religion and mental health might become more specialized in order to develop a broader base of consensually validated and clinically useful knowledge about the relationship between religion and mental health that avoids the bland generalizations that necessarily result from aggregating findings too broadly.

THE DIMENSIONS OF SPECIALIZATION

DIMENSION 1: RELIGIOUS INVOLVEMENT

The measurement of religion in the social sciences presents a perpetual challenge for researchers interested in religion and health (Gorsuch, 1984; Levin & Vanderpool, 1987; MacDonald, LeClair, Holland, Alter, & Friedman, 1995; Williams, 1994). Much of the measurement of religion in mental health has consisted of single-item measures of religious affiliation, religious attendance, or self-rated religiousness. While such single-item measures of religiousness are generally presumed to be indicators of a single underlying construct—"religiousness" or "religious commitment"—Levin and Vanderpool observerd that the amalgamation of such variables into single measures of religiousness tends to obfuscate the effects of religion on health since it is not clear what such a "metavariable" of religiousness might mean.

The Pitfalls of Taking the Measurement of Religion for Granted

Similarly, generalizations about the relationship between religion and mental health without respect for how religion is conceptualized or measured in these various studies also confuses the effects of religion on mental health; measures of religiousness are not necessarily interchangeable. For example, in Smith's (1996) investigation of 131 citizens of Missouri and Illinois who were affected by the 1993 Midwest flood, frequency of church attendance was inversely proportional to subjects' positive affect 5 months after the initial assessment. On the other hand, self-rated religiousness was directly proportional to positive affect 5 months after the initial assessment. Thus, these are two important findings for an at-risk population. The difference between these two results is important, but no adequate explanation for such discrepancies currently exists (although researchers commonly offer post hoc methodological explanations such as sampling error or restriction of range or measurement error in one or both variables). Should we conclude, then, that church attendance is risky and that "self-rated religiousness" is salutary in coping with natural disasters or should we conclude from Smith's study that, on balance, religiousness has no reliable longitudinal effect on positive affect following a natural disaster? Other studies (e.g., Ellison, 1995; Pressman, Lyons, Larson, & Strain, 1990) also find that the direction of the religion–mental health relationship is very much dependent on how religiousness is assessed. As a result of the field's inability to adequately predict which aspects of religion might be conducive (or deleterious) to mental health in a given circumstance, such studies are less helpful than they could be in helping to build a base of consensually validated knowledge. Moreover, no research-minded clinician could have felt comfortable in making a recommendation to a flood victim about how religion might assist or hinder him or her in efforts to cope (based on Smith's inconsistent findings). The lack of specificity in teasing out the effects of various measures of religion leads to an unfortunate bottleneck: If these practices are maintained our hard-won scientific data might never be translated into scientifically defensible clinical practices.

Specialized Measurement of Religion

Greater specialization with respect to the measurement of religion might lead to greater understanding of how aspects of religious involvement, such as religious attendance (Levin & Vanderpool, 1987), prayer (e.g., McCullough, 1995), or use of religious resources for coping with stress (Pargament, 1997), might influence mental health status (see Levin, 1996, for a helpful taxonomy of eight dimensions of religious involvement). Social scientists interested in religion from clinical and social science perspectives have invested tremendous energy in developing measures of religious beliefs, motivations, behaviors, and knowledge (Hall, Tisdale, & Brokaw, 1994; Hill & Hood, in press; Miller, 1997) as well as a wide variety of measures of spiritual experience and spiritual well-being (MacDonald et al., 1995). Use of such well-accepted measures of religious involvement and spirituality would add considerable depth to the broad range of studies on religion and mental health that currently involve a single-item measures of religiousness. They would also help us gain a greater understanding of which aspects of religiousness are particularly conducive or deleterious to mental health in specific clinical contexts and disorders.

Development of Clinical Measures

Another bottleneck related to the measurement of religion is that research-based tools for assessing mental health-relevant aspects of religion in the clinical setting are virtually nonexistent ((Strayhorn, Wiedman, & Larson,1990). For example Kehoe and Gutheil (1994) reviewed many scale-based measures of suicide assessment to determine how many assessment tools assessed aspects of clients' religious beliefs. They found not a single tool that included religious beliefs or religious involvement as an aspect of the assessment of suicide risk, even though the existing data suggest that some aspects of religious involvement could deter suicide (Bagley & Ramsay, 1989; Gartner et al., 1991; Stack, 1992).

Similarly, very little work has been done to develop clinically useful tools for assessing patients' religious lives and how various elements of their religious lives might be related to greater resiliency or greater risk for psychological difficulties. Pargament and Koenig (1998) are validating of a tool for assessing various dimensions of religious coping in a sample of medical patients. Other researchers in religion and mental health should examine the prospects for developing measures of religiousness that would enable clinicians to assess the religious components of clients' mental health difficulties or their risk for developing mental health difficulties in the face of stressful life circumstances. These assessment tools could be based on religious beliefs that have been linked to particular mental health outcomes (e.g., Bagley & Ramsay, 1989; Kroll & Sheehan, 1989). The development of such assessment tools would be a natural way to begin building a clinically useful science of religion and mental health.

In addition, research on the differential validity of psychological assessment tools for various religious groups, especially culturally distinct groups that might respond differently to the content of standardized measures of well-being and psychopathology, is needed to ensure that such tests are providing valid assessments for members of such groups (Hall et al., 1994; Larson, Lu, & Swyers,1996). The work of Richards and Davison (1992) illustrates the need for such psychometric research. They found that Rest's (1979) Defining Issues Test, an instrument for assessing Kohlbergian moral development, had a built-in bias against subjects from conservative religious groups (e.g., Latter-day Saints), who responded to some of the items differently than did subjects from nonconservative religious groups.

Given Richards and Davidson's (1992) results, it is not unreasonable to expect that other psychometric instruments are also plagued with differential validity problems for conservative religious groups (Gartner et al., 1991). Since a scientifically based approach to mental health treatment requires the accurate assessment of patients' well-being and symptomology, the need for systematic examination of the differential validity of psychological tests for religious groups could be a productive area of inquiry for research on religion and mental health.

DIMENSION 2: DIAGNOSTIC GROUPS

A second dimension on which researchers should concentrate is the dimension of diagnostic groups. Researchers rarely find that all measures of mental health and mental illness are related to measures of religiousness in the same way. For example, Kendler, Gardner, and Prescott (1997) conducted interviews with nearly 1000 pairs of female twins from the Virginia Twin Registry. They assessed the women on measures of personal religious devotion, religious conservatism, and the conservatism of the religious group with which the women were affiliated. Also, they assessed depression, panic disorder, phobia, bulimia, alcoholism, and generalized anxiety disorder according to *DSM-IV* (American Psychiatric Association [APA], 1994) criteria. While one or more of the measures of religion were inversely related to lifetime risk of major depression, alcoholism, and nicotine dependence, none of the religious measures were related to lifetime risk of generalized anxiety disorder, panic disorder, phobia, or bulimia. Such inconsistencies are not uncommon. Other researchers have found religious measures to predict some measures of well-being, psychopathology, and psychiatric symptoms but not others (e.g., Benson, Masters, & Larson, 1997; Strayhorn et al., 1990).

For the field to develop certainty about the disorders and conditions that are most heavily influenced by religion, individual researchers should commit themselves to programs of research on, for example, the effects of religion on anxiety disorders, on depressive disorders, or on drug use. While several scholars have clearly identified themselves with the study of religion on small clusters of clinical problems such as drug use (e.g., Gorsuch, 1995; Miller, 1997), few researchers have managed to specialize successfully in single disorders or sets of disorders.

A Natural History Approach to Studying Specific Disorders

Researchers might focus their programmatic research by using a "natural history" approach to studying religion and specific indexes of mental health. A natural history approach—a concept that Levin (1996) adapted from epidemiology—assumes that understanding how religion influences mental health or mental illness requires conceptualizing how the effects of religion on physical health might change across the various phases or stages through which a person (a) becomes vulnerable to a disease, (b) experiences a "full-blown illness," and (c) eventually recovers or is disabled by the illness. Levin argued that we must begin to investigate how religion influences health and illness by promoting (or interfering with) processes that move an organism toward vulnerability, dysfunction, illness, and disability or toward equilibrium and, eventually, recovery.

Were many researchers to adopt a natural history approach to the study of religion and mental health, we might one day have an integrated body of research on religion and depression, for instance, that elucidates the mechanisms by which religious involvement is associated with (a) genetic and biologic factors that affect one's vulnerability to major depression, (b) psychological and perceptual factors that influence the appraisal of stressful circumstances, (c) perceived social support during and effective coping with environmental stressors that often precede the onset of depression, (d) social support and coping during a full-blown major depressive episode, (e) effective treatment of depression, and (f) eventual recovery from depression. Currently, we know of no theoretical framework that incorporates all six of these points at which religious involvement might influence the natural history of major depressive illness.

The lack of specialization in conceptualizing the effects of religion using the natural history concept is unfortunate because data are available as building blocks for several of the stages. While little is known about how religion might influence biological vulnerabilities to major depression, research has revealed that religious commitment might endow some benefits through influencing how people appraise, seek social support during and cope with stressful events (e.g., Pargament et al., 1988, 1990; Pargament & Koenig, 1998; Pargament, Smith, & Koenig, 1996; Pressman et al., 1990).

In addition, at least seven studies have used experimental designs to explore the efficacy of religious approaches to treating depression in Christian and Muslim patients. These studies suggest that religious approaches to treatment might play a very small role in enhancing treatment outcomes (McCullough, 1998; Worthington et al., 1996).

Obviously, many gaps must be filled. However, a natural history approach to conceptualizing the effects of religion on depression holds much promise for helping to specify the relationship between religion and mental health.

DIMENSION 3: AGE GROUP

Just as it has been shown in the fields of medicine, psychiatry, and psychology that there is a need to develop specialties (e.g., pediatrics and geriatrics) to understand and treat the physical and mental health issues that accompany particular phases of life, the field of research on religion and mental health also needs specialists who concentrate their efforts on the relationship between religion and mental health for specific age groups (e.g., children, adolescents, adults, older adults, and the very old). While many researchers have conducted studies examining specific age groups (e.g., Shortz & Worthington, 1994), it does not appear that many researchers have focused programmatic efforts on specific age groups, though there are notable exceptions in the area of geriatrics (Sherrill, Larson, & Greenwold, 1993). Virtually no researchers, for instance, have focused on religion and mental health in children or adolescents (Benson et al., 1997).

There are two reasons why we must begin to develop specialists in certain age groups. First, as people age, changes occur in manifestations of religious involvement (Levin & Taylor, 1997). For example, the religious faith of children is obviously quite closely related to the religious faith of their parents and other adult figures in their lives (Benson et al., 1997; Shafranske, 1992). Also, since children often lack higher-order cognitive processes and abstract reasoning, approaches for assessing children's religious faith might need to be different from those that assess adults' religious faith (Bassett et al., 1990; Goldman, 1964). Second, as people age, their manifestations of mental health and mental illness change (e.g., Kohn, Westlake, Rasmussen, Marsland, & Norman, 1997; Rummans, Smith, Lin Waring, & Kokmen, 1997).

DIMENSION 4: GENDER (AND OTHER SUBJECT VARIABLES)

Certainly, researchers could specialize in other subject variables. For example, it would be quite appropriate for researchers to focus exclusively on the role that gender might play in the relationship between religion and mental health, especially since expressions of religious faith (Levin & Taylor, 1997; Strawbridge, Coen, Shema, & Kaplan, in press) and the prevalence and manifestations of many mental disorders (APA, 1994) differ between men and women. While several researchers have begun to examine the "gendered" aspects of the relationship between religion and mental health (e.g., McCullough, Worthington, Maxey, & Rachal, 1997), greater specialization could and should occur.

Another subject variable that might be an important dimension of specialization is ethnicity (Benson et al., 1997). It is quite clear that both religious faith and mental health manifest themselves in specific ways for particular ethnic groups. Again, some researchers have focused on the relationship between religion and mental health for specific ethnic groups (e.g., Herd & Grube, 1996; Stack & Wasserman, 1995) and on the differences between ethnic groups in the religion–mental health relationship (e.g., Ellison, 1995). However, in the next decade, it will be important to find ways to convert these findings into clinically useful knowledge about how the religion–mental health relationship manifests itself for specific age, gender, and ethnic groups.

THE ROLE OF QUANTITATIVE REVIEWS IN THE FORMATION OF SPECIALTIES

Two types of quantitative literature reviews could be immensely helpful in delineating the most productive areas in which specialization could begin to occur. First, systematic reviews (e.g., Larson et al., 1992; Sherrill et al., 1993) could be used to quantify how frequently (and with what methods) religious variables are addressed in the best journals within specific mental health specialties. For example, it would be enlightening to assess how frequently religious variables have occurred in the leading journals that address (a) child and adolescent psychology and psychotherapy, (b) psychology and psychotherapy with ethnic minorities, and (c) psychology and psychotherapy with women. These findings could help to estimate the extent to which researchers in the mental health specialties have begun to build specialized knowledge about religion and mental health.

Second, meta-analytic reviews could be useful in actually producing consensually validated and clinically useful knowledge about the relationship between religion and mental health for which we have been advocating in this chapter. While several meta-analytic reviews of research on religion and mental health have appeared in the literature (e.g., Bergin, 1983; Donahue, 1985; Witter, Stock, Okun, & Haring, 1985), we are unaware of any published meta-analytic review on religion and mental health in the past 10 years. This is most unfortunate since ample studies now exist for conducting meta-analytic reviews that would specify the nature of the relationship between religion and mental health along some of the dimensions that we have described.

In preparing this chapter, for example, we searched through PsycLIT and MEDLINE to survey the existing literature on religion and depression. We found dozens of published empirical studies that investigated the relationship between religion and depressive symptoms. We suspect that many others may have been conducted as masters theses or doctoral dissertations. Since the data are available for conducting a meta-analytic review of research on religion and depression, it is puzzling that more researchers have not used this methodology. Whereas earlier meta-analyses of research on religion and mental health might have only attempted to estimate the mean effect size for the relationship between religion and depression (Bergin, 1983; Donahue, 1985; Witter et al., 1985), many more interesting questions can be addressed as well, such as whether the relationship between religion and depression changes (a) according to which measures are used to assess religious involvement, (b) according to which measures are used to assess depression, (c) across the natural history of depression, and (d) as a function of subjects' characteristics, such as age, gender, and ethnicity.

Clearly, these are the very questions that need to be addressed in order to develop the kind of knowledge base we have been advocating for in this chapter. While many researchers in this area might recall that meta-analytic technology received criticism earlier in its development for conceptual and methodological shortcomings (e.g., Shapiro, 1994), many of these shortcomings have been remedied. Indeed, the meta-analytic technology available to researchers in the 1990s is quite robust (Cooper & Hedges, 1994; Hunter & Schmidt, 1990; Johnson, 1989). We hope meta-analyses will be performed on the relationship between religiousness and mental illnesses, such as depression, substance use, suicide, and anxiety disorder, in the years to come.

SUMMARY

The research on religion and mental health has been a source of sustained scientific interest for many researchers since the early 1980s. This vigorous activity has, almost through brute force, raised a general awareness among many scholars that a curious and perhaps important relationship exists between religious faith and mental health. However, for religion and mental health to become a scientific discipline, it is necessary to develop a strategic approach to conducting research so that we can accumulate a database of well-established, clinically useful knowledge. The approach that we have recommended here will probably require that researchers specialize. However, if the field of research on religion and mental health can meet the challenges of specialization, the field might not only continue to grow but also begin to mature and yield valid, clinically useful knowledge about the relationships between religion and mental health.

ACKNOWLEDGMENT

This chapter was made possible in part through the generosity of the John Templeton Foundation and King Pharmaceuticals, a division of Monarch Pharmaceuticals.

REFERENCES

American Psychiatric Association. (1994). *Diagnostic and statistical manual of mental disorders* (4th ed.). Washington DC: Author.

Bagley, C., & Ramsay, R. (1989). Attitudes toward suicide, religious values, and suicidal behavior. In R. F. W. Diekstra, R. Maris, S. Platt, A.Schmidtke, & G. Sonneck (Eds.), *Suicide and its prevention*. New York: Brill.

Bassett, R. L., Miller, S., Anstey, K., Crafts, K., Harmon, J., Lee, Y., Parks, J., Robinson, M., Smid, H., Sterner, W., Stevens, C., Wheeler, B., & Stevenson, D. H. (1990). Picturing God: A nonverbal measure of God concept for conservative protestants. *Journal of Psychology and Christianity, 9*, 73–81.

Benson, P. L., Masters, K. S., & Larson, D. B. (1997). Religious influences on child and adolescent development. In N. E. Alessi (Ed.), *Handbook of child and adolescent psychiatry* (pp. 206–219). New York: John Wiley.

Bergin, A. E. (1980). Psychotherapy and religious values. *Journal of Consulting and Clinical Psychology, 48*, 95–105.

Bergin, A. E. (1980). Religiosity and mental health: A critical reevaluation and meta-analysis. *Professional Psychology: Research and Practice, 14*, 170–184.

Cooper, H., & Hedges, L. V. (1994). *The handbook of research synthesis*. New York: Russell Sage.

Donahue, M. J. (1985). Intrinsic and extrinsic religiousness: Review and meta-analysis. *Journal of Personality and Social Psychology, 48*, 400–419.

Ellis, A. (1992). My current views on rational-emotive therapy and religiousness. *Journal of Rational-Emotive and Cognitive-Behavior Therapy, 10*, 37–40.

Ellison, C. G. (1995). Race, religious involvement, and depressive symptomatology in a southeastern U.S. community. *Social Science and Medicine, 40*, 1561–1572.

Gartner, J., Larson, D. B., & Allen, G. D. (1991). Religious commitment and mental health: A review of the empirical literature. *Journal of Psychology and Theology, 19*, 6–25.

Goldman, R. (1964). *Religious thinking from childhood to adolescence*. London: Routledge Kegan Paul.

Gorsuch, R. L. (1984). Measurement: The boon and bane of investigating religion. *American Psychologist, 39*, 228–236.

Gorsuch, R. L. (1995). Religious aspects of substance abuse and recovery. *Journal of Social Issues, 51*, 65–83.

Hall, T. W., Tisdale, T. C., & Brokaw, B. F. (1994). Assessment of religious dimensions in Christian clients: A review of selected instruments for research and clinical use. *Journal of Psychology and Theology, 22*, 395–421.

Herd, D., & Grube, J. (1996). Black identity and drinking in the US: A national study. *Addiction, 91*, 845–857.

Hill, P. C., & Hood, R. *Measures of religious behavior*. Chattanooga, TN: Religious Education Press (In press).

Hunter, J. E., & Schmidt, F. L. (1990). *Methods of meta-analysis: Correcting error and bias in research findings*. Newbury Park, CA: Sage.

Johnson, B. T. (1989). *DSTAT: Software for the meta-analytic review of scientific literatures*. Hillsdale, NJ: Lawrence Erlbaum.

Kehoe, N. C., & Gutheil, T. G. (1994). Neglect of religious issues in scale-based assessment of suicidal patients. *Hospital and Community Psychiatry, 45*, 366–369.

Kendler, K. S., Gardner, C. O., & Prescott, C. A. (1997). Religion, psychopathology, and substance use and abuse: A multimeasure, genetic–epidemiologic study. *American Journal of Psychiatry, 154*, 322–329.

Kohn, R., Westlake, R. J., Rasmussen, S. A., Marsland, R. T., & Norman, W. H. (1997). Clinical features of obsessive–compulsive disorder in elderly patients. *American Journal of Geriatric Psychiatry, 5*, 211–215.

Kroll, J., & Sheehan, W. (1989). Religious beliefs and practices among 52 psychiatric inpatients in Minnesota. *American Journal of Psychiatry, 146*, 57–72.

Larson, D. B., Lu, F. G., & Swyers, J. P. (1996). *Model curriculum for psychiatry residency training programs*. Rockville, MD: National Institute for Healthcare Research.

Larson, D. B., Pattison, E. M., Blazer, D. G., Omran, A. R., & Kaplan, B. H. (1986). Systematic analy-

sis of research on religious variables in four major psychiatric journals, 1978–1982. *American Journal of Psychiatry, 143,* 329–334.

Larson, D. B., Sherrill, K. A., Lyons, J. S., Craigie, F. C., Thielman, S. B., Greenwold, M. A., & Larson, S. S. (1992). Associations between dimensions of religious commitment and mental health reported in the *American Journal of Psychiatry* and *Archives of General Psychiatry:* 1978–1989. *American Journal of Psychiatry, 149,* 557–559.

Levin, J.S. (1994). Religion and health: Is there an association, is it valid, and is it causal? *Social Science and Medicine, 38,* 1475–1482.

Levin, J. S. (1996). How religion influences morbidity and health: Reflections on natural history, salutogenesis, and host resistance. *Social Science and Medicine, 43,* 849–864.

Levin, J. S., & Taylor, R. J. (1997). Age differences in patterns and correlates of the frequency of prayer. *The Gerontologist, 37,* 75–88.

Levin, J. S. & Vanderpool, H. Y. (1987). Is frequent religious attendance really conducive to better health? Toward an epidemiology of religion. *Social Science and Medicine, 24,* 589–600.

MacDonald, D. A., LeClair, L., Holland, C. J., Alter, A., & Friedman, H. L. (1995). A survey of measures of transpersonal constructs. *Journal of Transpersonal Psychology, 27,* 171–236.

McCullough, M. E. (1995). Prayer and health: Conceptual issues, research review, and research agenda. *Journal of Psychology and Theology, 23,* 15–29.

McCullough, M. E. (1998). *Religious counseling with religiously committed clients: Review and meta-analysis.* Submitted for publication.

McCullough, M. E., Worthington, E. L. Jr., Maxey, J., & Rachal, K. C. (1997). Gender in the context of supportive and challenging religious counseling interventions. *Journal of Counseling Psychology, 44,* 80–88

Miller, W. R. (1997). Spiritual aspects of addictions treatment and research. *Mind/Body Medicine, 2,* 37–43.

Pargament, K. I. (1997). *The psychology of religion and coping.* New York: Guilford.

Pargament, K. I.,Ensing, D. S., Falgout, K., Olsen, H., Reilly, B., VanHaitsma, K., & Warren, R. (1990). Rod help me (I): Religious coping efforts as predictors of th outcomes to significant life events. *American Journal of Community Psychology, 18,* 793–824.

Pargament, K. I., Kennel, J., Hathaway, W., Grevengoed, N., Newman, J., & Jones, W. (1988). Religion and the problem-solving process: Three styles of coping. *Journal for the Scientific Study of Religion, 27,* 90–104.

Pargament, K. I., & Koenig, H. G. (1998). *A comprehensive measure of religious coping: Development and initial validation of the RCOPE.* Unpublished manuscript, Bowling Green State University.

Pargament, K. I., Smith, B. W., & Koenig, H. G. (1996, August). *Religious coping with the Oklahoma City bombing: The brief RCOPE.* Paper presented at the annual meeting of the American Psychological Association, Toronto, Canada.

Pressman, P., Lyons, J. S., Larson, D. B., & Strain J. J. (1990). Religious belief, depression and ambulation status in elderly women with broken hips. *American Journal of Psychiatry, 147,* 758–760.

Rest, J. R. (1979). *Development in judging moral issues.* Minneapolis: University of Minnesota Press.

Richards, P. W., & Davison, J. L. (1992). Religious bias in moral development research: A psychometric investigation. *Journal for the Scientific Study of Religion, 31,* 467–485.

Rummans, R. A., Smith, G. E., Lin, S., Waring, S. C., & Kokmen, E. (1997). Comorbidity of dementia and psychiatric disorders in older persons. *American Journal of Geriatric Psychiatry, 5,* 261–267.

Schumaker, J. F. (1992). *Religion and mental health.* New York: Oxford University Press.

Shafranske, E. P. (1992). Religion and health in early life. In J. F. Schumaker (Ed.), *Religion and mental health* (pp. 163–176). New York: Oxford University Press.

Shafranske, E. P. (1997). *Religion and the clinical practice of psychology.* New York: American Psychological Association.

Shapiro, S. (1994). Meta-analysis/shmeta-analysis. *American Journal of Epidemiology, 140,* 771–778.

Sherrill, K. A., Larson, D. B., & Greenwold, M. (1993). Is religion taboo in gerontology? Systematic review of research on religion in three major gerontology journals, 1985–1991. *American Journal of Geriatric Psychiatry, 1*, 109–117.

Shortz, J. L., & Worthington, E. L. (1994). Young adults' recall of religiosity, attributions, and coping in parental divorce. *Journal for the Scientific Study of Religion, 33*, 172–179.

Smith, B. W. (1996). Coping as a predictor of outcomes following the 1993 Midwest flood. *Journal of Social Behavior and Personality, 11*, 225–239.

Stack, S. (1992). Religiosity, depression, and suicide. In J. F. Schumaker (Ed.), Religion and mental health (pp. 87–97). New York: Oxford University Press.

Stack, S., & Wasserman, I. (1995). The effect of marriage, family, and religious ties on African-American suicide ideology. *Journal of Marriage and the Family, 57*, 215–222.

Strawbridge, W. J., Cohen, R. D., Shema, S. J., & Kaplan, G. A. (1997). Frequent attendance at religious services and mortality over 28 years. *American Journal of Public Health*, 957–961.

Strayhorn, J. M., Wiedman, C. S., Larson, D. (1990). A measure of religiousness, and its relation to parent and child mental health variables. *Journal of Community Psychology, 18*, 34–43.

Watters, W. (1992). *Deadly doctrine*. Buffalo, NY: Prometheus.

Williams, D. R. (1994). The measurement of religion in epidemiologic studies: Problems and prospects. In J. S. Levin (Ed.), *Religion in aging and health* (pp. 125–148). Thousand Oaks, CA: Sage.

Witter, R. A. Stock, W. A., Okun, M. A., & Haring, M. J. (1985). Religion and subjective well-being in adulthood: A quantitative synthesis. *Review or religious Research, 26*, 332–342.

Worthington, E. L., Jr. (1986). Religious counseling: A review of the published empirical research. *Journal of Counseling and Development, 64*, 421–431.

Worthington, E. L., Jr., Kurusu, T. A., McCullough, M. E., & Sandage, S. J. (1996). Empirical research on religion and psychotherapeutic processes and outcomes: A ten-year review and research prospectus. *Psychological Bulletin, 119*, 448–487.

RELIGION AND MENTAL FUNCTIONING

8

RELIGION AND COPING

KENNETH I. PARGAMENT

Department of Psychology
Bowling Green State University
Bowling Green, Ohio 43403

CURTIS R. BRANT

Department of Psychology
Baldwin–Wallace College
Berea, Ohio 44017

The conclusion seems inescapable that religiosity is, on almost every conceivable count, opposed to the normal goals of mental health. . . . On the whole religious piety and dogma do much more harm than good; and the beneficent behaviors that they sometimes abet would most likely be more frequent and profound without their influence.
—Ellis (1986, pp. 42–43)

A world without God would be a flat, monochromatic world, a world without color or texture, a world in which all days would be the same. Marriage would be a matter of biology, not fidelity. Old age would seem as a time of weakness, not of wisdom. In a world like that, we would cast about desperately for any sort of diversion, for any distraction from the emptiness in our lives, because we would never have learned the magic of making some days and some hours special.
—Kushner (1989, p. 206)

People rarely take a neutral position when it comes to religion. Some, such as Albert Ellis, argue that religion hinders the struggle for growth, freedom, and actualization. From this perspective, religion contributes to human pathology by emphasizing magical thinking and superstition above reason and rationality. Others, such as Rabbi Harold Kushner, see religion in a much more positive light. Religion, it is said, is an essential element in the search for significance; only by looking beyond ourselves can we discover purpose in our lives, achieve intimacy with others, and find a sense of comfort in living. Only with the aid of the sacred can we understand the incomprehensible, manage the unmanageable, and endure the unbearable.

Differences in the assessment of the benefits and harms of religion extend beyond scholars' writings to people in times of crisis. One parent of a young child with developmental delays said, "I really feel that my faith and my trust in God have been the stronghold of being able to deal with all of this—I can't be mad at Him because He's given me a less than perfect child, healthwise" (cited in Weisner, Belzer, & Stolze, 1991, p. 659). Another parent dealing with a child in a similar situation says quite differently, "[Everyone says] God only gives special children to special people; and I say "I'm not special . . . I don't want any more problems!" and I'm kind of to the point where I'm bitter, I'm angry right now" (cited in Weisner et al., 1991, p. 659).

Given such differing views of religion, it may be tempting to bypass evaluations of religion entirely. However, the question cannot be ignored: How we evaluate religion shapes the way we behave toward it. Imagine, for instance, how Kushner and Ellis would handle clients who raise spiritual issues in counseling.

In this chapter, we consider the effectiveness of religion in the coping process. The following are among the questions we will address: Is religion related to the outcomes of stressful life events? If so, how? Is religious coping more helpful to some individuals than others? Is religious coping better suited for certain types of situations than others? and Are there unique benefits to using religious forms of coping compared to other nonreligious or secular coping efforts?

As a prelude to this chapter, it is important to note the following: (a) A traditional, broad definition of religion is used here, one that includes both personal–spiritual and institutional expressions of faith; and (b) this evaluation of the effects of religion on the coping process is not based on the ultimate truth of any religious creed. Scientist cannot determine whether there is a God, whether people really experience miracles, or the ultimate truth of religious teachings. What can be evaluated scientifically is whether religious methods of coping affect adjustment to difficult negative life circumstance and, if so, how (for an extended treatment of many of the points in this chapter, see Pargament, 1997).

SELF-REPORTED EVALUATIONS
OF RELIGION'S EFFECTS ON OUTCOMES

Is religion helpful, harmful, or irrelevant? A straightforward way to learn how people evaluate the efficacy of religion is to ask them. In fact, many researchers have done just that and their results clearly suggest that people do find religion helpful. For instance, in a study of patients who were about to undergo cardiac surgery, 73% reported that prayer was very helpful to them in preparing for the surgery (Saudia, Kinney, Brown, & Young-Ward, 1991). These results seem to generalize across a wide range of people, such as parents dealing with children with physical handicaps (Barsch, 1968), women coping with breast cancer (David, Ladd, & Spilka, 1992), and physically abused spouses (Horton,Wilkins, & Wright, 1988). Generally, between 50 and 85% of the participants in these studies reported that religion was helpful in coping with their situations.

From these studies, the results seem fairly conclusive: Religion does have a positive impact on the coping process. Before jumping to this conclusion too quickly, however, it should be noted that these researchers asked people directly how important religion was to them when coping. What if these participants were simply reluctant to make an unfavorable judgment about their religion and admit that their faith did not help them at all? It is possible that the relatively high proportion of individuals who reported that religion was helpful was a result of the way the question was phrased. How do people respond to a more open-ended question about the impact of religion on adjustment?

In response to this type of question, significant numbers of people still mention that religion was helpful to them in coping, although the percentages are generally lower. In one study, widows and widowers were asked an open-ended question about the sources of comfort they found during their grieving. Fifty-nine percent stated that their religious beliefs were a major source of comfort (Glick, Weiss, & Parkes, 1974). Similar results have been reported among people with chronic illness and cancer (Raleigh, 1992), elderly women and men with medical problems (Conway, 1985/1986; Koenig et al., 1992), and adults facing unhappy periods in their lives (Veroff, Douvan, & Kulka, 1981). Across these samples, anywhere from 18 to 69% of the participants spontaneously mentioned that their faith was helpful to them in coping.

Thus, even in response to more open-ended questions, religion emerges as a source of help in coping (Koenig, 1994). However, we should exercise caution in interpreting these results. People may report that religion was helpful to them because, in fact, it was. Favorable comments, however, may reflect a desire to "keep the faith," whether or not it was helpful to them in that particular circumstance. To suggest that religion was not a source of support may in itself be threatening to the individual. It may be better to evaluate one's faith favorably than to consider the alternative and the possibility that one's faith is limited.

To evaluate the efficacy of religion, stronger tests are needed. Rather than evaluate religious helpfulness or harmfulness in one summary assessment, it makes sense to measure religious involvement separately from its end result and examine the relationship between the two. Through statistical analyses we can then determine whether religion is a positive force, a negative force, or simply irrelevant to adjustment to negative life events.

So far, we have discussed religion's impact on adjustment in general terms. Before we proceed further, however, we briefly mention some of the specific types of outcomes that researchers have examined. Generally, these studies focus on three types of outcomes: physical health, mental health, and religious. Physical health outcomes of stressful life events include physical symptomology (e.g., changes in blood pressure), length of hospital stay, and mortality. Mental health outcomes include coping efficacy (e.g., how well the event was handled), life satisfaction, depression, and anxiety. Finally, religious outcomes include changes in the individual's perceived closeness to God or spiritual growth as a result of coping with the event. Each type of outcome captures something different about the efficacy of religious coping; by examining all of them, we paint a more complete picture of the coping process.

RELIGIOUS ORIENTATIONS AND OUTCOMES TO NEGATIVE LIFE EVENTS

We begin this review by focusing on macroanalytic studies of religion, in which religion is measured as a stable, global, personal disposition—a part of an individual's orienting system. By orienting system we mean a general way of perceiving and dealing with the world. It consists of values, habits, generalized beliefs, relationships, and personality (Pargament, 1997). It is not only a frame of reference that is used to anticipate and come to terms with events in one's life but also a resource drawn upon in times of stress. Depending on the nature of this system, it can be a help or a hindrance to the coping process. Long-standing religious beliefs, congregation attendance, faith in God, and a commitment to live according to a set of religious ideals are all ways that religion can be expressed in a person's orienting system. The basic question is, Do people who are more religious in this global sense experience more positive or negative outcomes of stressful life events than those who are less religious?

Generally, studies that focus on the relationship between religious orientations and outcomes of negative life events can be categorized into four types. The first type of study examines the relationship between personal expressions of religion and outcomes. Religion is measured in terms of beliefs, religious commitment, faith, religious salience, and frequency of prayer. The second type of study focuses on organizational rather than personal religious expressions. Here, religion is measured by participation in congregational services and activities. A third type makes use of the standard measures of religious orientation: intrinsic, extrinsic, quest, and indiscriminant proreligiousness (Hood, Spilka, Hunsberger, & Gorsuch, 1996). Finally, a few studies use "mixed measures" of religion that incorporate both personal and organizational indices.

What can we say about the relationship between religious orientations and the outcomes to critical life events? Table 8.1 summarizes the results of 46 studies that have examined this relationship. These studies target people faced with a variety of stressful life events, such as chronic illness, abortion, surgery, and the death of

TABLE 8.1 A Talley of the Results of Research on the Statistical Relationship between Measures of Religious Orientation and the Outcomes of Negative Events

Measure	% (N)		
	Significant positive relationships	Significant negative relationships	Nonsignificant relationships
Personal religious expressions (religious beliefs, religious salience, frequency of prayer, religious faith)	34 (47)	1 (1)	65 (88)
Organizational religious expressions (participation in worship services and other congregational activities)	37 (52)	1 (2)	62 (85)
Standard religious orientation measures (intrinsic extrinsic, quest, indiscriminate proreligious)	29 (27)	11 (10)	60 (55)
Mixed personal and organizational expression measures	40 (4)	10 (1)	50 (5)
Total	34 (130)	4 (14)	62 (233)

a child, spouse, or loved one. The statistical relationships between religious orientation and outcomes for each study were sorted into one of three categories: significant positive, significant negative, and nonsignificant. Notice that across all four types of studies, 34% of the statistical relationships between religious orientation and adjustment were significantly positive, whereas about 62% of the statistical relationships were nonsignificant. Only rarely were significant negative relationships found between religiousness and adjustment. Therefore, when significant effects were found, they were largely positive. Specifically, higher levels of church involvement, personal religious beliefs, faith, and a more intrinsic religious commitment were related to beneficial outcomes. For instance, O'Brien (1982) examined patients undergoing hemodialysis and found that those patients who were frequent church attenders were more compliant with their treatment programs, more sociable, less alienated, and, in general, better adjusted to their circumstances than those who attended fewer church services. However, recalling the high percentage of people who reported that religion was helpful to them in coping, the numbers of positive results seem to fall short of what we might have expected to find. As Table 8.1 indicates, in the majority of relationships, religiousness was, in fact, unrelated to adjustment. Furthermore, this general pattern was true no matter how religious orientation was assessed.

How can we explain the relatively modest nature of these findings? It is possible the results are a product of methodological flaws, such as inadequacies in the ways religiousness and adjustment were measured. However, the large number of studies and the consistency of the results across the range of religious orientations argue against dismissing these results entirely. The alternative is to take these findings as genuine and try to make sense of them.

A COPING FRAMEWORK

Coping theory provides one explanation. We cope in an effort to maximize what is of value or significance to us in difficult times. Significance can be something psychological, social, physical, material, or spiritual. It can vary from person to person and it can be good or bad. Regardless of how significance is defined, coping involves an attempt to maintain or transform those things that we care for deeply in times of stress (Pargament, 1997).

A religious orienting system, like a general orienting system, provides a general frame of reference during times of stress. Although it is important as a general guide, a religious orienting system is one step removed from the specific coping methods an individual might use in a given situation. Knowing that religious faith is a central part of an individual's orienting system tells us something about that person, but it does not tell us how that person's faith expresses itself in specific situations. From the perspective of coping theory, adjustment is likely to have more to do with the specific use of coping in that situation than with the orienting system. If this notion is correct, then measures of religious coping should predict the outcomes of coping more consistently than measures of general religious orienting systems. Next, we will spotlight microanalytic studies concerning the relationship between specific religious coping activities and adjustment to negative life events.

RELIGIOUS COPING AND OUTCOMES TO NEGATIVE LIFE EVENTS

In recent years, there have been hundreds of studies on the coping process. Interestingly, relatively few have made serious attempts to assess the impact of religion. Some, however, have examined the relationships between specific religious coping strategies and adjustment to negative life events. In contrast to the macroanalytic studies, in which religion is measured as a global construct, these studies examine specific, functionally oriented expressions of religion in times of stress. One such study was conducted by Dalal and Pande (1988). They examined the role of causal beliefs in patients faced with temporary or permanent disability in an Asian Indian, Hindu sample. Attributions of the accident to Karma or God's will, they found, were significantly correlated with psychological recovery.

How common are such findings? Table 8.2 presents a tally of the results of 40 studies that examined the statistical relationships between measures of specific types of religious coping and the outcomes of negative life events (Pargament, 1997). Most of these studies included more than one measure of religious coping and more than one measure of adjustment. Ignoring the distinctions among the different types of religious coping, overall 53% of the relationships between religious forms of coping and adjustment were statistically significant. This figure is higher than the 38% figure for studies of the relationship between religious orientations and adjustment. This increase is due not only to the higher percentage of significantly positive relationships but also because of a higher proportion of negative relationships between some forms of religious coping and adjustment.

A more direct comparison of measures of religious coping and measures of religious orientation was reported by Pargament et al. (1990). Working with several samples of people dealing with a variety of life crises, they asked participants to respond to both religious orientation and religious coping measures. Participants described the most serious negative event they had experienced within the past year and then indicated how they coped with the event. Three outcome measures were obtained: the religious outcome of the event, coping efficacy, and the recent mental health of the individual. Through statistical analyses the authors were able to assess the unique predictive power of the religious coping measures (controlling for the religious orientation measures) and the unique predictive power of the religious orientation measures (controlling for the effects of the religious coping measures). The religious coping variables were much better predictors of all three outcome measures than the religious orientation measures. Similar results have been reported in other studies (Pargament et al., 1994; Pargament, Smith, & Brant, 1995).

TABLE 8.2   Tally of the Results of Research on the Statistical Relationship between Measures
of Religious Coping and the Outcomes of Negative Events

Measure	% (N)		
	Significant positive relationships	Significant negative relationships	Nonsignificant relationships
Spiritual coping			
Spiritual support	46 (43)	2 (2)	52 (48)
Spiritual discontent	0 (0)	56 (5)	44 (4)
Congregational coping			
Congregational support	39 (16)	2 (1)	60 (26)
Congregational discontent	0 (0)	54 (26)	46 (22)
Religious reframing			
God's will and love	53 (19)	0 (0)	47 (17)
God's punishment	0 (0)	52 (11)	48 (10)
Religious agency			
Self-directing	4 (1)	31 (7)	65 (15)
Collaborative	46 (11)	8 (2)	46 (11)
Deferring	28 (9)	6 (2)	66 (21)
Pleading	19 (7)	59 (22)	22 (8)
Religious rituals	40 (30)	23 (17)	37 (18)
Patterns of religious coping	56 (15)	11 (3)	33 (9)
Total	32 (151)	21 (98)	47 (219)

We return to the question, Is religion helpful, harmful, or irrelevant in coping?
The answer is yes. Religious coping is all of these. This answer, quite obviously,
leaves much to be desired. The problem, however, is not with the answer but with
the question—whether religion is helpful, harmful, or irrelevant in coping seems
to assume that religion is only one thing. However, religious coping is not uni-
dimensional.

Religious coping is multipurpose. It may provide comfort, stimulate personal
growth, enhance a sense of intimacy with God, facilitate closeness with others, or
offer meaning and purpose in life (Pargament & Park, 1995). Religious coping is
also multiform. It may be passive (waiting for God to resolve the crisis), active (a
force that motivates individuals to better the world), personal (seeking God's love
and care), interpersonal (seeking support from clergy and congregation members),
problem focused (aiding in problem solving), or emotion focused (looking to God
for emotional reassurance).

Given that religious coping may serve many functions and take many forms, a
better question might be, What forms of religious coping are helpful, harmful,
or irrelevant? Furthermore, is religious coping equally effective for all kinds of
people in all kinds of situations? Does religious coping add anything special to the
coping process? In the following sections, we examine these questions in more detail.

WHAT FORMS OF RELIGIOUS COPING ARE HELPFUL, HARMFUL, OR IRRELEVANT?

In Table 8.2 the microanalytic studies have been broken down into six different types of religious coping: spiritual, congregational, religious reframing, religious approaches to agency and control, religious rituals, and combinations of religious coping methods. Scanning the table shows some striking differences.

HELPFUL FORMS OF RELIGIOUS COPING

Spiritual Support and Collaborative Religious Coping

Perceptions of support, a partnership with God, and guidance from God in times of stress appear to be helpful in coping. For instance, in one study several dimensions of spiritual support were assessed, such as emotional reassurance ("trusted that God would not let anything terrible happen to me"), a close spiritual relationship ("sought God's love and care"), and guidance in problem solving ("God showed me how to deal with the situation") (Pargament et al., 1990). Higher levels of spiritually based coping were associated with higher levels of psychological adjustment to a variety of stressors. Similar results have been reported in other studies (Cook & Wimberly, 1983; Harris et al., 1995).

Congregational Support

Empirical studies find that support from the congregation and clergy in stressful times is beneficial to its members. Although the 39% significant positive relationships for congregational support statistic in Table 8.2 may seem low, this percentage was heavily influenced by one study of people coping with the type of negative situation that is often problematic for many religious institutions—fetal or infant deaths (Lasker, Lohmann, & Toedter, 1989). Generally, positive outcomes seem to be the result of the support sought and received from the congregation/clergy and God (Gibbs & Achterberg-Lawlis, 1978).

Benevolent Religious Reframing

Attributions of the negative events to the will of God or to a loving God are generally tied to better outcomes. For instance, Jenkins and Pargament (1988) asked patients with various kinds of cancer how much they felt God was in control of their illnesses. Those who attributed more control over the illness to God reported higher self-esteem and better adjustment according to the ratings of nurses. Similar results have been reported in other studies (Brant & Pargament, 1995; Park & Cohen, 1993).

HARMFUL FORMS OF RELIGIOUS COPING

By looking more closely at the specific forms of religious coping presented in Table 8.2, it is clear that not all forms are helpful. Some religious coping methods are often tied to poorer outcomes.

Discontent with Congregation and God

When people do speak negatively of religion, their comments are often targeted at members of their congregation or clergy. Less often, people express negative feelings toward God as well. People who report dissatisfaction with the church, congregation, or God often experience poorer mental health status, more negative mood, and a poorer resolution to the negative life event. The feeling that God or the congregation has abandoned or let them down in their time of need seems to be associated with other feelings of despair, hopelessness, and resentment. Although expressions of religious anger are uncommon and often time limited (Croog & Levine, 1972; Pargament, et al., in press), we do not know whether the effects of such religious anger are long-lasting. Longitudinal studies of religious coping are needed to answer such questions.

Negative Religious Reframing: God's Punishment

The reframing of a negative event in terms of a punishment from God is also not very common. The cost of this form of coping in terms of guilt and fear of further repercussions might be too great. However, when such reframing does occur, poorer outcomes usually result. Specifically, studies have shown that those who report more negative religious reframing also report higher levels of distress and negative mood (Grevengoed, 1985; Pargament et al., in press).

FORMS OF RELIGIOUS COPING
WITH MIXED IMPLICATIONS

Not all forms of religious coping can be easily classified as helpful or harmful. Table 8.2 indicates that some religious coping methods are associated with positive and negative outcomes.

Religious Rituals in Response to Crisis

Religious rituals are related to positive outcomes in 40% of the statistical relationships and to poorer outcomes in 23% of the relationships. How can we explain such mixed results? One possibility may have to do with the design and measures of these studies. Cross-sectional studies make it difficult to know whether rituals are the cause or the effect of poorer mental health. Religious rituals may lead to distress. Conversely, distress may mobilize the enactment of religious rituals. The mixed results may also reflect the many different types of rituals (e.g., confession, mourning, and healing) assessed in these studies. Some religious rituals may simply be more helpful than others. Similarly, some religious rituals may be more helpful to some groups than others.

Self-Directing, Deferring, and Pleading Religious Coping

Religion provides its adherents with many ways to attain control in coping. For example, Pargament et al. (1988) tested three religious methods to gain control: self-directing, deferring, and collaborative. Each method involved a different reported relationship between God and the individual. The self-directing style emphasizes the individual's personal responsibility and active role in problem solving. God is said to give individuals the freedom and resources to direct their own lives. The deferring style places the responsibility of problem solving on God. Rather than actively solve problems themselves, people wait for solutions to emerge through the active efforts of God. The collaborative style reflects the joint responsibility for problem solving by God and the individual. Both participants are seen as active partners.

The three styles had different mental health implications (Pargament et al., 1988). The self-directing and collaborative approaches were related to higher levels of psychological competence (i.e., the general level of psychological and social resourcefulness the person brings to life situations), whereas the deferring style was related to lower levels of competence. Aside from one other study (Harris, Spilka, & Emrick, 1990), however, the self-directing approach has been associated with more negative than positive outcomes. Also, the deferring approach has been tied to positive rather than negative outcomes in some studies. The creators of the scales have suggested that these mixed results may be explained by differences in the controllability of situations. For instance, in situations in which the individual does indeed have very little control, the most appropriate thing to do may be to defer control to God. The self-directing style may be more helpful in more controllable situations.

A similar explanation may account for the mixed results regarding pleas for direct intervention. While pleading for a miracle may not be an effective way to deal with controllable situations, it may offer a sense of vicarious control and mastery through God in situations that fall outside of the person's control.

POSITIVE AND NEGATIVE PATTERNS OF RELIGIOUS COPING

We have examined specific religious coping methods and their implications for adjustment to negative life events. By closely examining these measures, we may have left the impression that each is used in isolation from the others. This does not appear to be the case. Modest to moderately high intercorrelations have been found among the various religious coping scales suggesting that people make use of religious coping methods in some combination with each other.

What are these combinations? Initial research suggests two patterns of religious coping methods: one composed of positive religious coping methods and one composed of negative religious coping methods (Koenig, Pargament, & Nielsen, in press; Pargament, Smith, & Koenig, 1996).

The tragedy of the Oklahoma City bombing provided one context for the study of these coping patterns. Six weeks after the explosion, 310 members of one Baptist and one Disciples of Christ church located near the blast site completed a religious coping measure, a measure of posttraumatic stress, and measures of adjustment to the tragedy. A factor analysis of the religious coping items resulted in

TABLE 8.3 Positive and Negative Religious Coping Subscales: Results from Members of Churches Near the Oklahoma City Bombing

Positive religious coping subscale items
  Thought about how my life is part of a larger physical force
  Worked together with God as partners to get through this hard time
  Looked to God for strength, support, and guidance in this crisis
  Thought about sacrificing my own well-being and living only for God
  Tried to find the lesson from God in this crisis
  Prayed for those who were killed in the bombing and for the well-being of their families and friends
  Looked for spiritual support from my church in this crisis
  Tried to give spiritual strength to other people
  Confessed my sins and asked for God's forgiveness
  Asked God to help me find a new purpose in living
  Reminded myself that the victims of the bombing are now at peace with God in heaven
  Prayed for the spiritual salvation of those who committed this bombing
Negative religious coping subscale items
  Disagreed with the way my church wanted me to understand and handle this situation
  Felt that the bombing was God's way of punishing me for my sins and lack of spirituality
  Wondered whether God had abandoned us
  Felt God was punishing the victims of the bombing for their sins and lack of spirituality
  Tried to make sense of the situation and decided what to do without relying on God
  Questioned whether God really exists
  Prayed to God to send those who were responsible for the bombing to Hell
  Expressed anger at God for letting such a terrible thing happen
  Thought about turning away from God and living for myself alone

two factors. The first factor, labeled positive religious coping, consisted of items that included spiritual support, collaborative religious coping, and benevolent religious reframing. The second factor, negative religious coping, included items that reflected discontent with the church and God, reframing the blast as a punishment from God, and prayers for divine retribution (Table 8.3; Pargament, 1997). Overall, people indicated that they used considerably more positive than negative religious coping. Those that made more use of the positive methods of religious coping also reportedly grew more as a result of the tragedy, both spiritually and psychologically. Negative religious coping, on the other hand, was associated with reports of greater callousness to others.

The question of whether these short-term effects on mental health hold up over a longer period of time must still be addressed. Perhaps the negative pattern of religious coping reflects a process of religious struggle that ultimately holds more beneficial implications for the individual. On the other hand, the positive pattern of religious coping may produce only short-term relief (or even longer term problems). Before reaching more definitive conclusions about the helpfulness or harmfulness of these patterns of religious coping, we need to extend these findings to other groups over longer periods of time.

In this section, we have examined the specifics of what people do with their religion and their effects on adjustment. We have, however, glossed over some variables that are potentially relevant, such as who is doing the coping and with what is the individual coping.

IS RELIGIOUS COPING MORE HELPFUL TO SOME PEOPLE THAN TO OTHERS?

Very few studies have compared the helpfulness of religion to different groups faced with negative life situations. One exception is a national survey of black Americans in which participants were asked to indicate the one coping response that helped them the most in dealing with a serious personal problem (Neighbors, Jackson, Bowman, & Gurin, 1983). Overall, 44% said the prayer was the one coping response that helped them the most. Specifically, a higher percentage of females, older individuals, and lower income people reported prayer as most helpful. In another national survey, Veroff et al. (1981) found that prayer was reportedly more helpful to those who were black, less educated, widowed, churchgoers, and fundamentalists. Similar results have been reported in other studies (Bijur, Wallston, Smith, Lifrak, & Friedman, 1993; Ellison, 1991; Koenig, George, & Siegler, 1988).

Why should religion be more helpful to some groups—elderly, poorer, less educated, blacks, widowed, and women—in coping? It may be no coincidence that the groups that find religion more helpful are the same groups that report higher levels of personal religiousness and more frequent use of religion in coping (Hood et al., 1996; Pargament, 1997). For them, religion has become a larger part of their orienting system—a framework more frequently called upon for coping with major crises. It appears that those who invest more in their religion gain more from it when coping. Drawing on a more deeply established system of beliefs, practicers, feelings, and relationships, these people may be in a better position to find compelling religious solutions (e.g., spiritual and congregational support or benevolent religious reframing) to fundamentally disturbing problems. But why? What do these groups have in common? In general, they often have less access to secular resources and power in our culture. Religion, for them, may represent an alternative resource that can be accessed more easily than others.

IS RELIGION MORE HELPFUL IN SOME SITUATIONS THAN OTHERS?

Although religious beliefs and practices are not reserved for times of loss and pain, people are more likely to turn to religion for help as situations become increasingly stressful. Many of the religious mechanisms of coping, as noted earlier, do seem to be specifically designed to help people through their most difficult times in their life, when significance is at greatest risk. Perhaps, it would not be altogether surprising to find that religion is particularly helpful in moments of greatest stress.

Several studies have indeed shown that religion has the capacity to moderate the effects of stress. Maton (1989), for example, asked recently bereaved parents (high stress) and parents who lost a child more than 2 years ago (low stress) to complete measures of religious coping and adjustment. While spiritual support was related to better adjustment (lower levels of depression) among both the high- and low-stress groups, spiritual support was more strongly related to adjustment for the high- than the low-stress group. Other researchers have also reported a stress-buffering role of religion (Brown & Gary, 1988; Ellison & Gay, 1990).

Does it follow that religion is less than helpful to people in nonstressful situations? Not necessarily. Several studies also suggest that religion can operate as a stress deterrent—that is, a source of help at lower as well as higher levels of stress. For example, Pollner (1989) surveyed a national sample of adults and found that those who reported a close relationship with God also indicated more happiness and life satisfaction, regardless of whether they had experienced up to four major life events.

Whether and how religion works as a stress buffer or stress deterrent seems to depend on several factors, including the type of religious coping, the sample, type of outcome, and the type of study. For instance, Park, Cohen, and Herb (1990) found that intrinsic religiousness buffered the effects of uncontrollable life events on measures of depression among Protestant college students. However, intrinsic religiousness buffered the effects of controllable events among Catholic college students. The authors suggested that Catholic and Protestants may rely on different types of religious coping to deal with similar events. Catholics might draw on guilt-reducing religious beliefs to resolve the distress associated with controllable negative life events, whereas Protestants might rely on their intrinsic religious orientation when confronted with uncontrollable events. Thus, religious coping may be helpful as a stress buffer or as a stress deterrent in different ways for particular groups faced with different events.

WHAT IS SO SPECIAL ABOUT RELIGION?

Religious coping appears to affect the outcomes to negative life events. Sometimes it is helpful and other times it may be harmful. However, an important question remains: Does religious coping add anything to the coping process above and beyond the effects of more traditional or nonreligious coping efforts? In other words, Does religious coping have anything unique to contribute to adjustment beyond secular methods of coping?

Generally, studies have shown that religious coping does predict outcomes to negative events above and beyond the effects of traditional measures of coping. Several studies have reported that religious coping added unique power to the prediction of adjustment after controlling for the effects of traditional or nonreligious forms of coping (Pargament et al., 1990, 1994, 1995). For instance, measures of spiritual support have predicted adjustment above and beyond the effects of general measures of social support (Kirkpatrick, 1993). Greater social involvement in the church has been tied to lower levels of loneliness (Johnson & Mullins, 1989) and greater life satisfaction (Ellison, Gay, & Glass, 1989) even after the effects of other social relationships are controlled.

What is it that religion is adding? Religion seems to offer a response to the problems of human insufficiency. Try as we might to maximize significance through our own experiences and insights or through those of others, we remain human, finite, and limited. At any time we may be pushed beyond our immediate resources, exposing our fundamental vulnerability. Religion provides some solutions. The solutions may come in the form of spiritual support when other sources of support are lacking, explanations when no other explanations seem convincing, a sense of control through the sacred when life seems out of control, or new objects of significance when old ones are no longer compelling. Religion complements nonreligious coping by offering responses to the limits of our personal powers. Perhaps that is why the sacred become most compelling for many when human powers are put to their greatest test.

CONCLUSIONS AND IMPLICATIONS FOR MENTAL HEALTH PROFESSIONALS

Research on the relationship between religion and adjustment has taken both macro- and microanalytic approaches—and we have learned something from each. However, the finer detail that can be gleaned from microanalytic studies seems particularly important in our efforts to identify the value of specific forms of religious coping. When we move beyond a global view of religion and adopt a more microanalytic approach, we see that religion can be helpful, harmful, or irrelevant to adjustment. The results seem to depend on several factors: the method of religious coping, the sample, the situation, and the time frame. Future microanalytic research should consider each of these factors in more detail. For instance, Pargament, Koenig, and Perez (1997) developed a comprehensive set of religious coping scales that assess efforts to find meaning, gain control, obtain comfort, gain intimacy, enhance spirituality, and transform life. Research using other populations, such as, African Americans, Asians, Latinos, Muslims, and Jews, should also help to identify the helpfulness and/or harmfulness of various religious coping methods among specific populations (e.g., Brant & Pargament, 1995). More detailed examinations of particular stressful events will help delineate the value of religious coping in different life circumstances. Finally longitudinal studies are needed to assess the long-term effects of religious coping on mental health (e.g., Koenig et al., 1992).

What do these findings mean for the mental health professional? First, it is clear that religion represents a resource for coping. Mental health professionals should be aware of this resource and feel more free to draw upon it in their efforts to help. In this vein, a few have already begun to integrate religious coping methods, such as spiritual support, religious reframing, rituals, and forgiveness, into their interventions with some promising results (Pargament, 1997).

Second, professionals need to be aware that some forms of religious coping may be problematic or, in fact, harmful to the coping process. Knowledge of these religious warning signs should be a standard part of the mental health professional's education. At a minimum, the professional should be aware of these "red flags" and their implications for the psychological well-being of the individual. These warning signs could also become issues for further discussion and possible change in helping relationships. Particular care must be taken to approach these issues with sensitivity and respect for the diversity of forms and functions religion serves in the lives of people.

Researchers and mental health professionals are likely to be less religious than those they work with and study (Shafranske & Malony, 1990). It is all too easy to overlook the religious dimension. However, for better or worse, religion is an integral part of the lives of many people in our society. By entering into and learning more about diverse religious worlds, we are likely to enhance our own understanding and ability to help others. If we ignore the religious side of life, then our theories and methods will remain incomplete.

REFERENCES

Barsch, R. H. (1968). *The parent of the handicapped child: The study of child-rearing practices.* Springfield, IL: Charles C. Thomas.

Bijur, P. E., Wallston, K. A., Smith, C. A., Lifrak, S., & Friedman, S. B. (1993, August). *Gender differences in turning to religion for coping.* Paper presented at the annual meeting of the American Psychological Association, Toronto, Ontario.

Brant, C. R., & Pargament, K. I. (1995, August). *Religious coping with racist and other negative life events among African Americans.* Paper presented at the annual meeting of the American Psychological Association, New York.

Brown, D. R., & Gary, L. E. (1988). Unemployment and psychological distress among black American women. *Sociological Focus, 21,* 209–221.

Conway, K. (1985/1986). Coping and stress of medical problems among black and white elderly. *International Journal of Aging and Human Development, 2,* 39–48.

Cook, J. A., & Wimberly, D. W. (1983). If I should die before I wake: Religious commitment and adjustment to the death of a child. *Journal for the Scientific Study of Religion, 22,* 222–238.

Croog, S. H., & Levine, S. (1972). Religious identity and response to serious illness: A report on heart patients. *Social Science & Medicine, 6,* 17–32.

Dalal, A. K., & Pande, N. (1988). Psychological recovery of accident victims with temporary and permanent disability. *International Journal of Psychology, 23,* 25–40.

David J. P., Ladd, K. & Spilka, B. (1992, August). *The multidimensionality of prayer and its role as a source of secondary control.* Paper presented at the annual meeting of the American Psychological Association, Washington, DC.

Ellis, A. (1986). *The case against religion: A psychotherapist's view and the case against religiosity.* Austin, TX: American Atheist Press.

Ellison, C. G. (1991). Religious involvement and subjective well-being. *Journal of Health and Social Behavior, 32,* 80–89.

Ellison, C. G., & Gay, D. A. (1990). Region, religious commitment, and life satisfaction among black American. *Sociological Quarterly, 31,* 123–147.

Ellison C. G., Gay, D. A., & Glass, T. A. (1989). Does religious commitment contribute to individual life satisfaction. *Social Forces, 68,* 100–123.

Gibbs, H. W., & Achterberg-Lawlis, J. (1978). Spiritual values and death anxiety; Implications for counseling with terminal cancer patients. *Journal of Counseling Psychology, 25,* 563–569.

Glick, I. O., Weiss, R. S., & Parkes, C. M. (1974). *The first year of bereavement.* New York: John Wiley.

Grevengoed, N. (1985). *Attributions for death: An examination of the role of religion and the relationship between attributions and mental health.* Unpublished master's thesis, Bowling Green State University, Bowling Green, OH.

Harris, N. A., Spilka, B., & Emrick, C. (1990, May). *The sense of control and coping with alcoholism: A multidimensional approach.* Paper presented at the annual meeting of the Rocky Mountain Psychological Association, Tuscon, AZ.

Harris, R. C., Dew, M. A., Lee, A., Amaya, M., Buches, L., Reetz, D., & Coleman, G. (1995). The role of religion in heart-transplant recipients' long-term health and well-being, *Journal of Religion and Health, 34,* 17–32.

Hood, R. W., Spilka, B., Hunsberger, B., & Gorsuch, R. (1996). *The psychology of religion: An empirical approach* (2nd ed.). New York: Guilford.

Horton, A. L., Wilkins, M. M., & Wright, W. (1988). Women who ended abuse: What religious leaders and religion did for these victims. In A. L. Horton & J. A. Williamson (Eds.), *Abuse and religion: When praying isn't enough* (pp. 235–246). Lexington, MA: Lexington Books.

Jenkins, R. A., & Pargament, K. I. (1988). Cognitive appraisals in cancer patients. *Social Science & Medicine, 26,* 625–633.

Johnson, D. P., & Mullins, L. C. (1989). Religiosity and loneliness among the elderly. *Journal of Applied Gerontology, 9,* 110–131.

Kirkpatrick, L. (1993, August). *Loneliness and perceptions of support from God.* Paper presented at the annual meeting of the American Psychological Association, Toronto.

Koenig, H. G. (1994). *Aging and God: Spiritual pathways to mental health in midlife and later years.* New York: Hawthorn.

Koenig, H. G., Cohen, H. J., Blazer, F. H., Pieper, C., Meador, K. G., Shelp, F., Goli, V., & DiPasquale, R. (1992). Religious coping and depression among elderly, hospitalized medically ill men. *American Journal of Psychiatry, 149,* 1693–1700.

Koenig, H. G., George, L. K., & Siegler, I. C. (1988). The use of religious and other emotion-regulating coping strategies among older adults. *Gerontologist, 28,* 303–310.

Koenig, H. G., Pargament, K. I., & Nielsen, J. (1998). Religious coping and health status in medically ill hospitalized older adults. *Journal of Nervous and Mental Diseases,* in press.

Kushner, H. S. (1989). *Who needs God.* New York: Summit.

Lasker, J. N., Lohmann, J., & Toedter, L. (1989, October). *The role of religion in bereavement: The case of pregnancy loss.* Paper presented at the annual meeting of the Society for the Scientific Study of Religion, Salt Lake City, UT.

Maton, K. I. (1989). The stress-buffering role of spiritual support: Cross-sectional and prospective investigations. *Journal for the Scientific Study of Religion, 28,* 310–323.

Neighbors,H. W., Jackson, J. S., Bowman, P. J., & Gurin, G. (1983). Stress, coping and black mental health: Preliminary findings from a national study. *Prevention in Human Services, 2,* 5–29.

O'Brien, M. E. (1982). Religious faith and adjustment to long-term hemodialysis. *Journal of Religion and Health, 21,* 68–80.

Pargament, K. I. (1997). *The psychology of religion and coping: Theory, research, practice.* New York: Guilford.

Pargament, K. I., Ensing, D. S., Falgout, K., Olsen, H., Reilly, B., Van Haitsma, K., & Warren, R.

(1990). God help me: (I) Religious coping efforts as predictors of the outcomes to significant negative life events. *American Journal of Community Psychology, 18,* 793–823.

Pargament, K. I., Ishler, K., Dubow, E., Stanik, P., Rouiller, R., Crowe, P., Cullman, E., Albert, M., & Royster, B. J. (1994). Methods of religious coping with the Gulf War: Cross-sectional and longitudinal analyses. *Journal for the Scientific Study of Religion, 33,* 347–361.

Pargament, K. I., Kennell, J., Hathaway, W., Grevengoed, N., Newman, J., & Jones, W. (1988). Religion and the problem-solving process: Three styles of coping. *Journal for the Scientific Study of Religion, 27,* 90–104.

Pargament, K. I., Koenig, H. G., & Perez, L. (1997). *A comprehensive measure of religious coping: Development and initial validation of the RCOPE.* Report to the Retirement Research Foundation, Bowling Green, OH.

Pargament, K. I., & Park, C. L. (1995). Merely a defense? The variety of religious means and ends. *Journal of Social Issues, 51,* 13–32.

Pargament, K. I., Smith, B., & Brant, C. R. (1995, November). *Religious and nonreligious coping methods with the 1993 Midwest flood.* Paper presented at the annual meeting of the Society for the Scientific Study of Religion, St. Louis, MO.

Pargament, K. I., Smith, B., & Koenig, H. G. (1996, August). *Religious coping with the Oklahoma City bombing: The brief RCOPE.* Paper presented at the annual meeting of the American Psychological Association, Toronto.

Pargament, K. I., Zinnbauer, B. J., Scott, A. B., Butter, E. M., Zerowin, J., & Stanik, P. (1998). Red flags and religious coping: Identifying some religious warning signs among people in crisis. *Journal of Clinical Psychology, 54,* 77–89

Park, C. L., & Cohen, L. H. (1993). Religious and nonreligious coping with the death of a friend. *Cognitive Therapy and Research, 17,* 561–577.

Park, C., Cohen, L., & Herb, L. (1990). Intrinsic religiousness and religious coping as life stress moderators for Catholics vs. Protestants. *Journal of Personality and Social Psychology, 59,* 562–574.

Pollner, M. (1989). Divine relations, social relations, and well-being. *Journal of Health and Social Behavior, 30,* 92–104.

Raleigh, E. D. H. (1992). Sources of hope in chronic illness. *Oncology Nursing Forum, 19,* 443–448.

Saudia, T. L., Kinney, M. R., Brown, K. C., & Young-Ward, L. (1991). Health locus of control and helpfulness of prayer. *Heart and Lung, 20,* 60–65.

Shafranske, E. P., & Malony, H. N. (1990). Clinical psychologists' religious and spiritual orientations and their practice of psychotherapy. *Psychotherapy, 27,* 72–78.

Veroff, J., Douvan. E., & Kulka, R. A. (1981). *Mental health in America: Patterns of help seeking from 1957 to 1976.* New York: Basic Books.

Weisner, T. S., Belzer, L., & Stolze, L. (1991). Religion and families of children with developmental delays. *American Journal of Mental Retardation, 95,* 647–662.

9

RELIGION AND
DEPRESSION

GARY J. KENNEDY

Division of Geriatric Psychiatry
Albert Einstein College of Medicine
New York, New York 10461

In 1995 the National Institute on Aging and the Fetzer Institute of Kalamazoo, Michigan, cosponsored a 2-day conference on Methodological Approaches to the Study of Aging and Health. A number of methodological and conceptual problems were identified in the summary report. Are simple measures of religious attendance and religious group or denomination adequate, or are more complex assessments of personal devotion or beliefs needed to determine the importance of religiousness to seniors' health? Should research focus on health attributes of individual religious groups or seek commonalities across faiths? If religiousness potentially prevents, buffers, or repairs the effects of stress, may it also have deleterious effects? If there are indeed health effects of religiousness, do they remain substantial after measures of tangible and intangible social supports are controlled?

Among the general conclusions, the report advised that "more involvement with clinical epidemiologic studies is needed." In this chapter we explore the relation of depressive symptoms to attendance at services and religious affiliation. More specifically, we examine antecedents and correlates of depressive symptoms in a sample of Catholic and Jewish community residents whose rates of depression vary considerably. Because older adults are more religious than younger adults and because depressive symptoms are more prevalent among the elderly, we expect a greater impact of religiousness upon depression if there is indeed a significant relationship. Data from the Norwood–Montefiore Aging Study offer one example of how the epidemiology of depression may be studied in the context of religious characteristics.

RELIGIOUS INVOLVEMENT AMONG
OLDER AMERICANS

With notable exceptions (Koenig, 1995; Levin, 1994; Meador et al., 1992), the importance of religion in the epidemiology of late life mental illness has received little recognition (Larson, Pattison, Blazer, Omran, & Kaplan, 1986). Yet religious institutions are widely available to the elderly (Palmore, 1980) and religion is an important source of support for older adults (Mechanic, 1974). More than 50% of elderly Americans attend services weekly, close to 80% within the last month, despite difficulties with transportation or physical disability. These figures have remained stable for more than a decade (Princeton Religion Research Center, 1994). Although religious practice decreases with age, personal devotion increases (Bergin, 1984; Young, & Dowling 1987). Both are positively related to life satisfaction (Markides, 1983) and morale (Koenig, Krale, & Ferrel, 1988). Also, a substantial number of older Americans say religion is a resource for coping (Koenig, 1994) or comfort (Princeton Religion Research Center, 1982). Older adults are more often involved in religious organizations than in any other (Payne, Pittard-Payne, & Reddy, 1972). However, only 13% of older persons identify clergy as a source of help for a suicidal friend (Gallup, 1992). Also, the mentally ill profess and practice less religious commitment (Bergin, 1984: Lindenthal, 1970; Stark, 1972).

THEORETICAL MODELS FOR THE
RELATIONSHIP BETWEEN RELIGIOUSNESS
AND HEALTH

Wheaton (1985) proposed several models of how social factors might buffer the effects of stress. Krause and Van Tran (1989) tested these models (the suppressor, distress-deterrent, and moderator models) to determine which might best account for the stress-buffering effects of religion. In the suppressor model, religious practice increases directly in response to stress to alleviate or buffer adverse effects. In the moderator model, religious practice reduces stress only at the extremes of experience, such as acute illness,onset of disability, or bereavement. In the distress-deterrent model, religious practice is independent of stress, i.e., it is not a response to stress but is beneficial nonetheless. Levin (1994) articulated the "prevention" model in which religious practices preempt stress by reducing stress-inducing behaviors such as divorce, unsafe sex, problems with diet, smoking, or alcohol. Ellison and George (1994) add that religion may have both direct and indirect effects on stress through association with "other resources" such as social supports. Idler (1987) theorizes that religious involvement may enhance health by reducing risky behaviors, increasing social cohesion, and providing coherent, consistent beliefs about coping and shared experience. Koenig (1994) and Kaplan, Monroe, Blum, and Blazer (1994) suggest that faith may have a palliative role in alleviating suffering. Although age and perceived mental and physical health largely account for the older person's declining sense of control over life, religiosity and religious preference may contribute positively to preserving one's sense of control (Wolinsky & Stump, 1996). Thus, whether the stress is psychological, physical, or social, the relationship to depression may be modeled for hypothesis testing. However, without adequate methodological controls, the "religious factor" in mental health might be dismissed as a proxy for sociodemographic status, social support, or personality (Levin & Schiller, 1987).

MENTAL HEALTH

Koenig and Fitterman (1995) reviewed 89 studies of religion and mental or physical health. Regarding the 12 studies of depression, most examined organizational rather than nonorganizational practices. Only 1 studied religious attitudes and only 2 were longitudinal in design. A number of the studies did not control for relevant covariables. Nonetheless, a significant inverse correlation between depression and religion emerged, more sizable with clinical than epidemiologic samples and more strongly in the relation of depression to physical disability. Though the overall correlation was small ($-.24$), it was substantial compared to other psychosocial measures. Of 7 studies examining anxiety and religion, the relation was less strong than that observed for depression and in a different direction with more anxious persons exhibiting more religiousness. Although 1 study found that elderly veterans with no religious affiliation were more likely to engage in life-threatening behaviors than their affiliated peers, no study has examined the relation of religion to suicidal thought or behavior in later life. Only 1 study (71 cancer patients) examined chronic pain in relation to religiousness and attendance at religious services. Religious variables were inversely related to pain but the analyses were not controlled for covariates. Two cross-sectional studies of caregiver distress showed significant relationships between religiousness and either lower caregiver burden or greater positive affect.

PHYSICAL DISABILITY AND HEALTH

There are a number of problems with studies of religiousness, health, and disability. First, poor health and disability are more sizable contributors to the dynamics of depressive symptoms in community-dwelling seniors than are social or demographic factors (Kennedy, Lowinger, & Metz, 1996). Changes in the use of social supports are more frequently influenced by baseline levels of health and disability than by social or economic factors (Kelman, Thomas, Kennedy, & Chen,

1994). Thus the contribution of self-assessed health and physical disability to depression may overwhelm the genuinely beneficial influences or religiousness. In their review Koenig and Fitterman (1995) found that cross-sectional studies tend to find greater subjective religiousness among persons with more severe medical illness, indicating that religion may be nothing more than a post hoc defense against illness rather than a means of mastering health. Also measures of objective religiousness such as church attendance may reflect little more than the person's freedom from disability (Levin & Schiller, 1987). Nonetheless, from the limited studies available, organizational religious activities such as attendance at services are truly associated with less physical disability and better self-assessed health as predicted by the prevention model.

As predicted by the suppressor model, nonorganizational religious activities such as prayer are associated with poorer objective health but not greater disability or poorer self-assessed health. The relation of disability and attendance at services is complicated by denominational issues as well. Attendance at religious services is a moral imperative for Catholics but is less so for some Jews and Protestants. Also, the major denominations within Judaism and within Protestant Christianity differ widely in both practices and beliefs (Glicksman, 1991). Elderly believers whose mobility is compromised by physical limitations or inadequate transportation may choose to forgo attendance if a synagogue or church from an unacceptable denomination is the only one nearby.

RELIGIOUS PREFERENCE AS A PROXY FOR RESPONSE BIAS OR HEALTH-SEEKING BEHAVIOR

Cross-cultural comparisons suggest that different religious groups have different social expectations (Lenski, 1961), attitudes toward mental illness (Guttmacher & Ellison, 1971; Suchman, 1969; Srole et al., 1962), expression of negative emotions (Glicksman, 1991), and forms of religious devotion. Kohn and Levav (1994) recount "over a century of clinical observations" from Kraepelin on, in which a larger than expected number of persons treated for depression were Jewish. Failure to account for difference in health-seeking behavior, frequency of readmission, diagnostic reliability, and the differential effects of other diagnoses, or to control for confounding variables, led to a biased view of Jewish vulnerability to depression. Conversely, a number of studies found that American Irish Catholics tend to deny feelings (McGoldrick & Pearce, 1981), to be stoic (Zborowski, 1952), and to be less likely to seek help (Zola, 1966). Jews, in contrast, reported more symptoms on the Cornell Medical Index than other ethnic groups of similar educational level (Croog, 1961).

Glicksman (1991) has also investigated differences in response styles and psychological well-being and suggests that Jews of Eastern European descent are much more likely than Irish or Italian Catholics to express negative affect. Similarly, the elevated prevalence of major depression among Pentecostals in the Duke

Epidemiologic Catchment Arena study may relate to greater emotionality as a group (Meador et al., 1992). What is not clear, however, is whether the differences in response styles are related to the development or course of mental disorders.

RELIGIOUS PREFERENCE, DEPRESSION, AND ALCOHOL ABUSE/DEPENDENCE

Reanalyzing data from the 4152 subjects of the Los Angeles and New Haven Epidemiologic Catchment Area studies, Levav, Kohn, Golding, and Weissman (1997) found higher period and lifetime prevalence of major affective disorder and dsythymia among Jews compared to others. Period and lifetime rates were 12.4 and 18.7% respectively for Jews, 9.0 and 16.0% for Catholics, and 8.6 and 16.0% for non-Jews, including Catholics. Symptoms of depression (dysphoria, insomnia, fatigue, and loss of concentration) among those who did not meet criteria for affective disorder were also more frequent among Jews. The higher prevalence of these symptoms, however, was accounted for by greater frequencies in Jewish males compared with non-Jewish males. Indeed, rates of depression approached a 1:1 male-to-female ratio within Jews. Lower rates of depression within other groups were made up for by a greater prevalence of alcohol abuse or dependence.

These findings confirmed those of other community surveys suggesting a greater vulnerability of Jews to depression (Yeung & Greenwald, 1992), with an equivalency of depression prevalence among men and women and lesser frequencies of alcoholism. Rates of depression were highest among the Jews from New Haven, whom the authors argued might be more traditional (Orthodox or Conservative) than their more secular counterparts in Los Angeles. In Los Angeles, the rates of alcohol abuse were higher and the ratio of depressive disorder reflected the more typical 2:1 female-to-male frequency of depression. Citing other studies, Levav and colleagues (1997) argue that the social constraints of less tolerance for alcohol abuse, also seen among the Amish, result in a compensatory increase in depression. When combined, the prevalence of alcohol abuse/dependence and major depression were not significantly greater among the Jews compared to other groups.

Frequency of attendance at religious services made no contribution to period or lifetime risk of depression in any of the religious groups. Only 170 of 431 Jewish respondents, however, were aged 65 or older. The relative youth of the sample suggested that this group may be less religious and less traumatized by the European Holocaust.

RELIGIOUS PREFERENCE AS A PROXY FOR TRAUMA OR SOCIAL SUPPORT

Although genetic factors may contribute to depression among Eastern European Jews (melancholia agitata Hebraica) (Hollingshead & Redlich, 1948), social factors seem more compelling. The immigrant status of a religious group may explain the relation of advanced age and depression (Vega, Bohda, Hough, & Figueroa, 1987). In-migration to a less diverse community may be less distressing than arrival in a mixed group (Rahav, Goodman, Pepper, & Lin, 1986). Life stressors—notably the European Holocaust and anti-Semitism—might also play a role in depression (Brown et al., 1978; Lin and Ensel, 1984) and posttraumatic stress syndrome (Yehuda, Kahana, Southwick, & Gilles, 1994).

In a nationwide randomized sample of Jews in Israel aged 75–94, Ruskin et al. (1996) found 43% with significant levels of depressive symptoms. Higher rates were found among women, those with lower educational or income status, and those who immigrated from the Middle East or northern Africa. Persons who were either born in Israel or came to Israel before age 20 experienced significantly lower rates of depression. More than 50% of those who arrived in Israel at age 40 or older were depressed. Holocaust survivorship, "religious adherence," and number of self-assessed past traumatic experiences were not significantly associated with depressive symptoms.

Neither survivor distress nor the definition of exposed individual, however, are easily quantified. The effects of trauma early in life may be compounded by late life events. Yehuda et al. (1995) found that the severity of posttraumatic stress syndrome among Holocaust survivors was related both to the original stressor and to subsequent events. Posttraumatic stress syndrome disorder, however, may not adequately capture the mental morbidity for this population. Krystal and Niederland (1971) described sequelae of Holocaust survivorship. First, they described an anxiety syndrome associated with insomnia and nightmares; a second syndrome was chronic depression characterized by social isolation.

The definition of Holocaust survivorship also varies. Of the 8.8 million Jews living in Europe before the war, 3 million remained afterwards. An estimated 500,000 survived in hiding, labor camps, or the resistance, but only 75,000 survived the death camps (Epstein, 1977). Porter (1981) delegates Holocaust survivorship to these 575,000 but includes those German and Austrian Jews who fled Europe in the 1930s and others from the displaced persons camps who immigrated during or after the 1940s. Finally, there may be an indirect effect of Holocaust trauma that extends beyond the camp survivors. All Jews may not be Holocaust survivors, but in some sense all are Holocaust victims.

THE NORWOOD AGING STUDY

Data from the Norwood Aging Study indicate that among older community residents simple measures of religious preference and practice correlate with depressive symptoms. These data are relevant to Gallup's call for religious institutions to take on a more prominent role in combating late-life suicide (Gallup, 1992), which is so frequently linked to depression. They are equally relevant to the primary health care of older Jewish and Catholic community residents in that disability is so intimately linked to the prevalence and prognosis of depression. Approximately 2480 Medicare households from the Norwood area of the North Bronx were sampled to yield 1855 randomly selected individuals who agreed to a baseline interview. The Norwood area differs from the Established Populations for the Epidemiologic Study of the Elderly (Cornoni-Huntley & Lafferty 1986), in that 39.6% express a Jewish religious preference compared to 13.9% in New Haven and 1% in the population samples of Iowa and Washington state, East Boston, and North Carolina. Nearly 48% of Norwood respondents express a Catholic religious preference compared to approximately 14% in Iowa and Washington state, 90% in East Boston and 54% in New Haven. Protestants made up 96% of the North Carolina site. Norwood respondents, in contrast to the national elderly population, were older, more often female, more often living alone, and had lower median incomes (Kelman, Thomas & Tanaka, 1994).

MEASURES

Respondents provided information on health, chronic illness, physical and cognitive functioning, utilization of and attitudes toward health care, interactions with family, friends,and social service agencies, and financial resources. They were also asked to indicate their religious preference as Catholic, Jewish, Protestant, none, or other and whether they attended religious services weekly, monthly, or less. The Center for Epidemiologic Studies Depression scale (CES-D) was used to measure the level of depressive symptoms experienced during the past week (Radloff, 1977). Roughly a third of persons meeting the 16-point criterion for a significant level of depressive symptoms also met diagnostic criteria for major depression. From 13 to 19% of older community samples score 16 or above on the CES-D (Kinsie, Lewinsohn, Maricle, & Teri, 1986; Lin & Ensel, 1984; Phifer & Murrel, 1986).

Twenty-four months after baseline, 85% of the original sample completed a second CES-D and provided information on changes in problems with activities of daily living, formal and informal support, and health. Persons scoring less than 16 on the CES-D at both baseline and the 24-month assessments were considered not depressed. Persons scoring 16 or greater at both the baseline and 24-month interviews were designated as persistently depressed. However, for those who scored between 12 and 20 at baseline, only a change of ±4 points (.5 standard deviation) across the criterion score of 16 was considered meaningful. We designated respondents whose scores increased by at least 4 points across the criterion to have an emergence of depressive symptoms and those declining by at least 4 points to have a remission of symptoms. Data from 15 respondents who changed by less than 4 points were censored from the longitudinal analysis.

DISTRIBUTION BY RELIGIOUS PREFERENCE

Of the 1855 respondents, 711 (39.6%) reported a Jewish religious preference, 880 (47.7%) Catholic, and Protestants numbered 185 (10%). Persons indicating no religious preference ($n = 35$), not specified ($n = 10$), or one other than Jewish,

Catholic, or Protestant ($n = 34$) makeup 3.5% of the sample and were added to the Protestants to create an Other category for the purposes of analysis. Respondents not completing the CES-D ($n = 160$) tended to be confused, disabled, or ill and were more characteristic of persons scoring as depressed (Thomas, 1989) but equally represented across the three religious groups.

DEMOGRAPHICS, HEALTH, AND DISABILITY

Jewish respondents were older and more educated than either the Catholics or Others. The level of income was more favorable for the Jewish than Other respondents but was not significantly different from that of the Catholics. The proportion of women, persons married, and persons living alone was equivalent across the groups. A higher percentage in the Other group were either separated or divorced compared to the Jewish or Catholics groups. The percentage who never married was larger among the Catholics. More of the Jewish respondents received both formal and informal social supports than the Catholics or Others. Although there were no significant differences for the number of problems with activities of daily living, more than half the Jewish respondents rated their health as no better than fair to poor compared to one-third of Catholics and 40% of Others.

Forty-one depressed respondents had visited a psychiatric social worker, psychologist, or psychiatrist within the previous 3 months, and more than half were Jewish. Cognitive impairment, defined by a score <18 on the Mini-Mental State Exam, and the use of psychotropic prescription medications were more prevalent among the Jewish respondents.

A sizable minority of the sample were foreign born ranging from nearly half the Jewish respondents to 40% of the Catholics and more than one-third of the Other group. Fifty-eight percent of the foreign-born Catholics were from Ireland, 12% from Italy, and 30% elsewhere. The majority of foreign-born Jewish respondents were from Eastern Europe (Russia, 34.5%; Poland, 30.2%) with the remainder from Hungary (8.6%), Austria (9.8%), or other areas (14%).

RELIGIOUS PREFERENCE AND PRACTICE

Of the 16.9% of the sample who evidenced a significant level of depressive symptoms, <10% of the Catholics, 12% of Others, and >20% of the Jews were depressed (Table 9.1). The odds of being depressed for the Catholics were less than half that of the sample as a whole. For the Jewish respondents the odds were more than twofold greater.

Of the Catholics, close to three-fourths reported having attended religious services within the last month compared to 20% of the Jews and 38% of Others. For Jewish respondents and Others, the rates of depression were higher among those who did not attend compared to those who did, but the rates did not reach statistical significance. Protestants made up the majority of persons labeled as Other. Eleven percent of Protestants were depressed. Of those who had not attended services, 14.2% were depressed compared to 7.9% who attended, but the differences

TABLE 9.1   Religious Preference, Practice, and Odds of Depression

Characteristic	N	Depressed	χ^2	Odds ratio	95% Confidence interval
Catholic	1075	9.5	37.904*	0.462	0.362–0.591
Jewish	900	20.7	49.505*	2.308	1.829–2.914
Other	307	12.3	1.148	—	ns
Attend service monthly					
Catholic					
Yes	798	7.0	23.498*	0.369	0.244–0.559
No	277	16.9			
Jewish					
Yes	189	17.9	1.130	—	ns
No	711	21.5			
Other					
Yes	125	8.0	3.726	—	ns
No	182	15.3			

Note. Chi-squares and odds ratios were based on data weighted by number of household members age 65 years or older. ns, not significant. Adapted with permission from Kennedy et al. (1996).
*$p < .0001$.

were not significant. However, the rate of depression among Catholics who did not attend services compared to those who did was more than doubled.

BASELINE CHARACTERISTICS EXPLAINING THE VARIANCE IN DEPRESSION

Logistic regression analyses of respondent characteristics identified seven variables significantly contributing to the explained variance in depression at $p < 0.01$ (Table 9.2). These included fair to poor health, problems with activities of daily

TABLE 9.2   Magnitude of Characteristics Associated with Depression

Characteristic	Parameter estimate	Standard error	Wald χ^2	p value	Odds ratio	Confidence interval
Health fair/poor	−1.16	0.14	66.65	.0001	3.21	2.78–3.70
PADL	−0.70	0.14	23.90	.0001	2.02	1.75–2.34
Lives alone	−0.58	0.13	18.59	.0001	1.79	1.57–2.05
Jewish	−0.55	0.14	14.69	.0001	1.75	1.51–2.02
Not attend service	0.47	0.14	9.84	.001	1.60	1.38–1.86
Female	−0.42	0.15	7.37	.006	1.52	1.30–1.78
Social support	−0.40	0.17	4.96	.02	1.49	1.25–1.78
Education ≥9 years	0.34	0.13	6.62	.01	1.42	1.24–1.62
≥2 Cardiovascular conditions	−0.32	0.14	4.71	.03	1.38	1.19–1.60

Note. PADL, one or more problems with activities of daily living. All missing values were replaced by mean values of the variables. Adapted with permission from Kennedy et al. (1996).

living, living alone, Jewish religious preference, nonattendance at religious services, female gender, and education $\geq$9 years. Receipt of formal and informal social support services and cardiovascular conditions were significant at $p < .02$ and $p < .03$, respectively, but other medical conditions, cognitive impairment, foreign birth, age, income, and receipt of Medicaid were not significant. Thus, both Jewish religious preference and failure to attend services contributed significantly to the variance even after measures of sociodemographic status, immigration, health and disability, and social support were controlled.

EMERGENCE, PERSISTENCE, AND REMISSION
OF DEPRESSION 24 MONTHS AFTER BASELINE

Table 9.3 shows the longitudinal course of depressive symptoms from baseline to 24 months by comparing respondents in whom depressive symptoms emerged, remitted, persisted, or never reached clinical significance. Significantly more Jewish respondents experienced an emergence of depression. Jewish respondents also made up a greater percentage of persons in whom depression persisted but the differences did not reach statistical significance. The percentage of persons not attending services was significantly greater in the groups in which depression emerged and depression persisted.

We used stepwise and canonical discriminant function analyses to identify characteristics which distinguished the never depressed from those in whom depression emerged and to determine if Jewish religious preference and attendance at services would remain significant once other variables were taken into account. Baseline measures of health and disability made up most of the characteristics included in the model and accounted for 15% (average squared canonical correla-

TABLE 9.3   Religious Preference and Practice of Respondents Whose Depression Emerged, Persisted, or Remitted after 24 Months

Characteristic	Never depressed (%) $n = 1223$	Depression emerged (%); $n = 142$	Depression persisted (%); $n = 93$	Depression remitted (%); $n = 116$
Jewish	397 (32.4)	72 (50.7)[a,b]	60 (64.5)	59 (50.8)
Catholic	643 (52.5)	53 (37.3)	26 (27.9)	41 (35.3)
Other	183 (14.9)	17 (11.9)	7 (7.5)	16 (14.0)
Attends services monthly	702 (57.4)[c]	55 (38.7)	22 (23.7)[d]	43 (37.1)

Note. Adapted with permission from Kennedy et al. (1996).
[a]Significant difference between Jews and Catholics ($\chi^2 = 17.51$, $df = 1$, $p < .0001$).
[b]Significant difference between Jews and others ($\chi^2 = 5.70$, $df = 1$, $p < .01$).
[c]Significant difference between the never depressed and the emergence groups ($\chi^2 = 17.94$, $df = 1$, $p < .0001$).
[d]Significant difference between the persistence and remission groups ($\chi^2 = 4.33$, $df = 1$, $p < .03$).

TABLE 9.4 Characteristics Distinguishing Respondents Who Were Never Depressed from Those in Whom Depression Emerged

Characterisitic	Partial R^2	F	p value
Increase in PADL at 24 months	.085	99.83	<.0001
Health worse at 24 months	.041	46.01	<.0001
Baseline health, fair/poor	.009	9.70	<.001
Jewish	.006	6.51	<.01
Education ≥ 9 years	.007	7.76	<.005
Cognitive impairment	.004	4.47	<.03
Baseline PADL	.004	4.50	<.03

Note. PADL, one or more problems with activities of daily living. All missing values were replaced by mean values of the variables. Adapted with permission from Kennedy et al. (1996).

tion $= .15$) of the explained variance (Table 9.4). Jewish religious preference was significant but age, gender, social support, and attendance at services were not. Similar analyses of the respondents who were depressed at baseline indicated that worsening health ($F = 1.61$; $p = .0001$), increased problems with activities of daily living ($F = 5.00$; $p = .002$) at 24 months, and advanced age ($F = 9.10$; $p = .002$) distinguished the persistently depressed from the remission group and accounted for 25% of the explained variance (average squared canonical correlation $= .25$). Religious preference and attendance at services were not distinguishing characteristics of depression status at 24 months.

DEPRESSION AMONG JEWISH RESPONDENTS

Because of the elevated prevalence of depressive symptoms among Jewish respondents, we examined characteristics which might distinguish the depressed from the not depressed Jews at baseline. Table 9.5 portrays the prevalence of depressive symptoms among foreign-born respondents which is higher across the board but higher still among Jewish persons born in Eastern Europe. Respondents born in Eastern Europe were older, less educated, and reported less income. They

TABLE 9.5 Prevalence of Depression by Birthplace among Foreign-Born Respondents

Birthplace	N (% depressed)
Russia	108 (31)
Poland	100 (30)
Hungary	30 (33)
UK + Ireland + Canada = 19, Germany + Austria = 38, Turkey + Czechoslovakia + Rumania = 30, Greece + Malaysia + unspecified = 3	90 (21)

TABLE 9.6 Stepwise Discriminant Analysis of Characteristics Distinguishing the Depressed ($N = 156$) from the Not Depressed ($N = 524$) Jewish Respondents at Baseline

Characteristic	F	p	Average squared canonical correlation[a]
Activites of daily living problem	44.86	.0001	.06
Fair/poor self-assessed health	24.05	.0001	.09
Lives alone	14.85	.0001	.11
Eastern European born	10.68	.001	.12
Gender	4.86	.02	.13

received more tangible social support, attended religious services more often, and experienced poorer health and greater physical disability. The prevalence of cognitive impairment was significantly greater among persons of Eastern European origin than other Jewish respondents. Immigration after the European Holocaust was not associated with depression among foreign-born respondents, including those from Eastern Europe, as shown in Table 9.6. Birth in Eastern Europe remained significant after the contribution of other characteristics to the variance in baseline depression among Jewish respondents was controlled.

CONCLUSIONS

Our findings are consistent with a number of hypotheses offered to explain why religious groups might differ in their expression of depressive symptoms. These include the sociodemographic hypothesis of ethnic density, the cultural trait hypothesis of response bias, and the heredity hypothesis of Eastern European Jewish origin. Lacking a measure to assess the traumatic effects of the European Holocaust on the Jewish respondents, we can only speculate that a relationship exists. Jewish respondents did not report excess cardiovascular conditions which more than any other illnesses outside the central nervous system have been associated with elevated rates of depression (Oxman, Freeman, & Manheimer, 1995) or problems with activities of daily living. However, the greater prevalence and incidence of depression was accompanied by greater use of mental health services, psychotropic medications, and greater prevalence of cognitive impairment, suggesting that the Jewish participants were responding and acting as though they were genuinely depressed.

The elevated prevalence of depressive symptoms among Jewish respondents from Eastern Europe appears genuine and not fully explained by differences in health, disability, age, gender, or disadvantaged socioeconomic status. Whether Eastern European Jews are demoralized as suggested by Gliksman (1991) or suffering from melancholia agitata Hebraica as reported by Hollingshead and Redlich (1958), the health significance of our findings remains to be explored.

Regarding religious practice, depression was more frequent among all respondents not attending religious services suggesting that the hypothesized preventive model may apply particularly to Catholics. The regression analysis indicated that social supports did not substitute for failure to attend services in the variance of depression. Neither did problems with activities of daily living which might have explained the relationship for respondents too disabled to attend services. Among Eastern European-born Jewish respondents, the stress deterrent model may be a better fit in that depression and greater attendance at services were significantly associated.

Finally, differences in sociodemographics, disability and illness, immigrant status, and social supports did not account for the relation of lack of attendance at religious services and Jewish religious preference to symptoms of depression at baseline. Although failure to attend services was associated with the emergence and persistence of depression at 24 months, only Jewish religious preference remained significant once age, disability, and social support were controlled.

FUTURE AVENUES OF RESEARCH

Inferences from our data are limited by the 2-year interval between assessments of depressive symptoms, the lack of diagnostic data which might clarify the relation of depressive symptoms to depressive and other mental disorders, the availability of only baseline data for cognitive impairment, and the lack of information on the depth and dynamics of religious practice which might be associated with changes in health and disability. It is also important to note that our measures captured tangible rather than emotional support and that we did not assess the perceived adequacy of support. Neither do we have data on suicidal thought, appointment of health care proxy, possession of a living will or advanced directives, personality traits, or history of traumatic events. Thus, the influence of religious preference and practice on a number of health outcomes (mental disorders, suicidal ideas, cognitive impairment, and physical disability) and practices (use of psychotropic medications, health care proxy, and living will) remains uncertain. Investigating hypothesized mechanisms as well as health outcomes among two groups, Jews and Catholics, who appear to have different vulnerabilities to depression, has implications for their health services as well as those of the majority of Americans.

ACKNOWLEDGMENTS

This work was supported in part by grants P01 AG03424, and R01 AG08125 from the National Institute on Aging, the Resnick Gerontology Center, and the Julia and Leo Forchheimer Foundation.

REFERENCES

Ainlay, S. C., & Smith, R. D. (1984). Aging and religious participation: Reconsidering the effects of health. *Journal of Gerontology, 39,* 357–363.

Allport, G. (1963). Behavioral science, religion and mental health. *Journal of Religion and Health, 2,* 87–92.

Allport, G. W., & Ross, J. M. (1967). Personal religious orientation and prejudice. *Journal of Personality and Social Psychology, 5,* 432–443.

Anonymous. (1995). Summary report from the Conference on Methodological Advances in the Study of Religion, Health and Aging, March 16–17, sponsored by the National Institute on Aging and Fetzer Institute, Kalamazoo, MI.

Bergin A. E. (19084). Religiosity and mental health; A critical re-evaluation and meta-analysis. *Professional Psychology: Research and Practice, 14,* 170–184.

Brown, G., & Tirril, H. (1978). Meaning. In G. Brown (Ed.), *Social origins of depression* (pp. 82–99). New York: Free Press.

Clark, D. (1992). Comments delivered December 10 at a conference titled "Too Young to Die at Any Age," sponsored by the Empire Blue Cross Blue Shield, The Gallup Organization and The American Association of Suicidology.

Cornoni-Huntley, J., & Lafferty, M. E. (Eds.). (1986). *Established populations for the epidemiologic study of the elderly; resource data book,* NIH Publication No. 86: 2443. Bethesda, MD: National Institutes of Health.

Croog, S. (1961). Ethnic origins, educational level, and responses to a health questionnaire. *Human Organization, 20,* 65–69.

Devanand, D. P., Sano, M., Tang, M., Taylor, S., Gurland, B. J., Wilder, D., Stern, Y., & Mayeus, R. (1996). Depressed mood and the incidence of Alzheimer's disease in the elderly living in the community. *Archives of General Psychiatry, 53,* 175–182.

Ellison, C. G., & George, L. K. (1994). Religious involvement, social ties, and social support in a southeastern community. *Journal for the Scientific Study of Religion, 33,* 46–61.

Epstein, H. (1977, June 19). The heirs of the Holocaust. *The New York Times Magazine,* 12–15, 74–75.

Friedlander, Y., Kaark, J. D., & Stein, Y. (1986). religious orthodoxy and myocardial infarction in Jerusalem—A case control study. *International Journal of Cardiology, 10,* 33–41.

Futterman, A., & Koenig, H. (1995). *Measuring religiosity in later life: What can gerontology learn from the sociology and psychology of religion?* Paper presented at the Conference on Methodological Advances in the Study of Religion, Health and Aging, March 16–17, sponsored by the National Institute on Aging and Fetzer Institute, Kalamazoo, MI.

Gallup, R. (1992). *Executive summary: Attitude and incidence of suicide among the elderly.* Princeton, NJ: The Gallup Organization; and comments delivered December 10, at a conference title "Too Young to Die at Any Age," sponsored by the Empire Blue Cross Blue Shield, The Gallup Organization, and the American Association of Suicidology.

Glicksman, A. (1991). *The new Jewish elderly,* New York: American Jewish Committee.

Goldbourt, U., Yaari, S., & Medalie, J. H. (1993). Factors predictive of long-term coronary heart disease mortality among 10,059 males Israeli civil servants and municipal employees: A 23-year mortality follow-up in the Israeli Ischemic Heart Disease Study. *Cardiology, 82,* 100–121.

Guttmacher, S., & Ellison. J. (1971). Ethno-religious variation in perceptions of illness. *Social Science and Medicine, 5,* 117–125.

Hollingshead, A. B., & Redlich, F. C. (1958). *Social class and mental illness.* New York: John Wiley.

Idler, E. L. (1987). Religious involvement and the health of the elderly: Some hypotheses and an initial test.*Social Forces, 66,* 226–238.

Kaplan, B. H. (1976). A note on religious beliefs and coronary heart disease. *Journal of the South Carolina Medical Association, 72* (Suppl). 60–64/

Kaplan, B. H., Munroe-Blum, H., & Blazer, D. G. (1994). Religion, health and forgiveness.. In J. S.

Levom (Ed.). *Religion, aging and health; Theoretical foundations and methodological frontiers* (pp. 52–77). Thousand Oaks, CA: Sage.

Katz, S., Ford, A. B., Moskowitz, R. W., Amasa, B. F., Jackson, B. A., Jaffe, M. W. (1963). Studies of illness in the aged; The index of ADL: A standardized measure of biological and psychological function. *Journal of the American Medical Association, 185,* 914–919.

Kelman, H. R., Thomas, C., Kennedy, G. J., & Chen J. (1994). Cognitive impairment and mortality in older community residents. *American Journal of Public Health, 84,* 1255–1260.

Kelman, H. R., Thomas, C., & Tanaka, J. S. (1994). Longitudinal patterns of formal and informal social support in an elderly population. *Social Science & Medicine, 38,* 905–914.

Kennedy, G. J., Colon, S., Louis, A., Smyth, C., & Sherlock, L. (1995). Mental disorders among dementia caregivers persist beyond nursing home entry. *The Gerontologist, 35,* 418.

Kennedy, G. J. Kelman, H. R., & Thomas, C. (1990). The emergence symptoms in late life: The importance of declining health and increasing disability. *Journal of Community Health, 15,* 93–104.

Kennedy, G. J., Kelman, H. R., & Thomas, C. (1991). Persistence and remission of depressive symptoms in late life. *American Journal of Psychiatry, 148,* 174–178.

Kennedy, G. J., Kelman, H. R., Thomas, C., Wisniewski, W., Metz, H., & Bijur, P. (1989). Hierarchy of characteristics associated with depressive symptoms in an urban elderly sample. *American Journal of Psychiatry, 148,* 174–178.

Kennedy, G. J., Kelman, H. R., Thomas, C., & Chen, J. (1996). Religious preference, practice and the prevalence of depression among 1855 older community residents. *Journals of Gerontology; Psychological Sciences, 51B,* 301–308.

Kennedy, G. J., Lowinger, R., & Metz, H. (1996). Epidemiology and inferences regarding the etiology of late life suicide. In G. J. Kennedy (Ed.), *Suicide and depression in late life; Critical issues in treatment, research and public policy.* (pp. 3–22). New York: John Wiley.

Kinsie, J. D., Lewinsohn, P., Maricle, R., & Teri, L. (1986). The relationship of depression to medical illness in an older community population. *Comprehensive Psychiatry, 27,* 241–246.

Koenig, H. G., (1994). Religion and hope for the disabled elderly. In J. S. Levin (Ed.), *Religion, aging and health: Theoretical foundations and methodological frontiers,* (pp. 18–51).Thousand Oaks, CA: Sage.

Koenig, H. G. (1995). Religion and older men in prison. *International Journal of Geriatric Psychiatry, 10,* 219–230.

Koenig, H. G., & Futterman, A. (1995). *Religion and health outcomes; A review and synthesis if the literature.* Paper presented at the Conference on Methodological Advances in the Study of Religion, Health and Aging, March 16–17, sponsored by the National Institute on Aging and Fetzer Institute, Kalamazoo, MI.

Koenig, H. G., Kvale, J. H., & Ferrel, C. (1988). Religion and well-being in later life. *The Gerontologist, 28,* 18–28.

Koenig, H. G., & Seeber, J. J. (1987). Religion, spirituality, and aging. *Journal of the American Geriatrics Society, 35,* 472. [Letter to the editor].

Koenig, H. G., Siegler, I. C., Meador, K. G., & George, L. K. (1990). Religious coping and personality in laater life. *International Journal of Geriatric Psychiatry, 5,* 123–131.

Kohn, R.,& Levav, I. (1994). Jews and their intraethnic differential vulnerability to affective disorders, fact or artifact? I: An overview of the literature. *Israel Journal of Psychiatry and Related Sciences, 31,* 261–270.

Krause, N. (1993). Measuring religiosity in later life. *Research on Aging, 15,* 170–197.

Krause, N., & Markides, K. (1990). Measuring social support among older adults. *International Journal of Aging and Human Development, 30,* 37–43.

Krause, N. & VanTran, T. (1989). Stress and religious involvement among old blacks. *Journal of Gerontology, 44,* S4–S13.

Krystal, H., & Niederland, W. (Eds.). (1971). *Psychic traumatization: After effects in individuals and communities.* Boston: Little, Brown.

Larson, D. B., Pattison, E. M., Blazer, D. G., Omran, A. R., & Kaplan, B. H. (1986). Systematic analy-

sis of research on religious variables in four major psychiatric journals, 1978–1982. *American Journal of Psychiatry, 143,* 329–334.

Levav, I., Kohn, R., Golding, J. M., & Weissman, M. M. (1997). Vulnerability of Jews to affective disorders. *American Journal of Psychiatry, 154,* 941–947.

Lenski, G. (1961). *The religious factor,* Garden City, NY: Doubleday.

Levin, J. S. (Ed.). (1994). *Religion, aging and health: Theoretical foundations and methodological frontiers.* Thousand Oaks, CA: Sage.

Levin, J. S., & Schiller, P. L. (1987). Is there a religious factor in health? *Journal of Religion and Health, 26,* 9–36.

Levin, J. S., Taylor, R. J., & Chatters, L. M. (1994). Race and gender differences in religiosity among older adults; Findings from national surveys. *Journal of Gerontology,49,* S137–S145.

Lin, N., & Ensel, W. M. (1984). Depression–mobility and its social etiology: The role of life events and social support. *Journal of Health, Society and Behavior, 25,* 176–188.

Lindenthal, J. J. (1970). Mental status and religious behavior. *Journal for the Scientific Study of Religion, 9,* 143–149.

Markides, K. S. (1983). Aging, religiosity, and adjustment: A longitudinal analysis. *Journal of Gerontology, 38,* 621–625.

McGoldrick, M., & Pearce, J. K. (1981). Family therapy with Irish-Americans. *Family Process, 20,* 223–241.

Meador, K. G., Koenig, H.G., Turnull, J., Blazer, D. G., George, L. K., & Hughes, D. (1992). Religious affiliation and major depression. *Hospital and Community Psychiatry, 43,* 1204–1208.

Mechanic, D. (1974). Social structure and personal adaptation: Some neglected dimensions. In J. Adams, G. Coelho, & D. Hamburg (Eds.), *Coping and Adaptation* (pp. 33–40). New York: Basic Books.

Mirand, A. L., & Welte, J. W. (1996). Alcohol consumption among the elderly in a general population, Erie County, New York. *American Journal of Public Health, 86,* 978–984.

Oxman, T. E., Freeman, D. H., & Manheimer, E. D. (1995). Lack of social participation and religious strength and comfort as risk factors for death after cardiac surgery in the elderly. *Psychosomatic Medicine, 47,* 5–15.

Palmore, E. (1980). The social factors in aging. In D. Blazer & E. Busse (Eds.), *Handbook of geriatric psychiatry* (pp. 222–248). New York: Van Nostrand Reinhold.

Payne, R., Pittard-Payne, B., & Reddy, R. D. (1972). Social background and role determinants of individual participation in organized voluntary action. In D. Horton Smith, B. R. Baldwins, & R. D. Reddy (Eds.), *Voluntary action research* (pp. 207–250). Boston: D. C. Health.

Phifer, J. F., & Murrel, S. A. (1986). Etiologic factors in the onset of depressive symptoms in older adults. *Journal of Abnormal Psychology, 95,* 282–291.

Porter, J. N. (1981). Is there a survivor's syndrome? Psychological and socio-political implications. *Journal of Psychology and Judaism, 6,* 33–52.

Princeton religion Research Center. (1982). *Religion in America.* Princeton, NJ: The Gallup Poll.

Princeton Religion Research Center. (1985). *Religion in America* (1994 Supplement) Princeton, NJ: The Gallup Poll.

Radloff, L. S. (1977). The CES-D Scale: A new self report depression scale for use in the general population. *Applied Psychological Measurement, 1,* 385–401.

Rahav, M., Goodman, A. B., Popper, M., & Lin, S. P. (1986). Distribution of treated mental illness in the neighborhoods of Jerusalem. *American Journal of Psychiatry, 143,* 1249–1254.

Rosowsky, E., & Gurian, B. (1991). Borderline personality in later life. *International Psychogeriatrics, 3,* 39–52.

Ruskin, P. E., Blumstein, Z., Walter-Ginzburg, A., Fuchs, V., Luskay, A., Novikov, I., & Modan, B. (1996). Depressive symptoms among community dwelling oldest old residents in Israel. *American Journal of Geriatric Psychiatry, 4,* 408–416.

Sadavoy, J., & Fogel, B. (1992). Personality disorders in old age. In J. E. Birren, R. B. Sloane, & G. D. Cohen (Eds.), *Handbook of mental health and aging* (pp. 433–463). San Diego: Academic Press.

Seeman, T. E., Kaplan, G. A., Knudsen, L., Cohen, R., & Guralnik, J. (1987). Social network ties and mortality among the elderly in Alameda County Study. *American Journal of Epidemiology, 126,* 714–723.

Skoog, IL, Aevarsson, O., Beskow, J., Larsson, L., Sigurdur, P., Waern, M., Landahl, S., & Ostling, S. (1996). Suicidal feelings in a population sample of nondemented 85-year olds. *American Journal of Psychiatry, 153,* 1015–1020.

Srole, L., Langer, T. S., Michael, S. T., Kirkpatrick, P., Opler, M. K., & Rennie, T. A. C. (1962). *Mental health in the metropolis: The Midtown Manhattan Study.* New York: McGraw-Hill.

Stark, R. ((1971). Psychopathology and religious commitment. *Review of Religious Research, 2,* 1165–176.

Suchman, E. A. (1969). Ethnic and social factors in medical care orientation. *Milbank Memorial Fund Quarterly, 47,* 69–77.

Thomas, C. (1989). The effect of nonresponse and attrition on samples of elderly people (DHHS Publication No.PHS 3447, pp. 121–127). Washington, DC: U.S. Government Printing Office.

Thomas C., Kelman, H., Kennedy, G. J., Ahn, C., Ynag, C. Y. (1992). Depressive symptoms and mortality in elderly persons. *Journals of Gerontology; Social Sciences, 47,* S80–S87.

Vega, W. A., Bohdan, K., Hough, R. L., & Figueroa, G. G. (1987). Depressive symptomatology in northern Mexico adults. *American Journal of Public Health, 77,* 1215–1218.

Wheaton, B. (1985). Models of the stress-buffering functions of coping resources. *Journal of Health and Social Behavior, 26,* 352–364.

Williams, D. R., (1994). The measurement of religion in epidemiologic studies. In J. S. Levin (Ed.), *Religion, aging and health: Theoretical foundations and methodological frontiers.* Thousand Oaks, CA: Sage.

Wolinsky, F. D., & Stump, T. E. (1996). Age and the sense of control among older adults. *Journals of Gerontology: Social Sciences, 51B,* S217–S220.

Yehuda, R.,Kahana, B., Schmeidler, J., Southwick, S. M., Wilson, S., & Giller, EL. L. (1995). Impact of cumulative lifetime trauma and recent stress on current post traumatic stress disorder symptoms in Holocaust survivors. *American Journal of Psychiatry, 152,* 1815–1818.

Yehuda, R., Kahana, B., Southwick, S. M., & Giller, E. L. (1994). Depressive features in Holocaust survivors with post-traumatic stress disorder. *Journal of Trauma and Stress, 7,* 699–704.

Yeung P. P., & Greenwald, S. (1992). Jewish Americans and mental health: Results of the NIMH Epidemiologic Catchment Area Study. *27:* 292–297.

Yong, G., & Dowling, W. (1987). Dimensions of religiosity in old age: Accounting for variation in types of participation. *Journal of Gerontology, 42,* 376–380.

Zborowski, M. (1952). Cultural components in response to pain. *Journal of Social Issues, 8,* 4–16.

Zola, I. K. (1996). Culture and symptoms—an analysis of patients' presenting complaints. *American Sociological Review, 31,*615–630.

Zuckerman, D. M., Kasl, S. V., & Ostfeld, A. M. (1984). Psychosocial predictors of mortality among the elderly poor. *American Journal of Epidemiology, 119,* 410–423.

10

RELIGION AND ANXIETY: WHICH ANXIETY? WHICH RELIGION?

JAMES A. THORSON

Department of Gerontology
University of Nebraska at Omaha
Omaha, Nebraska 68182

Of the many functions of religion, providing peace of mind may be desired more frequently on a day-to-day basis than any other. Whether individuals enjoy greater well-being because of the promise of a life beyond this one, because of their belief in the efficacy of prayer, the comfort of ritual, the opportunity to socialize with friends, the strength of a philosophical system of beliefs, or the sense of being a part of something greater than oneself, religious belief and practice doubtless provide vast levels of comfort to millions throughout the world. That this is not the case for everyone should come as no surprise. Many would argue that religion can be as much a source of anxiety as it is a balm, or that religion first creates and then relieves anxiety. One concept that will be explored in this chapter is that the direction of influence may very well depend on which anxiety one has in mind, as well as which religion.

ANXIETY DEFINED

Included within the *DSM-IV's* (American Psychiatric Association, 1994) section on anxiety disorders are agoraphobia and panic disorder with or without agoraphobia, panic attack, specific phobias and social phobias, obsessive–compulsive disorder, posttraumatic stress disorder, acute stress disorder, anxiety disorder due to a general medical condition, substance-induced anxiety disorder, and generalized anxiety disorder. Generalized anxiety disorder is characterized by at least 6 months of persistent and excessive anxiety and worry.

We might also understand anxiety as it is usually defined, consisting of (Webster's Ninth New Collegiate Dictionary, 1988):

A painful or apprehensive uneasiness of mind usually over an impending or anticipated ill; fearful concern or interest; an abnormal and overwhelming sense of apprehension and fear often marked by physiological signs (as sweating, tension, and increased pulse), by doubt concerning the reality and nature of the threat, and by self-doubt about one's capacity to cope with it.

The characteristic words here are worry and fear, compounded by doubt, often with physical symptoms.

Busse and Pfeiffer (1969) define anxiety as a state of dread anticipation in which the object of the dread is vaguely defined. It includes tenseness, restlessness, increased heart rate, and sweating, all of which indicate preparedness for fight or flight. It has been estimated that 10–20% of elderly hospital patients have anxiety symptoms; they may be a consequence of medical illness, psychiatric illness, or a response to stressful life events (Hocking & Koenig, 1995). Cavanaugh (1993) cites estimates of up to 10% of women and 5%of men in the general population have symptoms of anxiety.

RELIGION AND ANXIETY

It would seem that religion is good for one's physical as well as mental health. In a major epidemiological study, Zuckerman, Kasl, and Ostfeld (1984) followed 400 elderly residents of New Haven, Connecticut. Detailed health histories and sociodemographic data were gathered, along with various behavioral and psychological indices. Controlling for demographic variables and health status, they found that three psychosocial variables were significant predictors of lower mortality: religiosity, happiness, and having children. Religiousness and happiness in particular reduced the risk of mortality among people who were in poor health.

In a very different type of study, Atkinson and Malony (1994) analyzed religious maturity among 32 older women and found that it related negatively to the MMPI depression subscale and the Anxiety and Psychological Distress scale. There are numerous other such studies, which have been reviewed in detail by Shafranske (1992) and by Koenig (1992, 1993a, & 1993b).

Koenig, George, Meador, Blazer, and Cyck (1994) examined religion and general anxiety, as well as depression and any *DSM-III* disorder, in groups of mainline and conservative Protestants as well as Pentecostals. The Pentecostals had significantly higher 6-month and lifetime rates of depression, anxiety, and any *DSM-III* disorder. Mainline Protestants had the lowest 6-month and lifetime rates of anxiety disorder and the lowest rates of any *DSM-III* disorder, and conservative Protestants had the lowest 6-month and lifetime rates of depressive disorder. Koenig (1992), however, has pointed out that, "It is well known that depression and anxiety are more common among the lower classes, the poor, and the uneducated" (p. 183). One might speculate that these terms fairly describe many of the

Pentecostals studied in the 1994 article, and perhaps their higher rates of anxiety and depression had socioeconomic, rather than religious, explanations. Also, it could be possible that individuals with higher levels of anxiety for some reason gravitate toward Pentecostal denominations. In terms of speculation, it is of course possible that Pentecostal affiliation in some way causes anxiety.

In another study of anxiety and religion, Koenig, George, Blazer, Pritchett, and Meador (1993) found that once the variables of chronic illness, low socioeconomic status, and greater functional disability were controlled for, ostensible relationships between anxiety and measures of religiosity disappeared. Similarly, in another 1993 study Koenig and colleagues found relationships between anxiety and religion fell away once social support was controlled for.

A study by Park, Cohen, and Herb (1990) claims to demonstrate significant negative correlations between extrinsic religiousness and both anxiety and depression but found none with intrinsic religiousness. They fail to point out, however, that extrinsic factors are those that are made up of socialization elements—getting up and going out to church, meeting with others, and attending events—just the kinds of things that anxious and depressed people may not be prone to do. Also, here we begin to see the muddy water created by studies of religion. What exactly is being studied when one studies religion?

Gordon Allport (1950) had pointed out the difference between extrinsic religiosity (the outward signs of religious socialization, such as churchgoing) and intrinsic religiosity (inward depth of feeling) and concluded that they were two distinct parallel continua. Anxiety studies frequently ignore this fundamental concept. Koenig, et al. (1993) recognized this issue in studies of religion and general anxiety and recommended that future studies of religion and anxiety should use a measure of the intrinsic dimension of religiosity.

DEATH ANXIETY AND RELIGION

A number of researchers have reasoned that the fear of death is certainly among the most universal fears, and that religion in one way or another should have an influence on death anxiety. Definition problems abound in this area of the literature, with few researchers giving adequate descriptions of religiosity, which a priori is a multidimensional construct. Some measure religion with questions on churchgoing, Bible reading, or listening to religious broadcasts on television or the radio. Others use a Likert item asking respondents to rank themselves on depth of religious feeling relative to other people. Several use scales of spiritual well-being that have not been adequately validated, and many use no scales at all but rather a jumble of questions on both extrinsic and intrinsic religiosity with hopes for the best.

Examples include an article by Rasmussen and Johnson (1994) in which respondents completed a death anxiety scale and a spiritual well-being scale. While no significant overall relationships were found between religiosity and death anx-

iety, the authors suggest a negative association between death anxiety and spirituality. Spirituality was said to consist of the degree of certainty with respect to life
after death, level of life satisfaction, and degree of feeling of purpose in life, which
we suggest is certainly a unique definition of the concept of spirituality.

Similarly, Alvarado, Templer, Bresler, and Thomas-Dobson (1995) tested a
group using a death anxiety scale and several items of their own construction designed to probe for extrinsic and intrinsic religious factors. The only significant relationship with death anxiety was for the item, "How is the strength of your religious conviction when compared to those of others?" (p. 203), although what was
called "death distress" and "death depression" also correlated negatively with a
life after death item.

We also have thus sinned (Thorson, 1991), giving groups of students and adults
a valid death anxiety scale along with a number of made-up items on church attendance, belief in an afterlife, and self-rated religiosity. Scratching around for correlations, we ultimately found some and published the study.

PEOPLE ARE DIFFERENT, AND SOME PEOPLE
ARE REALLY DIFFERENT

While it has been shown that religious attitudes tend to remain quite stable
across the lifespan, it is important to note that there is a great deal of intraindividual variability in religious attitudes and beliefs. In a recent study, Kim, Nesselroade, and Featherman (1996) demonstrate that an individual's degree of religious
coping changes according to situational factors. While religious beliefs have the
capacity to influence many aspects of the coping process, they may be markedly
different within the same individuals at different times, depending in part on the
stimuli.

Given what Kim et al. (1996) have said about the variability of the coping response relative to religiosity, including both interindividual and intraindividual
manifestations, it would stand to reason that religiousness might act as a buffer
against some types of anxieties while serving no particular function relative to others. That is, the power of religion to ameliorate fears and dreads in some realms
might not be present in others. Furthermore, the buffering effect of religion no
doubt is present for some people but not for others.

In two studies measuring intrinsic religiosity and death anxiety (Powell &
Thorson, 1991; Thorson & Powell, 1990), we sought to focus the way religiousness was measured by using a scale with demonstrated reliability and validity—
Hoge's Intrinsic Religious Motivation scale (1972). We isolated the sectors of our
sample that represented the 40% highest and 40% lowest scores on Hoge's scale.
We also isolated those representing the 40% highest and lowest scores on Thorson and Powell's Revised Death Anxiety scale (1992). The results for two cells
were in the predicted direction. For those lowest in death anxiety, the correlation
between intrinsic religiosity and death anxiety was $-.31$ ($p < .001$); for those
highest in intrinsic religious motivation, the correlation was $-.36$ ($p < .001$).

There was a significant negative relationship demonstrated between death anxiety and religiosity for the highly religious as well as for the people with the least death anxiety.

However, there was no relationship for the remaining two cells: Those high in death anxiety demonstrated an insignificant correlation between religiosity and anxiety ($r = .08$). For those low in intrinsic religious motivation, the same was true: an insignificant correlation ($r = .11$). One might conclude from these data that the construct is missing for people who either have a high fear of death or who lack religiosity. High intrinsic religious motivation equals low death anxiety; equally, low death anxiety seemingly reflects higher religiosity. However, high death anxiety does not necessarily indicate low religiosity; nor does low religiosity reflect high death anxiety. Therefore, religion and death anxiety are seemingly related for some people but not everyone. Thus, it might be beneficial to remember that while it would seem to many that religiosity and well-being go together, Heath (1993) points out that mentally healthy persons need not be religious.

WHICH ANXIETY? WHICH RELIGION?

At this point we should note that just about all of the studies we have reviewed on death anxiety and religion are on samples in the United States or Great Britain. We argue that there is a pervasive Judeo-Christian system of beliefs in Western countries that is influential in terms of one's understanding of religion. That is, while allowing for individual and denominational differences, the great majority of Americans and, perhaps, Europeans, would recognize a similar understanding of the meaning of religion: that there is a God or Supreme Being, and this Being is not only a creator but also a sustainer and is essentially beneficent and may be called upon in times of trouble, and that goodness is rewarded in a life beyond death. While the details of this understanding differ (and have caused any number of conflicts and bloody wars), the understanding is basically similar within the culture. It has been demonstrated that most Americans, for example, believe in an afterlife, and among those who do, most believe in an afterlife of reward (Klenow & Bolin, 1989). Those who have this understanding would, like those we identified in our 1990 study who are higher in intrinsic religiosity, probably have somewhat lower death anxiety. Perhaps they might also have less anxiety in general. However, the ones identified who have little intrinsic religious feeling—those who do not buy into the cultural understanding that has been described—do not necessarily have high death anxiety. For them, the relationship of the two concepts is simply missing.

RELIGION AND DEATH ANXIETY
IN DIFFERENT CULTURES

What happens when we examine other cultures and other religions? Instead of the prospect of survival of the personality after death, some Eastern religions emphasize extinction of selfhood, perhaps with a unification with a cosmic consciousness (Pressman, Lyons, Larson, & Gartner, 1992). It might be the case that those with a different conceptualization of religion have a very different understanding of death anxiety.

It could be said that the Judeo-Christian tradition heavily influencing American thought on an afterlife has been present in Hebrew—and subsequently Christian—thought at least since the time of the exile of the Jews in Babylon (Noss, 1969):

> The older Jewish belief that the dead descend to a colorless existence in the pit of Sheol, a land of forgetfulness not unlike the Greek Hades and the Babylonia Aralu, was in large part superseded by a belief in the resurrection of the body to an afterlife of full mental vigor and awareness. (p. 404)

In contrast to somewhat vague, but nonetheless pleasant, biblical references to a promise of paradise in the afterlife in both the Hebrew Old Testament and the Christian New Testament, the Muslin Koran is very specific indeed about the last judgment and the separation of the unjust from the righteous, (the Koran as cited in Azberry, 1955):

> Lo, the Tree of Ez-Zakkoum is the food of the guilty, like molten copper, bubbling in the belly as boiling water bubbles. "Take him, and thrust him into the midst of Hell, then pour over his head the chastisement of boiling water." (XLIV.44–50).

While Muslims believe that death is God's will and for that reason should not be questioned, their conceptualization of the afterlife may have a great deal to do with relationships between religiosity and death anxiety. Abu-Lughod (1993) points out that wailing, even excessive wailing, characterizes funerals in Muslim villages:

> It is a truism of functionalist theories of religion that religion helps people cope with death. Yet in this Bedouin society, as I suspect in nearly all communities of Muslims, religiously inspired beliefs about death and appropriate religious responses are not the only ones invoked. . . .Since all Muslims hold that a person's time of death is determined in advance by God (some say written on his or her forehead), to wail and lament in grief might be seen as a kind of public defiance or protest against God's will. (pp. 188–189).

Cultural as well as religious factors influence death anxiety.

We have had the opportunity to compare Intrinsic Religious Motivation scale and Revised Death Anxiety Scale scores for samples from the United States and Kuwait (Thorson, Powell, Abdel-Khalek, & Beshai, 1997) and, in the present instance, Egypt. It is interesting to detect variations in conceptualizations of religiosity and death anxiety from these different cultural perspectives.

Muslims in Egypt are perhaps somewhat secularized in comparison to other Muslims. Most observers believe that it is fair to say that Muslims in more conservative countries view the predominantly Sunni population in Egypt as westernized and less religiously orthodox. Jonker (1996) notes that Shi'ite Muslims would consider themselves to be much more devout than their Sunnite brothers. Despite the fact that Egyptian Muslims are predominantly Sunni and are seen by other Muslims as more westernized and secular in their practices (certainly in comparison, for example, to those in Saudi Arabia or Iran), they remain committed practitioners. They turn toward Mecca to pray five times a day. Their lives are influenced greatly by their religion.

In addition to this difference from most Americans in the extrinsic practice of their religion, another cultural difference can be found in what Muslims believe takes place immediately after death. The Muslim ideal is to be buried, without embalming or display, within 24 hrs of death. Professor Moazziz Ali Beg of the Muslim University in Uttar Pradesh, India (personal communication, February 13, 1989), stated,

> What is interesting is the fact that Muslims fear death in relation to two things: (1) Immediate consequences of death arising out of the happenings in the grave when the burial is over. Two angels are believed to descend in the grave for making certain interrogations with the departed person about his faith, and a wavering faith brings horrible punishment known as *azab-e-qabr*. This is one source of death anxiety. The other pertains to (2) remote consequences, meaning thereby the rising from the grave on the day of judgment which would settle the fate of the soul—Hell or Heaven.

The data in Tables 10.1 and 10.2 present items and scores on Hoge's (1972) scale of Intrinsic Religious Motivation for samples of males and females in Egypt

TABLE 10.1   Intrinsic Religious Motivation: American and Egyptian Males

	Mean (SD)		
Scale item	Americans (N = 172)	Egyptians (N = 249)	t
1. My faith involves all of life.	2.56 (.92)	3.26 (.62)	8.05***
2. In my life I experience the presence of the Divine.	2.32 (.92)	3.37 (.59)	0.63
3. One should seek God's guidance when making every important decision.	2.41 (1.01)	3.44 (.69)	11.44***
4. My faith sometimes restricts my actions.	2.05 (1.02)	3.11 (.93)	10.81***
5. Nothing is as important to me as serving God as best as I know how.	2.12 (.93)	3.25 (.73)	13.23***
6. I try hard to carry my religion over into all my other dealings in life.	1.95 (1.00)	3.05 (.84)	11.94***
7. My religious beliefs are what really lie behind my whole approach to life.	1.93 (1.01)	2.74 (.93)	8.31***
8. It doesn't matter so much what I believe as long as I lead a moral life.	1.80 (1.10)	2.35 (1.25)	4.75***
9. I refuse to let religious considerations influence my everyday affairs.	1.95 (1.08)	2.93 (.94)	9.61***
10. I feel there are many more important things in life than religion.	2.05 (1.22)	3.01 (.99)	8.52***
Age	20.90 (1.84)	20.84 (1.28)	0.37
α Coefficient	.88	.59	
Total mean score	21.15 (7.15)	30.50 (4.05)	15.48***

***p < .001.

154

TABLE 10.2   Intrinsic Religious Motivation: American and Egyptian Females

	Mean (SD)		
Scale item	Americans ($N = 172$)	Egyptians ($N = 249$)	t
1. My faith involves all of life.	2.64 (.90)	3.21 (.59)	7.24***
2. In my life I experience the presence of the Divine.	2.47 (.94)	3.37 (.56)	11.17***
3. One should seek God's guidance when making every important decision.	2.60 (1.00)	3.53 (.62)	10.74***
4. My faith sometimes restricts my actions.	1.98 (1.12)	3.08 (1.03)	10.17***
5. Nothing is as important to me as serving God as best as I know how.	2.17 (.93)	3.40 (.65)	26.84***
6. I try hard to carry my religion over into all my other dealings in life.	2.18 (1.03)	3.19 (.76)	10.90***
7. My religious beliefs are what really lie behind my whole approach to life.	2.08 (1.04)	2.89 (.86)	8.35***
8. It doesn't matter so much what I believe as long as I lead a moral life.	1.77 (1.06)	2.32 (1.30)	5.49***
9. I refuse to let religious considerations influence my everyday affairs.	2.41 (1.07)	2.86 (.98)	3.86***
10. I feel there are many more important things in life than religion.	2.47 (1.15)	2.94 (.99)	4.48***
Age	20.85 (1.94)	21.02 (1.41)	0.98
α Coefficient	.88	.71	
Total mean score	22.76 (7.13)	30.79 (4.20)	14.56***

***$p < .001$.

and the United States. (Note that negatively phrased items are reversed in scoring; in every instance, a higher score indicates higher intrinsic religiosity.) Briefly, the predominantly Muslim respondents from Egypt show wide differences from their American counterparts in almost every aspect of intrinsic religiosity. The Egyptian females are significantly higher on every single scale item and the males are significantly higher on 9 of the 10. These data clearly demonstrate a much different understanding of religion in everyday life. Not only are the Muslims higher in extrinsic factors, such as daily worship, but also they are much higher in the intrinsic religious items contained in Hoge's scale. One might conclude that religion plays a much greater part in these respondents' lives than it does in the everyday life of most Americans.

From the totals in Tables 10.3 and 10.4, it would seem that death anxiety scores are in the expected direction: The Egyptians, who scored much higher in intrinsic religiosity, have lower total scores on the Revised Death Anxiety Scale. Interestingly, this was not the case for the Kuwaitis, whose scores are reported in Thorson et al. (1997); they had much higher death anxiety scores. They also had been in-

TABLE 10.3 Revised Death Anxiety Scale: American and Egyptian Males

Scale item	Mean (SD)		
	Americans (N = 172)	Egyptians (N = 249)	t
1. I fear dying a painful death.	2.56 (1.22)	2.26 (1.06)	1.65
2. Not knowing what the next world is like troubles me.	1.59 (1.17)	1.78 (1.10)	1.42
3. The idea of never thinking again after I die frightens me.	1.83 (1.23)	1.38 (1.02)	2.56*
4. I am not at all anxious about what happens to the body after burial.	1.87 (1.23)	2.61 (.97)	6.57***
5. Coffins make me anxious.	1.33 (1.05)	2.00 (.92)	6.73***
6. I hate to think about losing control over my affairs after I am gone.	1.76 (1.21)	2.00 (.96)	2.16*
7. Being totally immobile after death bothers me.	1.59 (1.19)	1.31 (.95)	2.57*
8. I dread to think about having an operation.	1.86 (1.21)	1.59 (1.08)	2.34*
9. The subject of life after death troubles me greatly.	1.27 (1.05)	1.30 (.94)	.30
10. I am not afraid of a long, slow dying.	2.72 (1.19)	2.15 (1.14)	4.90***
11. I do not mind the idea of being shut into a coffin when I die.	1.84 (1.15)	2.52 (1.10)	6.06***
12. I hate the idea that I will be helpless after I die.	1.61 (1.23)	1.71 (.97)	.89
13. I am not concerned over whether or not there is an afterlife.	2.70 (1.20)	2.16 (1.26)	4.44***
14. Never feeling anything again after I die upsets me.	1.61 (1.18)	1.38 (.96)	2.12*
15. The pain involved in dying frightens me.	1.99 (1.09)	1.58 (1.11)	3.78***
16. I am looking forward to a new life after I die.	1.39 (1.07)	2.52 (.97)	1.27
17. I am not worried about being helpless.	1.99 (1.15)	2.41 (1.11)	2.06*
18. I am troubled by the thought that my body will decompose in the grave.	1.41 (.98)	1.49 (.96)	.83
19. The feeling that I will be missing out on so much after I die disturbs me.	1.88 (1.16)	1.39 (.98)	4.51***
20. I am worried about what happens to us after we die.	1.77 (1.16)	1.86 (1.11)	.79
21. I am not at all concerned with being in control of things.	2.26 (1.08)	2.16 (1.13)	1.05
22. The total isolation of death is frightening to me.	1.64 (1.05)	1.70 (.95)	.19
23. I am not particularly afraid of getting cancer.	2.70 (1.10)	2.02 (1.14)	6.15***
24. I will leave careful instructions about how things should be done after I am gone.	2.23 (1.14)	2.16 (.94)	.66
25. What happens to my body after I die does not bother me.	1.78 (1.20)	2.16 (.89)	3.53***
Age	20.90 (1.84)	20.84 (.04)	
α Coefficient	.88	.76	
Total mean score	47.16 (4.55)	42.86 (9.40)	2.70**

*p < .05.
**p < .01.
***p < .001.

TABLE 10.4　Revised Death Anxiety Scale: American and Egyptian Females

Scale item	Americans (N = 172)	Egyptians (N = 249)	t
	Mean (SD)		
1. I fear dying a painful death.	3.00 (1.12)	2.50 (1.07)	5.08***
2. Not knowing what the next world is like troubles me.	1.82 (1.22)	1.88 (1.13)	.55
3. The idea of never thinking again after I die frightens me.	1.82 (1.23)	1.51 (1.09)	2.96**
4. I am not at all anxious about what happens to the body after burial.	2.19 (1.28)	1.59 (1.12)	5.64***
5. Coffins make me anxious.	1.53 (1.21)	2.18 (.94)	6.16***
6. I hate to think about losing control over my affairs after I am gone.	1.64 (1.19)	1.85 (.96)	2.15*
7. Being totally immobile after death bothers me.	1.74 (1.29)	1.20 (.96)	4.49***
8. I dread to think about having an operation.	2.34 (1.22)	1.63 (1.13)	6.89***
9. The subject of life after death troubles me greatly.	1.36 (1.12)	1.32 (.98)	.42
10. I am not afraid of a long, slow dying.	3.08 (1.10)	1.78 (1.15)	12.81***
11. I do not mind the idea of being shut into a coffin when I die.	2.23 (1.23)	1.44 (1.13)	7.43***
12. I hate the idea that I will be helpless after I die.	1.89 (1.26)	1.73 (1.02)	1.55
13. I am not concerned over whether or not there is an afterlife.	2.74 (1.17)	1.66 (1.21)	10.07***
14. Never feeling anything again after I die upsets me.	1.71 (1.25)	1.26 (.88)	4.62***
15. The pain involved in dying frightens me.	2.71 (1.16)	1.65 (1.14)	10.25***
16. I am looking forward to a new life after I die.	1.46 (1.11)	2.40 (.97)	10.08***
17. I am not worried about being helpless.	2.40 (1.14)	1.45 (1.09)	9.45***
18. I am troubled by the thought that my body will decompose in the grave.	1.73 (1.21)	1.34 (.96)	3.96***
19. The feeling that I will be missing out on so much after I die disturbs me.	1.96 (1.31)	1.36 (1.03)	5.67***
20. I am worried about what happens to us after we die.	2.06 (1.24)	1.77 (1.15)	2.69**
21. I am not at all concerned with being in control of things.	2.34 (1.13)	1.66 (1.09)	6.80***
22. The total isolation of death is frightening to me.	1.92 (1.22)	1.84 (1.08)	.77
23. I am not particularly afraid of getting cancer.	2.97 (1.13)	2.00 (1.13)	9.51***
24. I will leave careful instructions about how things should be done after I am gone.	2.46 (1.10)	1.97 (.91)	5.38***
25. What happens to my body after I die does not bother me.	2.28 (1.20)	1.83 (.92)	4.67***
Age	20.85 (1.94)	21.02 (1.41)	1.07
α Coefficient	.89	.77	
Total mean score	53.39 (15.71)	42.39 (9.82)	9.36**

*p < .05.
**p < .01.
***p < .001.

fluenced by the compounding situational variable of having had a major war in their homeland in 1991 and 1992. It is illustrative to examine the tables more carefully to determine where the differences in death anxiety for the American and Egyptians lie.

Specifically, in Table 10.3 there are minor differences between the Egyptian and American males in two control items (nos. 6 and 7); one group is higher than the other on either of these, and not much can be made of these data. The real differences lie in two other factors measured by this multidimensional scale; fear of pain, on the one hand, and fear of decomposition or what happens to the body after death, on the other hand. The American males indicate significantly higher anxiety on items dealing with the physical pain involved in the dying process (Nos. 10, 15, and 23). The Egyptians, on the other hand, score much higher on the items dealing with what happens to the body in the grave (Nos. 4, 5, and 25). Again, note that negatives are reversed in scoring, so a higher score in each instance indicates higher anxiety. When answering the item, "I am not at all anxious about what happens to the body after the burial," the Muslims' response is that they are very anxious indeed. They are not particularly concerned about whether there is an afterlife (No. 13); they know there is, and they are worried about it. The only other difference among the two groups of males might also be ascribed to a cultural difference: The Americans are concerned about missing out on things after they die (No. 19).

Therefore, what might be concluded from an analysis of the items in Table 10.3 is that the differences in anxiety may have a cultural explanation as well as a religious one. American men seemingly have less of a need to present a Mediterranean macho image; they feel freer to express fears of pain. The Egyptians appear to have a characteristically Muslim fear of what happens to the body in the grave, perhaps the *azab-e-qabr*, the punishment inflicted by the two angels that visit the body immediately after burial.

This is missing in the women's responses reported in Table 10.4 in which an entirely different picture of death anxiety is seen. The Muslim women are, as might have been expected, higher than their American counteparts on the "coffins make me anxious" item (No. 5) and the item concerning an afterlife (No. 16), but these are the only instances in which they are significantly higher. The American women, presumably feeling much more free to express anxiety, score significantly higher than the Egyptian women on virtually every element of death anxiety measured by the scale. They indicate higher levels of anxiety on the items dealing with fear of pain (Nos. 1, 8, 10, 15, and 23), on the items dealing with "not being" (Nos. 3, 14 and 19), on the loss of personal control associated with dying (Nos. 7, 11, 17, 21, and 24), and on one of the afterlife items (No. 13).

Most interestingly, however, is the wide difference between the American and the Egyptian women on the fear of decomposition and loss of bodily integrity (Nos. 4, 18, and 25). This is in the exact opposite direction from the data presented in Table 10.3 for the two groups of males. The American women are much higher than the Egyptian women in their fear of what happens to the body after burial.

In fact, the Egyptian women not only score lower than the American women on these "body" items but also score significantly lower on them than the Egyptian men.

Therefore, by examining four groups of people and what it is about death that they are anxious about, we have ample realm for speculation but ultimately produce more questions than answers. It would seem clear enough that Muslim males are more afraid of what happens to their bodies after burial. This may be the only aspect that seems to be clear. This construct does not seem to apply to Egyptian women. If this area of anxiety is rooted in religious belief, can we conclude that men in Egypt take religion more seriously? Does the fear of *azab-e-qabr* apply to men only?

Viewing these results from a different perspective: Are Americans more free to express vulnerability? This would seem to be the case, and within this cultural difference American women appear to be much more free to express anxiety than are American men. In our earlier studies of American samples, we found much higher death anxiety scores among female respondents,and the difference was clearly in the element of fear of decomposition and loss of bodily integrity (Thorson & Powell, 1988, 1990). Our explanation then, which still seems plausible, is that women in America are socialized, seemingly from birth, into the notion that they must look good. They are bombarded with messages from cosmetics and fashion industries that to look good is to *be* good, and that being plain or ordinary is somehow associated with unworthiness. Given that few people die in the peak of good health, it is exceedingly difficult to look good when one has died, and what happens to the body after death is horrific.

This evidently is a Western concept, and Muslim girls are socialized into modesty to a much greater degree. Indeed, fashionable dress and makeup among Muslim girls are proscribed by religious authorities and condemned as Western decadence, and they are exhorted to cover up to the eyeball by the time they enter their teens. These things are not as frequently practiced in a country such as Egypt as they are in other Muslim countries, but the ideals are present. Whether or not the Muslim women are concerned with being visited by angels in the grave after they die, the Americans apparently have a much more immediate fear of decomposition and all that aging and death imply, and this fear supercedes whatever the Egyptian women might express.

CONCLUSION

These data cannot be wrapped up into a neat package. What we think they imply though, is the paradox that, although culture and religion cannot be separated, culure may have as much or more to say about anxiety than does religion. Again, when looking for relationships between religion and anxiety, we must ask which anxiety and which religion. Depth of belief moderates anxiety, at least among some people. For those who are irreligioius, the construct may well be missing.

Finally, in a study in another Muslim country (Malaysia), Azhar, Varma and Charap (1994) examined the value of religious psychotherapy among patients with anxiety disorder. There were 62 patients, all of who were seen as religious people. All were given supportive psychotherapy and anxiolytic drugs, but half of the sample also received religious psychotherapy that consisted of discussions of religious issues. All of the patients completed a rating scale for anxiety at the beginning of treatment and again at 3 and 6 monhts. Those who received the religious psychotherapy had significantly more rapid improvement in terms of anxiety symptoms.

Treatment modalities capitalizing on religiosity may well make good sense for people who are high in religiosity. While it may be true that, depending on which religion and which anxiety, being religious may be the cause of anxiety, it seemingly is equally true that religion provides peace of mind for a great number of people. It is evident that religiosity is a potent intervention for those who are religious, and that it shapes and buffers our anxieties as we face what often is a hostile world.

ACKNOWLEDGMENT

We acknowledge the help of Professor Ahmed Abdel-Khalek of the Department of Psychology, Kuwait University, for his translation of the two scales into Arabic and for providing the data from the Egyptian samples. We also thank Dr. F. C. Powell for his assistance with the data analysis.

REFERENCES

Abu-Lughod, L. (1993). Islam and the gendered discourses of death. *International Journal of Middle Eastern Studies, 25,* 187–205.

Allport, G. W. (1950). *The individual and his religion.* New York: Macmillan.

Alvarado, K. A., Templer, D. I, Bresler, C., & Thomas-Dobson, S. (1995). The relationship of religious variables to death depression and death anxiety. *Journal of Clinical Psychology, 51,* 202–204.

American Psychiatric Association. (1994). *Diagnostic and statistical manual of mental disorders* (4th ed.). Washington, DC: American Psychiatric Press.

Arberry, A. J. (1955). *The Koran interpreted.* London: Allen & Unwin.

Atkinson, B. E., & Malony, H. N. (1994). Religious maturity and psychological distress among older Christian women. *Intenational Journal for the Psychology of Religion, 4,* 165–179.

Azhar, M. Z., Varma, S. L., & Dharap, A. S. (1994). Religious psychotherapy in anxiety disorder patients. *Acta Psychiatrica Scandinavica, 90,* 1–2.

Busse, E. W., & Pfeiffer, E. (1969). Functional psychiatric disorders in old age. In E. W. Busse & E. Pfeiffer (Eds.), *Behavior and adaptation in late life* (pp. 183–235). Boston: Little, Brown.

Cavanaugh, J. C. (1993). *Adult development and aging.* Pacific Grove, CA: Brooks/Cole.

Heath, D. H. (1993). Personality roots of well-being, religiosity, and its handmaiden—Virtue. *Journal of Religion and Health, 32,* 237–251.

Hocking L. B., & Koenig, H. G. (1995). Anxiety in medically ill older patients: A review and update. *International Journal of Psychiatry in Medicine, 25,* 221–238.

Hoge, D. R. (1972). A validated intrinsic religious motivation scale. *Journal for the Scientific Study of Religion, 11,* 369–376.

160 JAMES A. THORSON

Jonker, G. (1996). The knife's edge: Muslim burial in the diaspora. *Mortality, 1,* 27–43.

Kim, J. E., Nesselroade, J. R., & Featherman, D. L. (1996). The state component in self-reported worldviews and religious beliefs of older adults: The MacArthur Successful Aging Studies. *Psychology and Aging, 11,* 396–407.

Klenow, D. J., & Bolin, R. C. (1989). Belief in an afterlife: A national survey. *Omega, 20,* 63–74.

Koenig, H. G. (1992). Religion and mental health in later life. In J. F. Schumaker (Ed.), *Religion and mental health* (pp. 177–188). New York: Oxford University Press.

Koenig, H. G. (1993a). The relationship between Judeo-Christian religion and mental health among middle-aged and older adults. *Advances, 9*(4), 33–39.

Koenig, H. G. (1993b). Religion and aging. *Reviews in Clinical Gerontology, 3,* 194–203.

Koenig, H. G., Ford, S. M., George, L. K., Blazer, D., et al. (1993). Religion and anxiety disorder: An examination and comparison of associations in young, middle-aged, and elderly adults. *Journal of Anxiety Disorders, 7,* 321–342.

Koenig, H. G., George,L. K., Blazer, D. G., Pritchett, J. T., & Meador, K. G. (1993). The relationship between religion and anxiety in a sample of community-dwelling older adults. *Journal of Geriatric Psychiatry, 26,* 65–93.

Koenig, H. G., George, L. K., Meador, K. G., Blazer, D. G., & Dyck, P. B. (1994). Religious affiliation and psychiatric disorder among Protestant Baby Boomers. *Hospital and Community Psychiatry, 45,* 586–596.

Noss, J. B. (1969). *Man's religions* (4th ed.) New York: Macmillan.

Park, C., Cohen, L. H., & Herb, L. (1990). Intrinsic religiousness and religious coping as life stress moderators for Catholics versus Protestants. *Journal of Personality and Social Psychology, 59,* 562–574.

Powell, F. C., & Thorson, J. A. (1991). Constructions of death among those high in intrinsic religious motivation: A factor-analytic study. *Death Studies, 15,* 131–138.

Pressman, P., Lyons, J. S., Larson, D. B., & Garner, J. (1992). Religion, anxiety, and fear of death. In J.F. Schumaker (Ed.), *Religion and mental health* (pp. 98–109). New York: Oxford University Press.

Rasmussen, C. H.., & Johnson, M. D. (1994). Spirituality and religiosity: Relative relationships to death anxiety. *Omega, 29,* 313–318.

Shafranske, E. P. (1992). Religion and mental health in early life. In J. F. Schumaker (Ed.), *Religion and mental health* (pp. 163–176). New York: Oxford University Press.

Thorson, J. A. (1991). Afterlife constructs, death anxiety and life reviewing: The importance of religion as a moderating variable. *Journal of Psychology and Theology, 19,* 278–284.

Thorson, J. A., & Powell, F. C. (1988). Elements of death anxiety and meaning of death. *Journal of Clinical Psychology, 44,* 691–701.

Thorson, J. A., & Powell, F. C. (1990). Meanings of death and intrinsic religiosity. *Journal of Clinical Psychology, 46,* 279–391.

Thorson, J. A., & Powell, F. C. (1992). A revised death anxiety scale. *Death Studies, 16,* 417–531.

Thorson, J. A., Powell, F. C., Abdel-Khalek, A. M., & Beshai, J. A. (1997). Constructions of religiosity and death anxiety in two cultures. *Journal of Psychology and Theology, 25,* 374–383

Webster's ninth new collegiate dictionary. (1988). Springfield, MA: Merriam-Webster.

Zuckerman, D. M., Kasl, S. V., & Ostfeld, A. M. (1984). Psychosocial predictors of mortality among the elderly poor. *American Journal of Epidemiology, 119,* 410–423.

11

RELIGION

AND PSYCHOSES

WILLIAM P. WILSON

Duke University Medical Center
Durham, North Carolina 27705

In the past most psychiatrists thought of religion as psychopathology. The literature is replete with articles that commented on the psychopathology of religious people and the influence of faith on their illness. Even in the psychoses, religion was thought to have a deleterious effect. Unfortunately, those who held such views did not do systematic studies to document their beliefs. Their impressions arose out of observations made on a few patients encountered in their practice. Matthews, Larson, and Barry (1993), in their review of the literature on clinical research related to spiritual subjects, list only a few articles related to religion and the psychoses. Little else has been written since their review to provide increased understanding of the relationship.

This chapter, therefore, will review the meager relevant literature and supplement the data with clinical observations made during the author's 50 years of clinical experience in many different mental health settings. Most of these settings were in the Third World.

RELIGIOUS BELIEF, EXPERIENCE, AND PRACTICE

We need a comprehensive understanding of the relationship of religion to the psychoses. We should, therefore, ask ourselves how religious beliefs influence psychotic illness. On reflection we can discern that they may in some way be related etiologically, or that religion may influence the presenting symptomatology of psychosis. In this latter category we should look at influences on behavior, affectivity, and content of thought.

The patient's religious belief system is determined by several factors. The first is nurture. The most effective religious nurture in childhood is done by parents. Children go to church and Sunday school and get very little out of it. Children are quite sensitive to their parent's belief system, and if they are not nurtured in their faith at home, the things they learn outside the home (e.g., Sunday school) will usually not be as strongly introjected. If their parents are living an immoral life, it does not avail much to teach children morality in Sunday school or youth groups.

Religious experiences, as distinct from religious teachings or nurturance, have a more profound effect on the lives of those who have them. In the Christian belief system, Jesus commands an encounter with God as the sine qua non for true faith (John 3:3). Most of the early investigative work on the psychology of religion focused on such experiences (Ames, 1919; James, 1902; Pratt, 1907). Almost all the authors noted that religious experience pervasively affected the personality of the person who had the experience. Later investigations have corroborated these observations (Nicholi, 1974a; Wilson, 1972). Empirical evidence discovered by these early pioneers in the field demonstrated that religious experiences can be truly life changing, and even the Group for the Advancement of Psychiatry (1968) attested to the dramatic effects of religious conversion on the personality.

Religious practices also influence the belief systems of persons. I have stated previously that church attendance does not influence the faith of children as much as their parent's spiritual nurturance. I will qualify this statement, though by saying that having children practice their faith (i.e., praying, learning Bible verses, celebrating the Eucharist, and regularly worshiping in formal services) may have a lasting effect on a child's faith. This is particularly true when it is done in a warm, loving environment by genuinely caring people. If these practices continue into adulthood they will strongly influence the faith of the person.

I must point out that humans are more than biopsychosocial beings. They are biopsychosociospiritual beings. If humans have a spiritual component then it follows that they can have spiritual disease. This is indeed true for humans suffering with the disease of being unregenerate (Evans, 1984), with the disease of sin (MacKay, 1918), and with fanaticism and possession syndromes (Wilson, 1976). If we accept that these diseases are spiritual in etiology, it stands to reason that spiritual interventions might be of benefit in treating them. In the Christian tradition, these spiritual interventions are evangelism; prayer; bibliotherapy; confession, repentance, and forgiveness; worship, including the Eucharist; exhortation; inner healing; and affirmation.

THE PSYCHOSES

Developments in the past three decades have profoundly influenced our views of the etiology of the psychoses. Until the 1960s, the consensus of the profession was that psychological factors played a primary role in the etiology of all the psychoses. Fanciful formulations of the dynamics of schizophrenia and major affective disorders abounded and could be found in almost all psychiatric textbooks and journals. One can understand, then, why religion was considered by many to be intimately involved in the etiology of the psychoses. There were many who did not believe these hypothetical formulations, but there were many who did, and they taught their formulations in most medical schools as verities. Today most physicians believe that the psychoses have a biological etiology with strong genetic links. The beneficial effect of electroconvulsive treatment and psychoactive drugs on these disorders has helped confirm their largely biological origins.

If psychotic disorders are largely biological in origin, it follows logically that religion could not play a major role in the etiology of schizophrenia, the major affective disorders, delirium, dementia, or other illnesses with psychotic symptoms. We can then eliminate this factor from our inquiry concerning the relationship of religion to the psychoses. What, then, is the relationship?

RELIGIOUS NURTURANCE IN THE CHILDHOOD OF SCHIZOPHRENICS

The family dynamics of schizophrenics before the onset of their illness are often distorted. Based on early research in this area, these distortions have been summarized elsewhere (Wilson et al., 1983). Mothers were often cold and aloof, with little physical contact. Fathers were frequently suspicious and paranoid. Discipline was often lacking or inconsistent. The mothers of schizophrenic patients are more often the disciplinarians than are their fathers. Parental sex roles were often blurred in other ways as well.

Religious nurturance in the homes of schizophrenic patients was also distorted. Parents rarely practiced family devotions. Values regarding sex, money, and family were presented negatively. Parents' attitudes were especially negative about sex and family. There was very little emphasis on generosity. God was presented most often as punitive and harsh, and the religious teachings were authoritarian (Wilson et al., 1983). The schizophrenic patient was much more likely to show an increased or decreased interest in religion as the child approached adolescence. This was in contrast to a control group in which religious interest was more often unchanged. The incidence of religious experience was essentially the same for schizophrenics and normals.

RELIGIOUS NURTURANCE IN CHILDHOOD IN MAJOR AFFECTIVE DISORDERS

The religious lives of patients with major affective disorders did not differ significantly from the religious lives of psychologically healthy individuals (Gallemore, Wilson, & Rhoads, 1969). The patients grew up in families that regularly practiced devotions. Parental roles were appropriate, and discipline was fair and appropriately applied. Father and mother taught conventional values authoritatively. Both parents possessed values about sex, money, and family that were conventional. The parents lived by them and served as good role models as they taught their children. Religious nurturance in childhood was similar to that of psychologically healthy individuals. Frequency of church attendance and the incidence of family devotions was essentially the same. The change in adolescent interest in religion was also similar for the two groups.

Only in the area of salvation experiences was there a significant difference,with affective disorder patients more likely to have such experiences. Interestingly, these experiences were not usually temporally related to the patient's illness. They most often occurred in adolescence long before the patient developed affective illness.

RELIGIOUS NURTURANCE IN CHILDHOOD IN DELIRIUM AND DEMENTIA

Since deliria are disturbances of brain function due to physiological or anatomical dysfunction secondary to exogenously determined etiologies, religious nurturance in childhood is unrelated to such disease. In delirium related to substance abuse, however, religion has an effect on the decision to indulge in the addictive substances and, as such, is etiologic (Cancellaro, Larson, & Wilson, 1982; Larson, 1980). Spiritual interventions play a major role in recovery from the drug and alcohol addiction. Because the subject of substance abuse appears elsewhere in detail in this book, I refer the reader to that chapter.

Since dementia is caused by physical deterioration of the brain, religious nurturance probably does not have a etiologic role, nor is it likely to significantly influence the psychopathology of the disease.

EFFECT OF RELIGION ON PSYCHOPATHOLOGY IN SCHIZOPHRENIA

Since schizophrenia is largely biologically determined, it appears that religion has little or no etiologic significance. Religion can, however, have profound effects on symptomatology. Schizophrenia is a disease that has global psychological effects (Bleuler, 1950). Although the most obvious effect is on thinking, schizophrenia also profoundly affects both behavior and emotion.

The behavioral effects of schizophrenia are usually consistent with the disordered thinking. Schizophrenics may develop a messiah complex believing that they are the Christ who has returned. If their disease process is not too debilitating, they may actually develop a sizeable group of followers who believe their claims. Their behavior is then altered to mimic what they believe Jesus did. Some will preach on the streets where their sermons reflect the religious delusions that motivate their behavior. Their sermons may consist of dissociated thoughts that make little sense or may be limited to a few phrases. I observed one woman who walked the streets, repetitively saying "My Lord told me to tell the world that Jesus is soon coming." She did this for at least 20 years rain or shine. The messiah or prophetic complex occurs rarely but does attract much attention.

Schizophrenics for the most part withdraw from the world and decrease their interactions with others. Commonly, they will read their Bible continuously. Others will pray and may even put on sackcloth and ashes in response to their understanding of scripture. Others have been known to follow the biblical injunction to "cut off their hand" and "pluck out their eye" if it "offends them" (Matt. 5:29, 30). I have known patients who cut their penis off or castrated themselves following this delusional directive. The concreteness of their thinking drives them to do this. Waugh (1986) and Culliford (1987) reported cases of young men who removed their genitals because of religious delusions arising from their interpretation of Matthew 19:12. Culliford's patient also cut out his tongue to atone for his obscene language. Waugh (1986) reviewed the literature that reported more than 50 such cases. The author had seen four patients who attempted to pluck out their eyes in response to their delusion that their eye offends them (Matt. 5:29) because they had looked lustfully on persons of the opposite sex. Self-mutilation is a very malignant symptom and is usually associated with a rapidly deteriorating form of schizophrenia.

A few schizophrenic patients develop stereotypes that they claim have religious significance. Most often the symbolism is unrecognizable or distorted or highly exaggerated when it occurs.

Affective expression and feeling is profoundly altered in the schizophrenic patient. The most common affective change is a loss of affective tone. In simple schizophrenia, loss of affect and motivation is the primary symptom of the disorder. The patient loses all drive to do anything. In its most pervasive form, the patient may not even attend to his or her elimination of bodily wastes, often urinating or defecating wherever he or she happens to be. This loss of affective tone mutes all of the patient's affective reflexes. Thus, the patient is, for the most part, expressionless and shows few if any emotional responses to external stimuli. Since the Christian religion requires an emotional response, the patient with loss of emotional tone and reflexes is almost incapable of religious passion. If the patient professes to be religious, he or she often does little to participate in or practice his or her faith.

Not all patients with schizophrenia are emotionless. Many have inappropriate emotional responses, especially paranoid schizophrenics. Their emotional reflexes may be exaggerated or inappropriate. Schizophrenic religious zealotry or fanaticism develop out of a synthesis of their distorted thinking and exaggerated and/or inappropriate emotion. Our previous observations of affective disorder patients (Gallemore et al., 1969) suggested that those who had increased emotionality had a higher incidence of salvation experiences compared to normal controls. For this reason, we expect schizophrenic patients to be less likely to have religious salvation experiences. We did not observe this, however, in our studies. Schizophrenics had an incidence equal to that of normal controls. Another interesting observation was that salvation experiences often occurred before the onset of clinically apparent symptoms (Wilson et al., 1983).

After the development of clinical symptoms,a few schizophrenics—mostly paranoid subtype—can have genuine religious experiences unconnected with their illness. The experience of baptism in the Holy Spirit (in the Christian tradition), however, occurs only rarely in these patients. Wootton and Allen (1983), reviewing the literature on this subject, concluded that in some instances decompensation can be similar to religious conversion. They describe a case in which the onset of the illness was accompanied by religious turmoil and an experience that was intense but was not a true conversion experience if one uses the criteria of James (1902).

I now discuss possession syndromes. Possession by evil spirits is commonly reported in Third World countries. The manifestations of such evil spirits are usually patterned along those depicted in the Christian Bible. Nevius (1968) cataloged the primary symptoms as follows:

The chief differentiating mark of so-called demon possession is the automatic presentation and the persistent and consistent acting out of a new personality. The new personality says he is a demon.
He or she uses personal pronouns: first person for the demon and third person for the possessed.
The demon uses titles or names.
The demon has sentiments, facial expressions, and physical manifestations that harmonize with the above.
The demon gives of knowledge and intellectual power not possessed by the subject.
With the change there is a complete change of moral character (aversion and hatred to God and especially to Jesus, in the Christian tradition).

As is evident from the previous list, the basic symptoms of schizophrenia as described by Bleuler (1950) are quite different from those of demon possession. The demonized person does not have the affective changes (blunting), disturbances of association, or ambivalence commonly seen in schizophrenia. The only symptoms that mimic those of schizophrenia are behavioral excitement and, occasionally, hallucinations.

When it occurs in the Western world, demonic possession often does not have the classic presentation described previously. The Christian Bible describes possession states as simulating mental disease (Luke 8:27-30), epilepsy (Luke 4:35), or other physical illness with mutism, blindness, excessive menstrual flow, or other problems. I have observed schizophreniform illnesses caused by demon possession in Madagascar and Zimbabwe on several occasions. Epileptiform manifestations are also common. These differ in many ways from conversion phenomena and are easily differentiated.

McAll (1976) reported a high incidence of possession states in patients with schizophrenia. When demons were cast out, the patient remained schizophrenic but many of the more dramatic or violent manifestations of the illness disappeared. These patients still require pharmacological treatment.

The effect of religion on the content of thought of schizophrenic patients has been the subject of considerable investigation. This is not to say that there is a plethora of information available, but most investigators have focused on the more common symptoms. Both Kraepelin (1904) and Bleuler (1950) described delusions, illusions, and hallucinations with religious content. Their descriptions, however, were quite limited. Sin and sex were closely linked. Other schizophrenics were harassed by the devil or his demons. One of our patients believed 40 demons were constantly accusing her of immoral acts that she had not performed. Many schizophrenics see or misidentify persons in the environment as God. Others patients with Christian backgrounds believe they are the reincarnation of Jesus or are married to the Holy Ghost.

Recent studies have described similar phenomena. One of the better studies is that of Tateyama et al. (1993), who analyzed the content of delusions in German and Japanese schizophrenic patients. There was no significant difference in the incidence of delusions in the two groups (87 vs 89%). German patients, however, had significantly more religious delusions than did patients in Japan. The incidence of religious delusions in German patients was 21.3%, whereas it was only 6.8% in Japanese. The authors attributed this to cultural differences, a conclusion that is in keeping with the idea that the content of delusions is always affected by culture. Persecutory delusions are found with the same incidence in schizophrenics in all cultures, but the specific persecutors differ according to the culture. Grandiose delusions occur in all cultures, but the delusional personage chosen by the patient is determined by the culture. Religious content occurs in these delusions.

An excellent literature review relating to this subject was performed by Cothran and Harvey (1968). The authors evaluated both manics and schizophrenics to determine the incidence of religious delusions in the two diagnostic groups. The report did not address the thematic aspects of delusions except to determine whether they were religious or not. Unfortunately, the sample of patients was small, making the paper of dubious validity. Cothran and Harvey did not find any difference in the incidence of religious delusions in manics and schizophrenics. The religiosity of the patient also did not correlate with the occurrence of religious delusions.

In summary, it can be said that religion or religious experiences do not play a significant role in the etiology of schizophrenia. Religion can and does influence behavior as a result of its effect on the content of the patients thinking. Because of the blunted affect associated with schizophrenia, religious experiences are uncommon once the psychopathology has developed. They do, however, occur fre-

quently in the prepsychotic state. It can be hypothesized that this increased incidence is a result of the patient's search for something to ameliorate the sense of
impending disintegration that he or she feels.

Demonization is described in the Christian Bible on at least one occasion with
schizophrenic-like symptoms, making the two somewhat difficult to distinguish. I
have observed that demon possession still occurs frequently in Third World Countries, although it is not common in the Western world. Demon possession has also
been reported in schizophrenic patients. Deliverance alters their secondary symptomatology, but the basic symptoms of the disease persist.

Religion does affect the schizophrenic illness symptomatically. Patients may
act out their delusions behaviorally. Thus, there are schizophrenics who mutilate
themselves in response to the biblical injunction to cut off an offending part of their
body, preach on the streets, or constantly read their Bibles or pray. Many with messianic complexes may attract followings and organize them into cults. Schizophrenics do not have religious experiences as often as normal or affectively disordered patients. Prior to the onset of their illness, however, schizophrenics do
have religious experiences at the same frequency as normal persons and those with
affective disorders. Some paranoid schizophrenics may act on their religious delusions.

Content of schizophrenic thought frequently includes religious themes. These
are quite variable but fall into three major categories: persecutory (often involving the devil), grandiose (messianic complex), and belittlement (commission of
unpardonable sins). Spiritual interventions do not significantly influence the symptoms and course of schizophrenia except in rare cases. In patients with paranoid
delusions, spiritual interventions are contraindicated since these persons can mis-
interpret efforts to influence their spirituality as having a malevolent purpose.

EFFECT OF RELIGION ON
PSYCHOPATHOLOGY IN MAJOR
AFFECTIVE DISORDERS

Although the major affective disorders are of biological origin, religion can
play a prominent role in the illness. Religious experiences may precipitate an attack of mania or may end a major depressive episode. Religious conflicts are a
stress and, as such, can play a role in the precipitation of a major depression. Religious beliefs, however, are not etiologic in either mania or depression.

Symptomatically, religion colors the illness of both manic and depressed patients. Religious beliefs can profoundly color the behavior of manic patients who,
because of their increased affective tone and energy, may act on their religious
delusions. The delusions are exaggerations of normal religious beliefs and impulses, in contrast to those of schizophrenics that are bizarre and autistic. Manic
patients are often moved to preach, pray long prayers, indulge in exaggerated litur-

gical exercises, and are witness to the marvels of their religious experiences to any and all who will listen.

Manics have surges of elation that they interpret as religious experiences. One of my patients reported five salvation experiences in 1 day. He said that the last one lifted him 3 feet off the bed. In the same way, the cyclic variations in the severity of depressive affect may intensify the patient's feelings of guilt and shame or heighten obsessive thinking concerning their sinfulness.

Content of thought is often markedly affected in these patients by their religious beliefs and experiences. Manic patients with pervasive feelings of power and facile thinking translate these into grandiose delusions. As with schizophrenics, these patients may begin to think that they are important New Testament biblical characters or Jesus or God. For example, I once had as a patient an English graduate student who had a salvation experience at the beginning of his manic attack. A day later he thought he was the Apostle Paul, the next day he was Jesus, and finally he ascended to be God. He proudly presented his physician with a check signed by God for 300 trillion dollars drawn on the Bank of Heaven. Treatment with lithium resulted in a rapid descent through the various personages to being an English graduate student again.

Delusions of patients with psychotic depression often center on hopelessness, unworthiness, shame, and guilt. Many such patients from Christian backgrounds will doubt their salvation. Despite being presented with evidence that refutes their argument, they persist in believing that they are unsaved. These patients may argue that they were insincere when they gave their lives to the Lord. They cite some unconfessed sin that they believe prevented them from really committing their lives to God. Others will feel estranged from God and are convinced that God has condemned them because of their failure to live perfect lives. This is often true of patients who have had abortions or have had extramarital affairs. They consider these sins as unforgivable and consequently feel forever condemned. One patient of mine, a veteran of World War II, believed he had committed an unpardonable sin because he had hired a prostitute to perform oral sex on him in London during the war. He believed that this act had brought unforgivable condemnation on him and his whole household. No argument to the contrary could convince him that he could be and was forgiven.

Obsessional thinking is frequent in patients with psychotic depression. Patients may feel compelled to curse God. They are often tortured by obscene thoughts concerning God or Jesus. Many will spend hours in prayer confessing and repenting. They do not, however, feel forgiven because there is no relief from the suffering. Patients often complain that God has turned away from them because God does not answer their prayers. They beg for relief and promise any and everything if God will just relieve the pain. When relief does not come, they look for reasons why God does not heal them. They can easily find sins that condemn them.

Suicide does occur occasionally in patients with strong religious faith. In many instances these persons have legalistic, fundamentalist backgrounds. On the other hand, a strong faith tends to restrain suicidal impulses. It has been my experience that the hope that is inherent in Christianity and the belief that suicide is a sin are the factors that inhibit suicidal impulses in persons from this faith tradition.

Spiritual interventions can be useful in the treatment of affective disorders. For patients with mania, spiritual interventions can be risky since religion can influence the psychopathology manifested by the patient. This is especially true of their grandiose delusions or their impulsive behavior. Praying with a manic patient is best avoided, and if the person is reading the Bible constantly, it is best to allow him or her only limited access to it. Taking the Bible from the patient completely may cause the patient to believe that he or she is being mistreated, which may interfere with the positive rapport that the physician has with the person.

Spiritual interventions can be safely used in manic patients who are in remission. Many have feelings of shame and/or guilt related to their illnesses. Others may have neurotic problems that need to be treated psychotherapeutically. In many instances, these patients can have other psychospiritual problems, such as unresolved grief or low self-esteem, which they need help resolving.

In contrast to patients with mania, those with depression can benefit markedly from the use of spiritual interventions. Exhortation (encouragement) is particularly useful. Since the patient is discouraged, exhortation can give the person hope until somatic treatment has begun to relieve his or her symptoms. Patients with faith receive great encouragement if prayers for healing are offered. Forgiveness should be given for real or imagined sins. Even though such prayers may not relieve the feelings of guilt and shame the patient suffers, they will provide the person with positive belief to counteract dysfunctional cognitions as part of cognitive restructuring (Beck, 1976). In the Christian tradition, this is especially true when the patient is told that forgiveness is based on Jesus' deputization of him or her to pass the forgiveness on to others (John 20:23).

For Christians, the use of the Bible in therapy may provide an authoritative source to help the patient restructure his or her thinking. Use of scripture quotes to counteract the notion that the patient's sin cannot be forgiven can be very helpful. Most patients do not know what a genuine unpardonable sin really is. When the biblical version of the unpardonable sin (Matt. 12:31) is presented and explained, the person may often begin to see the fallacy of his or her thinking. In the same way, the belief of unforgiveness can be refuted when the person is told that if he or she confesses his or her sins to God, God is faithful and just to forgive him or her (I John 1:9). Depression almost always gives rise to low self-esteem. For Christians, the Bible offers many affirmative statements that refute the self-accusatory ideation of the patient. Neil Anderson lists and discusses affirmative statement of this kind in his book *Living Free in Christ* (1993), which I recommend.

Since the Bible in the Christian tradition is considered to be revealed truth, scripture carries great weight when it is used in the cognitive therapy of the depressed patient (Backus, 1985). Most Christian patients view scripture as far more authoritative than the utterances of the therapist, for he or she is human and is no more authoritative than any of the other persons who have offered correction prior to entering treatment.

In summary, our research suggests that the religious nurturance of patients with major affective disorders is similar to that of normal controls. There is one major difference, however, in their religious lives. They have a significantly higher incidence of religious experience than schizophrenics and normal controls, which may be related to the former's increased affectivity. Manics have a high incidence of religious delusions. They differ from schizophrenic delusions, however, in that they are not autistic or bizarre but are exaggerated normal beliefs. Feelings of power result in delusions of grandeur. These delusions result in behavior that is again an exaggeration of normal religious behavior.

Depressive psychoses can have a pervasive effect on the patient's religious belief. Profound depression results in delusions of unworthiness and hopelessness, which may be assigned religious significance by the patient. Patients may attribute the pain they feel to God, who is punishing them for past sins. They exaggerate the significance of these sins and assign greater weight to them than they deserve and may even believe that they are unforgivable.

Severely depressed patients may feel their prayers are not heard, since their suffering seems endless. They have low self-esteem because they feel so sinful and unworthy. Obsessional thinking is common. Patients will doubt their salvation or will feel compelled to silently curse God. Some have obscene thoughts about God. They will confess these over and over, but no relief comes because as soon as they have finished confessing, they think the same thoughts over again.

Spiritual intervention should not be used with patients who are manic but can be selectively used in severe depressions. Spiritual interventions are especially useful in the cognitive treatments for depression.

EFFECT OF RELIGION ON PSYCHOPATHOLOGY IN DELIRIUM AND DEMENTIA

Religion does not play a significant role in the etiology or treatment of delirium or dementia since these conditions are known to be caused by altered physiological processes in the brain. In delirium, the brain dysfunction is often caused by exogenous agents or medical conditions; in dementia, brain dysfunction results from progressive degeneration of the brain itself. Both of these disorders globally affect all aspects of the patient's thought life. Demented persons can have religious experience. I had on patient who was sent to the hospital for evaluation and the appointment of a guardian. A friend had told her about me and about her own religious experience that occurred while under my care. She suggested that the patient ask me about God.

During her first days in the hospital it was obvious that the patient had severe dementia. She was disoriented to time, place, and person. She had severe recent and remote memory loss. She also had almost no retention or recall of new information. Other signs of a disturbed sensorium were present. Even so, she said to me several times that she was supposed to ask me something, but did not know what it was. When I asked her if it had to do with her faith, she replied "Yes!"

I know she had never been religious, so I told her that faith had to do with a relationship with Christ. I then asked her if she would like to have him for her Lord and master. She answered that she would. When she had prayed a prayer of commitment, she was filled with joy. During the next few days she went around the ward weeping. When the ward personnel asked her what she was weeping about, she said she did not know, but she was so happy she had to cry. Another patient who was confused from electroconvulsive treatment (ECT) was able to understand the plan of salvation and to accept Christ when her roommate read to her from the Gideon Bible in French. The girl was fluent in French, and despite her confusion clearly understood what was read to her and was able to accept the message contained within the Bible. This salvation experience lasted and was remembered despite five more ECT treatments.

COMMENT

The relationship of religion to psychoses is a subject that has not yet been adequately researched. What is known is that the religious beliefs of the patient may color the expression of symptoms. Religion, like any other cultural influence, affects behavior, delusions, and hallucinations in patients with both schizophrenia and major affective disorders. Religion is only one of the factors that influence the content of symptoms. Religion has little etiological influence, although it may serve as a precipitating factor in certain affective disorders. Salvation experiences among Christians are common in both schizophrenia and affective disorders. There is a higher incidence in patients with affective disorders, however, than in active schizophrenia. Salvation experiences can occur in patients who have delirium or dementia but they are relatively uncommon.

REFERENCES

Ames, S. (1910). *The psychology of religious experiences.* New York: Houghton Mifflin.
Anderson, N. (1993) *Living free in Christ.* Ventura, CA: Regal Books.
Backus, W. (1985). *Telling the truth to troubled people.* Minneapolis, MN: Bethany House.
Beck, A. (1976). *Cognitive therapy of emotional disorders.* New York: International Universities Press.
Bleuler, E. (1950). *Dementia Praecox or the Group of Schizophrenias.* New York: International Universities Press.
Cancellaro, L. A., Larson, D. B., & Wilson, W. P. (1982). Religious life of narcotic addicts. *Southern Medical Journal, 75,* 1166–1168.
Cothran, M. M., & Harvey, P. D. (1968). Delusional thinking in psychotics: Correlates of religious content. *Psychological Reports, 58,* 191–199.

Culliford, L. (1987). Autocastration and Biblical delusions in schizophrenia. *British Journal of Psychiatry, 150,* 407–412.

Evans, C. S. (1984). *Existentialism.* Grand Rapids, MI: Zondervan.

Gallemore, J. L., Jr., Wilson, W. P., & Rhoads, J. M. (1969). The religious life of patients with affective disorders. *diseases of the Nervous System, 30,* 483–486.

Gallup, G., & Castelli, J. (1989). *The people's religion.* New York: MacMillan.

Group for the Advancement of Psychiatry. (1968, January). *The psychic function of religion in mental health,* GAP Report N. 67, New York:

James, W. (1902). *The varieties of religious experience: A study in human nature.* New York: Longmans Green.

Kraepelin, E. (1904). *Lectures on clinical psychiatry.* New York: W. Wood.

Larson, D. B. (1980). Religious life of alcoholics. *Southern Medical Journal, 73,* 723–727.

MacKay, W. M. (1918). *The disease and remedy of sin.* London: Hodder & Stoughton.

Matthews, D. A., Larson, D. B., & Barry, C. P. (1993). *The faith factor: An annotated bibliography of clinical research on spiritual subjects.* Washington, DC: National Institute for Healthcare Research.

McAll, R. K. (1982). *Healing the family tree.* London: Sheldon Press.

McAll, R. K. (1976). Personal Communication.

Nevius, J. L. (1968). *Demon possession.* Grand Rapids, MI: Kregel.

Nicholi, A. (1974). A new dimension of the youth culture. *American Journal of Psychiatry, 131,* 396–401.

Pratt, J. B. (1907). *The psychology of religious Belief.* New York: MacMillan.

Tateyama, J., Asai, M., Kamisada, M., Hashimoto, M., Bartels, M., & Heimann, H. (1993). Comparison of schizophrenic delusions between Japan and Germany. *Psychopathology, 26,* 151–158.

Waugh, A. C. (1986). Autocastration and biblical delusions in schizophrenia. *British Journal of Psychiatry, q149,* 656–659.

Wilson, W. P. (1972). Mental health benefits of religious salvation. *Diseases of the Nervous System, 33,* 382–386.

Wilson, W. P. (1976). Hysteria and demons, depression and oppression, good and evil. In J. W. Montgomery (Ed.), *Demon possession* (pp. 223–231). Minneapolis, MN: Bethany Fellowship.

Wilson, W. P., Larson, D. B., & Meier, P. D. (1983). Religious life of schizophrenics. *Southern Medical Journal, 78,* 1096–1100.

Wooton, R. J. & Allen, D. F.(1983). Dramatic religious conversion and schizophrenic decompensation. *Journal of Religion and Health, 22,* 212–220.

12

SPIRITUAL AND RELIGIOUS

FACTORS IN SUBSTANCE

USE, DEPENDENCE,

AND RECOVERY

JENNIFER BOOTH AND JOHN E. MARTIN

San Diego State University
San Diego, California 92120
and
University of California at San Diego School of Medicine
San Diego, California 92093

This chapter examines the clinical research and programmatic interventions addressing the influence of religiousness and spirituality on substance use, abuse, and recovery. Harmful substance use targeted in this chapter includes alcohol, drugs of abuse, and tobacco. Following our review and summary of what is known about the relationship between spiritual and religious factors and problematic substance use, abuse/dependence, and recovery, we provide recommendations for future intervention and clinical/research investigation in this important and growing field.

OVERVIEW AND CURRENT STATUS
OF THE FIELD

Despite inconsistent assessment measures with poor psychometrics, and the traditional putative view of "religiousness" by psychology, the literature has consistently revealed an inverse relationship between religiousness and substance use, abuse, and recovery (Burkett & White, 1974; Gorsuch, 1995; Larson & Wilson, 1979; Parfrey, 1976). Studies indicate that a variety of religious practices (e.g., church/synagogue attendance, prayer, and scripture reading), as well as religious affiliation and/or denomination, tend to be inversely associated with psychoactive substance use, abuse, and dependence. The relationship between spiritual and

---

religious factors and recovery from addictive behavior/substance dependence has received less attention, although this situation appears to be rapidly changing as more and better studies are conducted addressing spiritual and religious factors as independent (i.e., treatment) and not just dependent variables. Research on use and abuse has historically tended to take a more religious factor approach, whereas the research conducted on recovery predictors tends more to the spirituality dimensions. Finally, the connection between religious and spiritual beliefs, practices and community, and positive outcomes (lower use, abuse, and negative health and recovery outcomes) are among the stronger results in the addictions field as well as the behavioral health area in general—and therefore worthy of considerably more clinical and research attention. The following sections focus on this growing body of research, beginning with a summary of the findings for the association with drug and alcohol use and abuse followed by a discussion of spiritual and religious factors in treatment and recovery.

GENERAL RELIGIOUSNESS: PERSONAL FACTORS

The first section provides an overview of the phenomenon, examining the role of religiousness in substance use, abuse, and dependence across a span of developmental stages and clinical subtypes, including adolescents, college students, adults, and inpatient and outpatient populations. General substance use, alcoholism, and smoking literature are discussed accordingly, and we rely on the mainly religious perspectives and measures that were more commonly used when these associations were explored. Finally, causal models for this reputed relationship will be addressed.

ADOLESCENTS AND COLLEGE STUDENTS

General Substance Use

General religiousness, measured using a variety of religious practices and preferences questionnaires, is inversely related to substance use and abuse. In a longitudinal prediction of substance abuse using religiousness as a predictor, seven of eight studies examined suggest a positive role of religion in substance abuse. In these studies, religious activity measured at one point in time predicted substance nonabuse at later points ranging from 1 to 15 years. For example, in a prospective study, teenage boys from France who were more religious smoked less at 5-year follow-up (Weill & Le Bourhis, 1994).

Family and peers also influence substance use. Religion has been shown to have an indirect inhibitory effect on adolescent marijuana use through encouraging associations with peers who do not use drugs (Burkett & Warren, 1987), whereas maternal religiousness, as measured by worship attendance and perceived importance of attendance, was predictive of lower rates of adolescent alcohol use (Foshee & Hollinger, 1996). In the latter study, worship attendance and importance of religion were more predictive of decreased levels of alcoholic use than adolescent religious commitment. Higher levels of family religiousness have similarly been related to lower perceived use of elicit drugs among adolescent peers (Hardy & Kirby, 1995). Family religiousness significantly increased the variance accounted for by a model associating peer drug use with ethnicity, gender, and family social climate for 6 of 10 drugs (beer, alcohol, marijuana, cocaine, crack, and amphetamine) identified by Hardy and Kirby. Finally, church and synagogue attendance has been consistently inversely related to substance use (Coombs, Wellisch, & Fawzy, 1985).

Alcohol Use

Overall, religiousness and attendance at religious services are inversely associated with beliefs and consumption of the primary drug of concern, alcohol, among adolescents and college students. In one study, respondents who did not attend church regularly, but whose parents did, had increased alcohol consumption. This effect of religious service attendance may well be at least partly dose–response related, although the causal link must only be cautiously considered. For example, Humphry et al. (1989) found that individuals who attended religious services regularly were significantly more likely to abstain and less likely to be dual users of intoxicants than were occasional religious service attendees. Also, high school students who rarely attended church were more likely to drink two or more times a week and drink hard liquor than students who attended church more often (Turner et al., 1994).

The general effect of religion on alcohol use and abuse is also apparent. In several studies, more religious subjects reported lower rates of alcohol use (Amoateng & Bahr, 1986) but not perceived misuse of alcohol (Cochran, Beeghley, & Bock, 1988). One study found that more religious subjects had increased antialcohol attitudes; however, none of these correlations were statistically significant. More religious subjects were also more likely to change their attitudes about alcohol and to increase their knowledge of the deleterious effects of alcohol after 4 weeks of alcoholism treatment (Zucker et al., 1987). Lorch and Hughes (1985) found slightly stronger inverse correlations between perceived importance of religion and alcohol use than for drug use among adolescents. Interestingly, gender may also be a determining factor in the strength and direction of this relationship. Bliss and Crown (1994), for example, found that males who reported that religion was very important in their lives consumed more alcohol than those who reported that religion was not important to them, whereas females who reported that religion was not important to them consumed more alcohol than females who reported that religion was very important to them. In addition, males who rarely participated in religious services were found to consume more alcohol than females who attended services more than once a week (Bliss & Crown, 1994).

ADULTS

General Substance Use

Given the relatively strong and consistent evidence linking religiousness with drug and alcohol use and abuse in younger people, it is not too surprising to find a similar relationship among adults. Indeed, religious involvement in adults has been inversely related to substance use and abuse with few exceptions, although one study found that religious conservatism was negatively associated with alcohol use but not drug use. In addition, this inverse relationship between spiritual/religious involvement and less problems with alcohol, tobacco, and illicit drugs has been extended to other cultures and ethnicities (Adelekan et al., 1993).

Overall, adults who view themselves as "very religious" consumed less alcohol and used less psychoactive drugs when compared to subjects who consider themselves "not religious at all" (Khavari & Harmon, 1982). Furthermore, elevated use of alcohol, tobacco, marijuana, hashish, and amphetamines was associated more with the reported "not religious at all" group (Khavari & Harmon, 1982). Finally, homeless women who relied on prayer to cope were less likely to drink in the previous 6 months or use cocaine recently than those who did not use prayer to cope (Shuler, Gelberg, & Brown, 1994).

Alcohol Use

As with adolescents and college students, frequent church attendance is related to lower levels of alcohol consumption. Koenig et al. (1994) found that individuals who attended church at least weekly were one-third less likely to report alcohol abuse and dependence than those who attended church less frequently. Furthermore those who prayed and read the Bible several times a week were 42% less likely to have a diagnosed alcoholic disorder within the prior 6 months compared to the rest of the sample (Koenig et al., 1994). Interestingly, alcoholism was two times greater among those who frequently watched or listened to religious television and/or radio. However, perceived importance of religion was unrelated to either recent (i.e., 6 month) or lifetime alcoholic disorders (Koenig et al., 1994). Strengthening this finding, a national sample concluded that persons for whom religion is important are less likely to have drinking problems (Midanik & Clark, 1995). Subjects surveyed in this sample were overall less likely to have social problems associated with alcohol use and abuse. As noted by Gorsuch (1995), all religious groups have fewer alcohol abusers than are found in nonreligious groups, and religious groups with more antialcohol norms produce fewer abusers.

Smoking/Tobacco Use

Smoking and tobacco use and dependence has received relatively less research attention despite the fact that it more negatively impacts morbidity and mortality statistics (e.g., prevalence, incidence, and association with negative health outcomes), per se, than the other substances or even lifestyle factors. Consequently, we will pay particular attention to this relatively neglected area of smoking and also tobacco use, as we evaluate overall spirituality and religiousness effects on addictive behavior and related health outcomes.

From a general health standpoint, any level of smoking is considered substance abuse, whereas it is generally believed that an average use of over about 10 cigarettes (one-half of a pack) a day is likely to be associated with nicotine dependence. Importantly, many (80–95%) of those who abuse alcohol also are smokers (Bobo, 1989; Istvan & Matarazzo, 1984), and tobacco use in alcohol abusers synergistically potentiates risk of oral cancers (Blot, McLaughlin, & Winn, 1988) and cardiovascular diseases (Criqui, Wallace, Mishkel, Barrett-Connor, & Hess, 1981; Vaillant, Schnurr, Barron, & Gerber, 1991) among other diseases (DHHS, 1988). Therefore, any protective variable that reduces the risk of this combined threat is worthy of careful study.

Statistics on tobacco use indicate that it is inversely related to religiousness. For example, African American men who frequently attended church were only two-thirds as likely to be a current smoker than those who attended less frequently (Brown & Gary, 1994). Neither denomination nor overall religiousness were associated with smoking behavior in this sample (Brown & Gary, 1994), although a subsequent portion of this chapter will provide evidence for its association with particular religious denominations and overall affiliation.

INPATIENTS AND OUTPATIENTS

General Substance Use

In one study of outpatients with a high level of religious involvement, 15% abused alcohol and 4% of these subjects abused other drugs. Even narcotics users were significantly less likely than controls to read their Bible, engage in prayer before meals, or tell others about their religious commitment than abstinent controls. However, Hater, Singh, and Simpson (1984) found that recovering opioid users who were more religious tended to be more satisfied with life than those who were nonreligious, although there were no statistical differences in long-term treatment outcome. In a study suggesting that more religious individuals may have greater motivation for treatment, Zucker et al. (1987) found that higher religiousness scores were associated with elevated numbers of admissions for detoxification and more antialcohol attitudes on admission.

Alcohol Use

In another study, psychiatric inpatient alcoholics more frequently lost their interest in religion as adolescents than abstinent controls (Larson & Wilson, 1980). These subjects also reported that they rarely (a) shared their faith with others, (b) read the Bible daily, (c) prayed several times per day, or (d) experienced salvation. Individuals who reported an experience of religious salvation, however, reported that their "deliverance" from alcohol dependence was not long-lasting. Although 38% reported sobriety for 6 months or longer after salvation, all had resumed drinking on subsequent follow-up (Larson & Wilson, 1980). In another study supporting this relationship, adult psychiatric outpatients and inpatients recovering from chemical dependence reported that they were both more likely to avoid drinking because of their religion and more likely to "help run the church" than were controls (Brizer, 1993).

Although not all research supports the religiousness–substance use relationship, religiousness is inversely associated with a variety of substance abuse problems for both in- and outpatients in much of the literature. The following section will examine specific religious affiliation rather than just religiousness in general.

RELIGIOUS AFFILIATION FACTORS

General Substance Use

Research suggests that religious affiliation and/or denomination strongly influence substance use, abuse, and dependence. For example, Divine Light Mission converts significantly reduced alcohol use upon religious conversion. Data are available primarily for the Christian faith, individual denominations focusing on Jesus Christ as the "Higher Power," followed by studies of persons of the Jewish faith. Denominations and Christian affiliations primarily examined in this relationship have included Catholics, Latter-day Saints (LDS) (Enstrom, 1978; Hawks & Bahr, 1992), Protestants (Koenig et al., 1994), and other Pentecostals (Koenig et al., 1994). Information on other world religions, such as the Muslim faith, will be incorporated as studies are reported.

Not surprisingly, the general finding is that denominations such as LDS that proscribe any use of substances have fewer instances of substance use and dependence than denominations that simply proscribe the abuse of substances. For example, substance use is proscribed in Muslim, some Baptist denominations (Miller, 1996), Mormon, the Christian Union (Jolly & Orford, 1983), and Seventh-day Adventists. Pentecostal Christians are opposed to the sale, distribution, and consumption of alcohol.

Other Judeo-Christian affiliations also warn against excess use of alcohol and drugs; however, the use of these substances is not proscribed (Miller, 1996). For example, Jews and Catholics do not oppose the use of alcohol but are opposed to drunkenness and most Protestants tend to share a similar position. Nevertheless, in cases in which official doctrine proscribes alcohol and substance use, the inverse relationship between religiousness and substance use is strongest (Cochran, 1991).

As with alcohol abuse, the inverse association between religious involvement and drug use is strong, and the relationship is particularly strong among members of religious groups that teach abstinence. In a study of high school seniors, overall drug use tended to be highest among subjects reporting "no religion," followed by Jews, Catholics, Mainline Protestants, Methodists, Fundamental Protestants, Fundamental Baptists, and the Other Religious group (including Christian denominations). Mormons had the lowest percentage of drug users.

Adlaf and Smart (1985) found that more religious Roman Catholic students used fewer drugs (cannabis, nonmedical substances, and hallucinogens) than less religious Catholics. Females in particular showed an inverse relationship between religiousness and these nonprescription drugs of abuse. Furthermore, there was also an overall inverse relationship between church attendance and both medical and nonmedical substances, cannabis, hallucinogens, and polydrug use. Finally, tobacco, marijuana, and alcohol use were inversely related to religious behavior such as church attendance and choir or youth group involvement, with a stronger inverse relationship found among females.

Alcohol Use

Hawks and Bahr (1992) found that 31% of Utah LDS consumed alcohol in the past 30 days as opposed to 62.3% in the "other religion" group and 68.3% in the "no religion" group. There were no significant differences in the number of drinks consumed in the past 30 days for those who reported drinking during this time. In addition, the no religion group reported an earlier first consumption of alcohol than both the other religion and the LDS affiliations. The authors suggest that religious affiliation has a tendency to delay first alcohol use and influence the frequency of alcohol intake (Hawks & Bahr, 1992). Similarly, Bliss and Crown (1994) found that Catholic undergraduates with *higher* levels of religiousness consumed *more* alcohol than Catholic undergraduates with lower levels of religiousness (primarily among the males in the sample). This finding, however, is inconsistent with that of Adlaf and Smart (1985).

Other studies have supported the notion that denominations and religious affiliations differentially predict substance use and abuse. In one study examining the role of religious affiliation on alcohol use, Turner et al. (1994) found that students with no religious affiliation were more likely than others to drink twice a week or more, to drink hard liquor, and to have consumed more than five drinks on one occasion in the previous month. In addition, Catholics were more likely to report having consumed five or more drinks on four or more occasions during the past month than were Protestants (Turnet et al., 1994). Although Koenig et al. (1994) did not find a relationship between religious affiliation and 6-month rates of alcohol disorders, they did find that lifetime rates of alcoholic disorders were highest among Pentecostal religions (17.4%) and lowest among conservative Protestants (8.6%). Also, both 6-month and lifetime rates of alcoholic disorders were lower among born-again Christians than among those who were not born-again Christians (Koenig et al., 1994).

Smoking

With respect to its association with religious affiliation, smoking is comparable to alcohol abuse and dependence. In their study of African American women, Ahmed, Brown, Gary, and Saadatmand (1994) found that non-Pentecostal women had a 3.6 times higher odds ratio of current smoking than Pentecostal women. The Pentecostal women in their sample were nearly 10 times more likely to quit smoking than non-Pentecostal women. Nevertheless, despite previous research that suggests that religiousness is associated with smoking behavior, this study failed to find a statistically significant relationship between current smoking/quitting and religiousness. Another study found that for smoking-related cancers, religiously active Mormons in California have a standard mortality rate (SMR) of 26, whereas less religiously active Mormons have a SMR of 73 (Enstrom, 1978). Furthermore, the expected death rate for total cancer in religiously active Mormons in California is 50% that of the general U.S. population (SMR = 50) (Enstrom, 1978).

ATTITUDES AND BELIEFS REGARDING SUBSTANCE USE

General Substance Use

Most of the literature described previously involved substance behavior patterns as they relate to the role of religiousness. Few studies have actually examined how beliefs and attitudes regarding substance use relate to religiousness. In one study arranging various religious groups across a fundamentalist–liberalist continuum, fundamentalist groups were more likely to consider alcohol and drug abuse to be "sins," whereas more liberal groups considered alcoholism and drug addiction as "illnesses" (Lorch & Hughes, 1985). Unfortunately, research on the role of attitudes and beliefs of addicts and substance users has not received much research attention which would provide important insight into subjective attitudes regarding religious factors in substance use and dependence.

Alcohol Use

In addition to literature on church attendance, religiousness, and denominational affiliation, attitudes have also been examined as they relate to alcohol use and abuse. Teachers' attitudes regarding alcohol use have also been examined. Weiss and Moore (1992) found that Jewish teachers were less likely to view alcoholism as a moral issue than Moslems and Christians, whereas Jewish and Moslem teachers were more likely to view alcoholism as a disease than Christians.

Smoking

In their examination of childrens' attitudes toward smoking, Francis and Mullen (1993) found that unaffiliated atheists (41%) were the least likely to agree that smoking was wrong compared to affiliated atheists (47%), unaffiliated agnostics (47%), and affiliated agnostics (46%). Also, unaffiliated believers in God who did not attend church were the least likely to agree that smoking behavior was wrong compared to affiliated believers not attending (47%), believers attending occasionally (45%), and believers attending regularly (56%). Across denomination and religiosity, half of the sample reported that it is wrong to smoke cigarettes (Francis & Mullen, 1993).

PARADOXICAL ALCOHOL USE

Sometimes a paradoxical drinking pattern exists among members of religions that teach abstinence from alcohol (Skolnick, 1958). This pattern suggests that although most members of abstinence-promoting religions remain abstinent, the small percentage who do consume alcohol tend to consume large amounts and on a frequent basis. The per capita rate of alcoholism among those who drink tends to be higher in the denominations that strongly proscribe alcohol use (Royce, 1985). "Dry" sects have the largest per capita rate of alcoholism. This paradoxical alcohol pattern is hypothesized to exist among Muslims, Buddhists, (conservative/Southern) Baptists, Mormons, and Seven-day Adventists. Research support for this hypothesis has been found for Jewish men (Calahan, Cisin, & Crossley, 1969; Mulford, 1964; Skolnick, 1958; Snyder, 1958) and Protestants but not for Mormons (Hawks & Bahr, 1992). More research in this area would be beneficial.

Paradoxical alcohol use may result from punishing or abusive forms of religiousness (Booth, 1992); in which alcoholics report experiencing a negativistic, punishing religion. A number of alcoholics consistently report presentation and experience of a judging, condemning, vindictive deity (Gorsuch, 1995). Religious-based social control using punishment (i.e., rigid "thou shalt not"-focused religiosity) may not serve to reduce substance abuse but rather potentiate it (Gorsuch, 1995).

SUBSTANCE ABUSE PREVENTION: RELIGIOUS AFFILIATION/INVOLVEMENT

Regardless of whether one's religious affiliation proscribes or permits substance use, one's level of religious involvement per se may strongly influence psychoactive substance initiation. Clearly, religion is a multifaceted institution with differing norms about substance use, and not all individuals who ascribe to a denomination are similarly involved in or committed to their denomination's religious practices and preferences (Gorsuch, 1995). These factors may, in turn, account for some of the variance in the role of denominational influence on substance use patterns. A better understanding of denominational influence on substance prevention might be facilitated through a categorization of abstinence, ambivalence, and substance abuse promotion.

Religion Influences Abstinence

Several studies have examined reasons for drinking abstinence, even among those denominations that do not proscribe the use of alcohol. In one study, Jewish subjects abstained because of disliking the taste and/or smell of alcohol and because they did not care for it (Moore & Weiss, 1995). Christian subjects abstained mainly because of the harmful effects of alcohol on health and the dislike of taste and/or smell (Moore & Weiss, 1995). Muslim and Druze subjects avoided alcohol because of harmful health consequences of alcohol use and because of religious injunction (Moore & Weiss, 1995). Other research suggests that Pentecostals believe that alcoholism is the devil's work (Mariz, 1991) so it makes sense that they would abstain from alcohol. While Hindus and Islamic adherents forbid alcohol, cannabis and hashish are widely used (Royce, 1985). Similarly, opium is widely used in Oriental societies that prohibit alcohol use (Royce, 1985).

It might be suggested, however, that religion influences substance abuse through more general features of the religion since there is little evidence that religious groups spend a significant amount of time teaching against substance abuse (Gorsuch, 1995). Another possible reason for this inverse relationship may simply be that religious people respond to questionnaires in ways to make their religion "look good" and therefore give socially acceptable responses regarding drug use (Gorsuch, 1995).

Religion Influences Ambivalence

Ambivalence has been found to be a central feature of individuals "stuck" in maladaptive patterns of substance use (Miller & Rollnick, 1991). Not surprising, then, is the idea that ambivalent teachings and practices stemming from religious traditions regarding substance use might affect their congregations' use of substances. Fundamentalist religious groups have the lowest percentages of substance abuse in general, whereas more liberal types of religious groups have the lowest percentages of heavy substance abuse (Lorch & Hughes, 1985). Carlucci et al. (1993) found that Catholics reported more drinking-related problem behaviors than Protestant and Jewish subjects. Furthermore, drinking behavior was unrelated in this study to the frequency of church attendance but it was related to denominational identity. Finally, members of the Free churches in England who frequently attend church have less liberal attitudes regarding drinking behavior and are less likely to engage in drinking than Anglicans, Roman Catholics, or individuals who claimed no denominational identity.

Some Religions Promote Substance Use and Abuse

There are religious groups that promote the use of certain drugs for a variety of reasons. Miller (1996) discusses religions which use drugs in search of transcendence and divine contact. Some native Hawaiians and other Polynesian religions advocate chewing khat root, and hashish is used to worship in India (Albaugh & Anderson, 1974). Another religious tribe encourages a ritual of collective drunkenness in the temple in order to experience the kingdom of death (Pages Larraya, 1978). Some Native American religious groups even encourage the use of peyote to treat alcoholism. Finally, worshippers of Bacchus celebrate with drunkenness, whereas some "cults" of the 1960s and 1970s used LSD ritualistically (Gorsuch, 1995).

CAUSAL MODELS FOR THE
RELIGIOUSNESS–SUBSTANCE USE RELATIONSHIP

Based on the general evidence, there appears to be a relatively robust inverse relationship between substance use and overall religiousness. Is it causal? Most of the research is descriptive or correlational since research designs and ethical barriers prevent experimental manipulation or randomization necessary to objectively determine causality with respect to the role of religion in substance use, abuse, dependency, and recovery. However, Gorsuch (1976) posed several important causal models for investigation.

First, an experiential model suggests that one's personal religious experience may influence behavior (Gorsuch, 1976). For example, worship, the feeling of being loved by God, and other personal experience may produce a general change in behavior, perhaps by meeting needs which are not otherwise met. An individual having had some essential need filled by spirituality/religion rather than by chemical mood alteration will experience a decreased need for and use of drugs.

Gorsuch's (1976) second model is based on the cognitive consistency model of psychology in which consistent exposure to church doctrines through participation in settings of worship constantly reminds one of ideals. This need to see behaviors as consistent with ideals, rather than cognitively dissonant, constantly supports the maintenance of these norms and hence substance use/abuse avoidance.

Gorsuch (1976) also proposes an indirect role of the religion–substance use/abuse and use relationship: Religious people in a constant social environment associate together and thus form a mutually supportive subgroup. Group pressure provides reinforcement for a particular style of behavior—substance use or disuse—depending on the norms and values of that particular subgroup.

Koenig et al. (1994) provide a fourth model in an effort to explain possible causality. Perhaps religion prevents the onset or persistence of alcoholism with doctrines that prohibit the use of alcohol through a religious environment that is uniquely supportive, especially by offering alternative cognitive and behavioral means of coping with painful emotions and feelings that may precipitate alcohol consumption and drug use.

Each of these causal models provides important insight into the antecedents and consequences of religiousness on substance use and abuse. They serve not only to explain outcome as well as process variance but also, in turn, as heuristics for further empirical exploration and validation (e.g., through path analysis) of causal links between religiousness, religious behavior, affiliation/denominational contrasts, and substance use and abuse. These models may also promote the development and testing of primary interventions (i.e., school-based and general population education programs) and secondary interventions (i.e., reducing the likelihood of development in high-risk groups such as minorities). This is in contrast to the historical research emphasis on tertiary intervention for addictions, especially 12-step programs.

SUBSTANCE DEPENDENCE RECOVERY

The focus of this chapter has been on the relationship between substance use, abuse/dependence, and religiousness. The following sections will describe and contrast recovery programs for substance and alcohol abusers, including nonreligious spiritual 12-step programs, religious 12-step programs, and secular 12-step programs. Suggestions for future interventions, including matching, will also be discussed.

NONRELIGIOUS SPIRITUAL INTERVENTIONS

Spiritual Meditation and Recovery

Some of the strongest evidence in support of nonreligious spiritual interventions (NRSI) comes from the field of behavioral medicine in which meditation, meditative relaxation, and biofeedback have been employed in an effort to directly produce or enhance recovery from alcohol/drug use and associated problems. Several studies (Alexander et al., 1994; Gelderloos et al., 1991; Taub, Steiner, Weingarten, & Walton, 1994) have reported on the therapeutic potential of transcendental meditation, and to a lesser extent biofeedback, in improving clinical outcomes in the prevention and particularly the treatment of alcohol and illicit substance use/abuse and dependence.

The 12-Step Program of Recovery

The primary therapeutic vehicle for most individuals' recovery from alcohol and substance abuse, however, has been through the NRSI 12-step programs. Although Alcoholics Anonymous (AA) is the prototype of 12-step programs, a variety of other 12-step programs have subsequently developed for substance dependency, including Narcotics Anonymous (NA), Cocaine Anonymous, Marijuana Anonymous, Nicotine (formerly Smokers) Anonymous, and Pills Anonymous, all of which are in high demand (Buxton, Smith, & Seymour, 1987). Twelve-step treatment remains one of the most effective ways to establish and maintain sobriety (Project MATCH Research Group, 1997), while complementing medical, psychiatric, and psychological treatment (Chappel, 1990). Clergymen also look to AA as a treatment complement rather than a formal religion (Royce, 1985). Positive spiritual values replace feelings of guilt and punishment, feelings which may encourage the alcoholic to drink again (Royce, 1985).

Overall Efficacy of 12-Step Programs

Every week, 15 million Americans attend more than 500 self-help group assemblies (Bailey, 1991). Its chief representatives, AA, NA, and related 12-step "self-help" programs, make up the predominant NRSI substance dependence therapy in the United States (Ellis & Schoenfeld, 1990). Twelve-step programs have helped millions of people overcome substance dependence (Alford, Koehler, & Leonard, 1991; Ellis & Schoenfeld, 1990; Kus, 1995) and AA's 60-year record of success gives validity to this spiritual approach (Twerski, 1990). At least 15 questionnaire surveys of members attending AA meetings show that 40–50% of alcoholics who join AA become long-term members, and 60–68% of these long-term members remain abstinent or at least decrease the amount of time they spend drinking. In an average AA meeting, approximately 35% of members have been sober for less than 1 year, 35% between 1 and 5 years, and the remaining have been sober for more than 5 years (Gorski, 1991).

Alford and associates (1991) evaluated the outcome of 12-step intervention in adolescent inpatients. These researchers found that 75% of adolescents who completed the 12-step-oriented treatment were abstinent at the end of treatment compared to only 35% of noncompleters. In addition, regardless of completion of the program, subjects who attended NA/AA less often were less likely to be abstinent than those inpatients attending meetings more frequently (Alford et al., 1991). Other studies also show a positive association between AA attendance and abstinence (Alford, 1980; Hoffman, Harrison, & Belille, 1983; Sheeren, 1988), and NA attendance is associated with less drug use for patients in residential care (Christo & Franey, 1995).

The overall effectiveness of AA and NA in altering substance abuse has been largely attributed by researchers to their spiritual tenants and practices. This consistent finding by those exploring spirituality as an independent variable further reinforces the putative relationship between spiritual factors and recovery from substance abuse and dependence (Ellis & Schoenfeld, 1990). Although this research provides empirical support for the efficacy of 12-step programs, specific components of NA/AA that facilitate treatment are not explicitly known. Investigations have nevertheless addressed the individual factors that may drive this apparent therapeutic linkage.

One body of evidence reveals that AA involvement may be generally more beneficial than clinical treatment, including detoxification and antabuse, in maintaining total abstinence (Fry, 1985; Sheeren, 1988). Vaillant (1983), in a prospective treatment study, found that 28% of the variance of good clinical outcome of 12-step programs could be attributed to attendance at AA meetings, whereas only 7% was due to miscellaneous (positive premorbid status) variables, including stable adjustment, married, employed, and never having been detoxified. Furthermore, AA involvement was more important in the long term than professional treatment, and psychotherapy did not contribute to good clinical outcome (Vaillant, 1983). This and other similar findings have led to the use of psychotherapy in conjunction with AA after stable recovery has been achieved (Chappel, 1990).

Although AA alone appears to be an effective treatment for alcoholism, AA combined with professional treatment may be the most effective form of help (Gorski, 1991; Project MATCH Research Group, 1997). About 50–60% of the alcoholics who attend AA will drop out in the first 90 days (Gorski, 1991). This dropout rate, however, is cut in half for alcoholics referred to treatment as part of professional treatment (Gorski, 1991). Twelve-step programs do advise that members should be willing to go to any lengths to achieve sobriety and remain sober, which often includes additional help from psychologists, doctors, and/or counselors (Gorski, 1991), as well as returning to their religion of origin (Alcoholics Anonymous [AA], 1976). There is also empirical support to show that AA members who asked for help from other AA members were less likely to relapse, and further formalization, by having a sponsor, was even more effective (Sheeren, 1988). While these studies suggest that 12-step programs are more efficacious than more secular programs, additional research is needed to expand knowledge in this area and to suggest ways to enhance the effectiveness of current clinical as well as naturalistic substance dependence treatment and maintenance methods. The following section addresses more of the specifics of spiritually oriented 12-step processes, especially with regard to nonabstinence-related outcomes.

Other Outcomes of 12-Step Programs in Addition to Abstinence

Influence of the Individual 12 Steps.

Brown and Peterson (1991) have examined the use of spiritual practices endorsed by 12-step programs among successfully recovering alcoholics. In their sample, 100% of the participants reported having admitted powerlessness over the dependency (step 1). Also, 94% reported that they conducted a "searching and fearless moral inventory" (step 4) and "told their life story to another person" (step 5). Ninety-seven percent reported practicing self-evaluation daily (step 10). Other spiritual practices endorsed include practicing meditation/quiet time/relaxing (100%), engaging in the practice of prayer (100%), and regular reading of spiritual literature or personal growth books (91%). Significantly, Brown and Peterson discovered that frequent use of the broad range of spiritual practices endorsed by the 12-step program (e.g., admitting powerlessness, turning over to a higher power, making amends for past wrongs, prayer, and mediation) predicted successful recovery among alcoholics. Although this study included a small sample ($N = 35$), its preliminary data provide rare process information on those aspects of 12-step programs that contribute to their efficacy (Brown & Peterson, 1991).

Carroll (1993) has also reported that prayer and meditation (step 11) along with regular AA attendance are positively associated with length of sobriety and purpose in life in AA members. Significant positive relationships were also uncovered between the practice of step 11 and both purpose of life scores and length of sobriety. Finally, the number of AA meetings attended was significantly associated with purpose in life scores and length of sobriety (Carroll, 1993).

Psychosocial Outcomes.

While recognizing how the religious connotations of the 12-step program have remained an obstacle for many potential participants and clinicians, Peteet (1993) examined the positive effects of the 12 steps in recovery from addictive behaviors. He points out that 12-step programs provide accessible group support and a clear ideology regarding addiction, and they support the individual's search for identity, integrity, inner life, and interdependence within a social, moral, and spiritual connection (Peteet, 1993). Active involvement in AA (e.g., regular meeting attendance) has also been associated with overall stress attenuation, increased spirituality, and increased contentment with life among studied subjects (Corrington, 1989). Purpose in life, self-actualization, and internal locus of control also have been reported to increase over the course of 12-step spiritual treatment for alcoholism (Giannetti, 1987). Finally, Briggman and McQueen (1987) examined how non-Christian members of AA change since AA does not emphasize a religious relationship with Jesus Christ. They concluded that the alcoholics changed from an internal to an external locus of control regarding drinking behaviors. That is, alcoholics were more internal with respect to drinking at baseline but shifted to an external locus of control across treatment and successful follow-up.

Spiritual Outcomes.

The effects of the 12-step process on spirituality have been another area of fruitful investigation, in which spiritual factors appear to exert a positive influence on recovery. In a retrospective study of the concept of spirituality as understood by substance abusers, recovering individuals showed highly significant prerecovery to postrecovery increases in spirituality and change in cognitive patterns (Mathew, Georgi, Wilson, & Mathew, 1996). Emphasizing the spiritual rather than religious/dogmatic aspects of recovery, substance abusers were able to build on an inner experience using visualization techniques as a way to develop resources in their recovery (Krystal & Zweben, 1988). In an even less religiously oriented examination of 12-step recovery, Mathew et al. (1995) attributed successful recovery from drug addiction to mystical changes that take place as a result of participation in 12-step programs of AA and NA.

In contrast, not all studies have found the spiritual aspects of 12-step programs to be efficacious. For example, methadone programs with spiritual/religious components were no more effective than methadone programs without spiritual/religious ingredients (5 vs 5%; Desmond & Maddux, 1981). Furthermore, 12-step programs showed greater increases in alcohol use from posttreatment to 6-month follow-up than did relapse prevention participants (Desmond & Maddux, 1981). Finally, in the Brown and Peterson (1991) study in which spiritual/AA practices were associated with positive outcomes, length of sobriety was not associated with increased spiritual practices endorsed by 12-step programs.

DO 12-STEP PROGRAMS NEED TO INCORPORATE SPIRITUAL/RELIGIOUS FACTORS?

Critics of Spiritual Components in 12-Step Programs

Many spiritual aspects of 12-step programs are difficult for many clinicians and researchers to accept (Keller, 1994). The difficulty some mental health counselors have in accepting 12-step programs as a viable form of therapeutic change may be due to counselors' lack of familiarity with relevant literature (Hanna, 1992). Some researchers argue that 12-step programs' religious emphasis cannot be substantiated, criticize its sectarian emphasis, and view the spiritual component to recovery as a rejection of psychology and psychiatry (Keller, 1990). Others suggest that the belief that one can only recover through the intervention of a Higher Power may undermine the client's confidence to change and control himself or herself (Ellis & Schoenfeld, 1990). Still others have argued that individuals with sub-

stance abuse/dependence have rejected treatment through 12-step programs because of a rejection of spiritual influences of the programs (Twerski, 1990). Fem-
inists, among others, have argued that the concept of a Higher Power as a plan for
life may not be comfortable for women from different cultural or religious backgrounds.

Support for Spiritual Components in 12-Step Programs

In addition to the growing body of evidence suggesting the overall beneficial
role of spiritual factors in substance abuse/dependence treatment and recovery,
there are several reasons why spiritually oriented interventions should be strongly considered as part of an optimal intervention package as well as included in clinical investigational studies. First, and perhaps of crucial importance, 12-step programs are not religions (Chappel, 1990). They make concerted efforts to remain
both religiously and spiritually "neutral" so as to attract as many who meet the single criterion for "membership": "A desire to stop drinking/using drugs" (AA,
1976). Although 12-step programs may appear to be a form of religion, they do
not have strict dogma, demanding rituals, or clergy (Chappel, 1990) that are inherent in a religion. Furthermore, AA does not require that its participants believe
in God, although it suggests that the individuals accept a higher power, or "God of
their understanding," defined as anything outside of the individual to which the individual can turn over his or her problems (AA, 1976). Additional evidence that
AA is not a religion is that atheists and agnostics can work comfortably within AA
once they understand the need to acknowledge something other than themselves,
or other human beings, which helps facilitate treatment (Chappel, 1990). Most 12-
step programs merely require attendance at NA or AA, emphasize the need to give
up the strong will ("self-will run riot") to the individual's Higher Power (Mansky,
1984)/"God of their understanding," or their home fellowship/group, and encourage the following of the 12-step principles, practices, and traditions and fellowship (AA, 1976). Although there is no religious orientation in 12-step programs,
spirituality is an integral component in the success of these programs (AA, 1976).

While some researchers maintain their claim that more dependent substance
abusers could be helped if the need for a Higher Power was eliminated (Buxton et
al., 1987; Ellis & Schoenfeld, 1990; Reinert, Estadt, Fenzel, Allen, & Gilroy,
1995), not all alcoholics who reject 12-step-oriented treatment do so because of
the spiritual influence of AA. Rather, some researchers contend that the only element that deters individuals from AA is its disease-model message that alcoholics
can never drink safely again (Twerski, 1990).

Critics may also be opposed to spiritual treatment in substance abuse due to a
different understanding of abuse/dependency etiology. Substance dependence and
alcoholism have been viewed etiologically by some as a spiritual decay, in which
mood-altering substances are substituted for true spiritual nourishment and subsequent moral development. Relatedly, the biblical perspective of alcoholism is
concerned with its spiritual and moral aspects (Mathew, 1992), and therefore it
makes sense that treatment for these individuals would be facilitated if it includ-

ed the spiritual aspects of their lives and problems in living. In other words, there is a clear spiritual component to human health. Alcoholism is seen by many within the 12-step program and portions of the religious community as a "spiritual disease" requiring spiritual recovery (Royce, 1995). Some have even claimed that the "etiology of alcoholism is an attempt to satisfy religious needs by non-religious means—alcohol" (Clinebell, 1963, p. 476).

If "negative spirituality" underlies and sustains alcoholics and other addictions, it follows that a secure recovery is not possible without a "spiritual awakening" (AA, 1976; Warfield & Goldstein, 1996), either gradual as many note or sudden, such as experienced by Bill Wilson, cofounder of AA (AA *Big Book;* AA, 1976), or in a "leap of faith" (Clinebell, 1963)—all of which may be best achieved through 12-step program involvement. Some would even go as far to say that "Spirituality is the treatment" (Booth, 1992, p. 139). Since lack of purpose in life and perceived powerlessness over circumstances are related to alcoholism, the recovering alcoholic makes a leap of faith out of the hopelessness of the alcohol situation (Clinebell, 1963). In this respect, there is a spiritual recovery process from alcoholism inherent in AA (Clinebell, 1963).

One question, posed especially by the religious community, is whether this "healing spirituality" must eventually be expressed or realized through religious faith processes. For example, an intriguing recent study has indicated the importance of religion in predicting substance dependence recovery outcome. Craig, Krishna, and Poniarski (1997) compared successful and unsuccessful outcome at 1-year follow-up in a sample of 101 VA inpatients who participated in a combined 12-step facilitation/relapse prevention treatment program. They found that self-reported absence of a mainstream Christian religious preference strongly predicted poor outcome. The following section will address this critical question: Is religious spirituality per se necessary or sufficient for recovery from alcoholism/substance abuse?

"RELIGIOUS SPIRITUALITY": A NECESSARY OR SUFFICIENT CONDITION IN RECOVERY?

Efficacy of Religiously Tailored 12-Step Programs

Despite the debate surrounding spiritual 12-step programs, many studies have supported the efficacy of religiously oriented 12-step programs (Brown & Peterson, 1991; Muffler, Langrod, & Larson, 1995). In their examination of four religiously based programs (two mainline churches and two conservative churches) for substance dependence, Muffler et al. found that religiously based programs had better outcomes than secular interventions, although few studies have compared these interventions. Also, treatment attendance was negatively related to cocaine use at posttreatment and cocaine and marijuana use at 6-month follow-up. In addition, patients who attended spiritually based programs were much more likely to report abstinence from opiods 1 year after the program (45 vs 5%; Desmond & Maddux, 1981). Similarly, data from Teen Challenge, a large Christian-based drug and alcohol treatment program, support this positive outcome link. Thompson (1994) reported anecdotally that 80% of subjects in the Teen Challenge recovery program for drug addicts credited their developing relationship with Jesus Christ as a major influence in helping them stay off drugs.

Bahr and Hawks (1995) discuss additional religiously tailored 12-step programs. Several Christian-tailored support groups have been modeled after AA. For example, Alcoholics for Christ (AC) is a nondenominational, nonprofit lay-Christian fellowship for substance abusers and their families. In addition to the 12-step program, AC also includes Bible study, a 12-step recovery workbook with scriptural examples, and support groups for family members. Overcomers Outreach is another Christian support group for individuals and families in evangelical Christian churches who suffer from chemical addiction. Also, Substance Abuse Volunteers Efforts was patterned after the 12-step programs in 1983 and tailored to Mormon substance abusers. Unfortunately, little or no data have been published concerning the efficacy of these interventions, but our hope is that these studies will be forthcoming given the heightened interest in and funding for investigations of spiritual and religious factors in the fields of medicine, psychology, and psychiatry (i.e., behavioral medicine/health psychology).

SECULAR ALTERNATIVES TO SPIRITUAL/RELIGIOUS INTERVENTION

Many secular interventions have attempted to provide effective alternatives to the spiritually and religiously guided 12-step programs. Interventions have consequently been adapted to suit a variety of needs for drug and alcohol addictions (Brady, 1995). Some of these programs, for example, have emphasized social support (Brady, 1995) or nontraditional interventions such as acupuncture. Others have attempted to add components to traditional 12-step programs such as a token economy for dually diagnosed psychiatric inpatients (Franco, Galanter, Castaneda, & Patterson, 1995) or a combination of 12-step program, therapeutic community, and reality therapy concepts.

For 40 years after its inception in 1935, AA was the only national self-help organization for alcoholics; however, this nearly exclusive grip on self-help intervention in the addictions was broken in the mid-1970s. Three new groups that emphasize behavior modification through reliance on self rather than a higher power include Rational Recovery (RR), Save Our Selves/Secular Organization for Sobriety (SOS), and Women for Sobriety (WFS). These groups employ similar peer-counseling formats and attract, not surprisingly, many patients dissatisfied with AA.

In 1975, Jean Kirkpatrik established a set of 13 steps in the "New Life Program" while searching for concepts conducive to personal growth and recovery for women dissatisfied with traditional 12-step programs. In 1985, Jim Christopher developed SOS, the largest secular alternative to AA. SOS does not have a structured recovery program as do AA, WFS, and RR. Instead of a formal alternative to the 12 steps, SOS has "Suggested Guidelines for Sobriety," which places emphasis on overcoming denial and simultaneously making sobriety one's most important priority in life. Finally, the third alternative to spiritually focused 12-step programs, RR, was founded in 1985 by Jack Trimpey with the aim of enabling alcoholics to remain sober independent of any professional involvement. Instead, RR teaches alcoholics the basics of Albert Ellis' Rational Emotive Therapy. Rather than having a set of steps to follow, RR has a set of irrational concepts, "Central Ideas to Alcoholism," and their rational counterparts. In 1991, RR established the first nationwide nonreligious residential alcoholism treatment program. Unfortunately, there are no reliable studies comparing these three interventions with AA (Uva, 1991).

However, one study (Reinert et al., 1995) did examine the relationship between high AA, low AA, and RR involvement. Results indicated that there were statistically significant differences in length of continuous sobriety (HiAA, 77.4 months; LoAA; 38.3 months; RR, 16.9 months). There were also differences in the number of meetings attended (15.4, 12.9, and 5.9, respectively) and degree of alcohol dependence on the Alcohol Dependency Scale (26.3, 22.0, and 14.8, respectively). This study suggests that increased spiritual components in AA help to increase length of sobriety more than less spiritual, secular treatment, although considerably more investigation is warranted before any reliable conclusions might be drawn from these differences.

Hence, we turn now to the obvious question of whether it is necessary or sufficient to include spiritual and/or religious approaches in the (cost-)effective prevention, early intervention, tertiary treatment, and recovery/maintenance of psychoactive substance use/abuse/dependence. Perhaps the most obvious solution, mirroring a movement in the field of psychology over the past 20–25 years, is patient/therapist/therapy matching.

MATCHING: ONE APPROACH TO END THIS DEBATE?

"Matching" suggests that clients who are matched to most appropriate treatments based on their religious and spiritual orientations, alcoholism/drug dependence "disease" concepts, and other individual characteristics will exhibit superior outcomes compared to those who were mismatched (Keisler, 1966). Fortunately, a recent large cooperative study has provided some timely evidence in this regard.

Project MATCH (1997) is a large-scale, randomized, clinical trial which assessed the benefits of matching alcohol-dependent clients to three 12-week treatments: Cognitive Behavioral Coping Skills therapy (CBT), Motivational Enhancement Therapy, or Twelve-step Facilitation Therapy (TSF). At 1-year posttreatment, there was little difference on outcomes by type of treatment. Only one client attribute had an overall matching effect that was not time dependent. Specifically, outpatients with psychopathology had significantly more abstinence when treated in TSF than with the CBT, but as psychiatric severity increased, the TSF advantage over CBT disappeared. Therefore, while there is some advantage

194 BOOTH AND MARTIN

to assigning outpatient clients with psychopathology to TSF treatment, definitive client–treatment matching recommendations for outpatient clients with moderate to high psychiatric severity cannot be made at this time.

Perhaps Project MATCH results may have been different if certain variables would have been controlled, such as the number of AA meetings attended. Project MATCH (1997) has shown that increased attendance at 12-step programs has yielded increased rates of abstinence. Also, while TSF encourages AA attendance and the working of the 12 steps, TSF is clearly distinguished from AA. On the other hand, it is important to note that the TSF was conducted by experienced 12-step facilitators and followed the spiritual program of AA, and the results should not be entirely discounted as dissimilar to what might happen in AA self-help groups. Nevertheless, given this essential difference between TSF and community-based 12-step group processes, results may well have been different if the AA 12-step program was one of the three treatment modalities instead of TSF. This hypothesis is particularly important given the popularity of AA for alcoholism treatment.

Despite the somewhat disappointing, perhaps even equivocal, results of the large MATCH study, continued research in client–intervention matching may facilitate an end to the debate of whether spiritual factors in 12-step programs are efficacious and/or ethical. Rather than randomly assigning all addicted subjects to either the secular or the spiritual intervention, one may instead assess the client for level of spiritual practice and belief and then randomly assign the client to either the secular or the spiritual intervention and examine differences in treatment outcome for spiritually oriented and nonspiritual clients. Perhaps this design may help to determine whether spiritual interventions are more efficacious for spiritual individuals. Also, treating a substance abuser who is religious may entail helping the person shift from a harsh and condemning religiousness to a caring and supporting one (Gorsuch, 1995). Further research in this area might increase the generalizability of the results with respect to the effects of interventions with spiritual or nonspiritual patients and thereby suggest combinations and contexts of treatments that may best serve their needs and ethical rights.

CONCLUSIONS AND FUTURE DIRECTIONS

There exists relatively reliable, if not robust, evidence suggesting the important positive role of (a) religiousness factors in substance use, abuse, dependency and (b) spiritual factors in recovery from addictions. The strongest evidence for the religiousness–substance nonabuse relationship is at the initial and continued substance abuse stages (Gorsuch, 1995). In general, the more religious a person is, irrespective of their age or substance of abuse/dependence, and the more spiritually or religiously oriented the treatment approach or system, the more positive the outcome. Some important exceptions and caveats include the paradoxical effect of certain religious and spiritual systems, especially those that are overly authoritarian or promoting of ambivalent messages about substance use and abuse and that seem to enhance problematic substance use and recovery. Secular alternatives to the spiritual 12-step programs, particularly to AA and NA, have not yet demonstrated their efficacy or differential superiority to the spiritually and religiously integrated interventions, and more research is clearly warranted.

Research is also needed with respect to the role of specific spiritual factors and processes in substance use and abuse. In particular, prospective case-control studies should be considered in which participants are randomly assigning to secular and spiritual 12-step programs. Furthermore, interventions other than 12-step programs that encourage spiritual practices may also be important areas of study and replication, such as the spiritual smoking intervention conducted by Voorhess *et al.* (1996) in African Americans. In this regard, we know relatively little about cultural and ethnic factors that will legislate different spiritual, religious, or secular approaches to chemical/substance dependence, and it is hoped that studies on these factors will be forthcoming as well.

Also needed are examinations of efficacious interventions which do not explicitly suggest the incorporation of spiritual components in order to increase the understanding of spiritually efficacious factors in treatment. One example might include cost-effective, well-validated brief therapies such as motivational interviewing (Miller & Rollick, 1993) or the directive, client-centered counseling approach for initiating behavior change by helping clients to resolve ambivalence in their addiction (Miller, 1996). Although there is evidence to support the utility of this intervention (Bien, Miller, & Tonigan, 1993; Miller, Benefield, & Tonigan, 1993), the underlying reasons and mechanisms for change are unknown (Miller, 1996). Even if mechanisms of effect are not spiritually related, they still may provide important insight into the factors associated with efficacious, secular interventions. Additional importance is lent to the determination of effective treatment outcomes due to the spiritual aspects of 12-step programs versus social/group support (Hanna, 1992) versus strategic encouragement of a motivational therapist (Miller, 1996).

For any of these studies to be comparable, researchers should attempt to develop consistent measures of spiritual and religious components. Inconsistent definitions and interpretations of spirituality as well as different models of recovery reinforce the debate (Cook, 1988) while perhaps further muddying the waters. The challenge is to gather scientifically appropriate data in order to gain a better understanding of what spirituality means in terms of recovery from drugs of abuse (Johnsen, 1993). Contrary to the claims of Bakken (1995), it would appear quite possible to scientifically quantify such concepts as belief and faith in God or a higher power, and spiritual processes, in addition to religious affiliation and practice. With better operational definitions of spirituality, religiousness, and substance use, we will be better able to provide the empirical support for the development of more proficient and cost-effective treatment interventions.

Finally, it is fairly evident that religious and spiritual factors play an important role in substance abuse and recovery. Rather than continue this debate, it is time to conduct research on what factors and specific processes (whether spiritual or secular) or combinations of factors and processes will promote abstinence and reduction of harm from substance abuse and, ultimately, apply this research-born knowledge to the clinical setting.

REFERENCES

Adelekan, M. L., et al. (1993). Psychosocial correlates of alcohol, tobacco, and cannabis use: Findings from a Nigerian university. *Drug and Alcohol Dependence, 33,* 247–256.

Adlaf, E. M., & Smart, R. G. (1985). Drug use and religious affiliation, feelings, and behaviour. *British Journal of Addiction, 8,* 163–171.

Ahmed, F., Brown, D. R., Gary, L. E., & Saadatmand, F. (1994). Religious predictors of cigarette smoking: Findings for African American women of childbearing age. *Behavioral Medicine, 20,* 34–43.

Albaugh, B. J., & Anderson, P. O. (1974). Peyote in the treatment of alcoholism among American Indians. *American Journal of Psychiatry, 131,* 1247–1250.

Alcoholics Anonymous. (1976). *Alcoholics Anonymous* (3rd. ed.). New York: Alcoholics Anonymous World Series.

Alexander, C. N., et al. (1994). Treating and preventing alcohol, nicotine, and drug abuse through transcendental meditation: A review and statistical meta-analysis. *Alcoholism Treatment Quarterly, 11,* 13–87.

Alford, G. S. (1980). Alcoholics Anonymous: An empirical outcome study. *Addictive Behaviors, 5,* 359–370.

Alford, G. S., Koehler, R. A., & Leonard, J. (1991). Alcoholics Anonymous–Narcotics Anonymous model inpatient treatment of chemically-dependent adolescents: A two year outcome study. *Journal of Studies on Alcohol, 52,* 118–126.

Amoateng, A. Y., & Bahr, S. J. (1986). Religion, family, and adolescent drug use. *Sociological Perspectives, 29,* 53–76.

Bahr, S. H., & Hawks, R. D. (1995). In R. H. Coombs & D. M. Ziedonis (Eds.). *Handbook on drug abuse prevention: A comprehensive strategy to prevent the abuse of alcohol and other drugs.* Boston: Allyn & Bacon.

Bailey, J. (1991). The spirituality of 12-step programs. *St. Anthony Messenger,* 23–27.

Bien, T. H., Miller, W. R., & Tonigan, J. S. (1993). Brief interventions for alcohol problems: A review. *Addiction, 88,* 315–336.

Bliss, S. K., & Crown, C. L. (1994). Concern for appropriateness, religiosity, and gender as predictors of alcohol and marijuana use. *Social Behavior and Personality, 22,* 227–238.

Blot, W. J., McLaughlin, J. K., & Winn, D. M. (1988). Smoking and drinking in relation to oral and pharyngeal cancer. *Cancer Research, 48,* 3282–3287.

Bobo, J. K. (1989). Nicotine dependence and alcoholism epidemiology and treatment. *Journal of Psychoactive Drugs, 21,* 323–329.

Booth, L. (1984). Aspects of spirituality in San Pedro Peninsula Hospital. *Alcoholism Treatment Quarterly, 1,* 121–123.

Booth, L. (1987). Alcoholism and the 4th and 5th Steps of Alcoholics Anonymous. *Journal of Psychoactive Drugs, 19,* 269–274.

Booth, L. (1992). The stages of religious addiction. *Creation Spirituality, 8,* 22–25.

Briggman, L. P., & McQueen, W. M. (1987). The success of Alcoholics Anonymous: Locus of control and God's general revelation. *Journal of Psychology and Theology, 15,* 124–131.

Brizer, D. A. (1993). Relgiosity and drug abuse among psychiatric inpatients. *American Journal of Drug and Alcohol Abuse, 19,* 337–345.

Brown, D. R., & Gary, L. E. (1994). Religious involvement and health status among African American males. *Journal of the National Medical Association, 86,* 825–831.

Brown, H. P., & Peterson, J. H. (1991). Assessing spirituality in addition to treatment and follow-up: Development of the Brown–Peterson Recovery Progress Inventory (B-PRPI). *Alcoholism Treatment Quarterly, 8,* 21–50.

Burkett, S. R., & White, M. (1974). Hellfire and delinquency: Another look. *Journal for the Scientific Study of Religion, 13,* 455–462.

Burkett, S. R., & Warren, B. O. (1987). Religiosity, peer association, and adolescent marijuana use: A panel study of underlying causal structures. *Criminology, 25,* 109–131.

Burns, C. M., & Smith, L. L. (1991). Evaluating spiritual well-being among drug and alcohol dependent patients: A pilot study examining the effects of supportive/educative nursing interventions. *Addictions Nursing Network, 3,* 89–94.

Buxton, M. E., Smith, D. E., & Seymour, R. B. (1987). Spirituality and other points of resistance to 12-step recovery process. *Journal of Psychoactive Drugs, 19,* 275–186.

Cancellaro, L. A., Larson, D. B., & Wilson, W. P. (1982). Religious life of narcotic addicts. *Southern Medical Journal, 75,* 1166–1168.

Carlucci, K., Genova, J., Rubackin, F., Rubackin, R., et al. (1993). Effects of sex, religion, and amount of alcohol consumption on self-reported drinking-related problem behaviors. *Psychological Reports, 72,* 983–987.

Carroll, S. (1993). Spirituality and purpose in life in alcoholism recovery. *Journal of Studies on Alcohol, 54,* 297–301.

Chappel, J. N. (1990). Spirituality is not necessarily religion: A commentary on "Divine Intervention and the Treatment of Chemical Dependency." *Journal of Substance Abuse, 2,* 481–483.

Christo, G., & Franey, C. (1995). Drug users' spiritual beliefs, locus of control and the disease concept in relation to Narcotics Anonymous attendance and six month outcomes. *Drug and Alcohol Dependence, 38,* 51–56.

Clinebell, H. J. (1963). Philosophical–religious factors in the etiology and treatment of alcoholism. *Quarterly Journal of Studies on Alcohol, 24,* 473–487.

Cochran, J. K. (1991). The effects of religiosity on adolescent self-reported frequency of drug and alcohol use. *Journal of Drug Issues, 22,* 91–104.

Cochran, J. K., Beeghley, L., & Bock, E. (1988). Religiosity and alcohol behavior: An exploration of reference group theory. *Sociological Forum, 3,* 256–276.

Cook, C. H. (1988). The Minnesota model in the management of drug and alcohol dependency: Miracle, method or myth? Part I. The philosophy and the programme. *British Journal of the Addictions, 83,* 625–634.

Coombs, R. H., Wellisch, D. K., & Fawzy, F. (1985). Drinking patterns and problems among female children and adolescents: A comparison of abstainers, past users, and current users. *American Journal of Drugs and Alcohol Abuse, 11,* 315–348.

Corrington, J. E. (1989). Spirituality and recovery: Relationships between levels of spirituality, contentment, and stress during recovery from alcoholism in AA. *Alcoholism Treatment Quarterly, 6,* 151–165.

Craig, T. J., Krishna, G., & Poniarski, R. (1997). Predictors of successful vs. unsuccessful outcome of a 12-step inpatient alcohol rehabilitation program. *American Journal of Addictions, 6,* 232–236.

Criqui, M. H., Wallace, R. B., Mishkel, M., Barrett-Connor, E., & Hess, G. (1981). Alcohol consumption and blood pressure: The lipid research clinics prevalence study. *Hypertension, 3,* 557–569.

Desmond, D. P., & Maddux, J. F. (1981). Religious programs and careers of chronic heroin users. *American Journal of Drug and Alcohol Abuse, 8,* 71–83.

Ellis, A., & Schoenfeld, E. (1990). Divine intervention and the treatment of chemical dependency. *Journal of Substance Abuse, 2,* 459–468.

Engs, R. C. (1980). The drug-use patterns of helping-profession students in Brisbane, Australia. *Drug and Alcohol Dependence, 6,* 231–246.

Enstrom, J. E. (1978). Cancer and total mortality among Mormons. *Cancer, 42,* 1943–1951.

Foshee, V. A., & Hollinger, B. R. (1996). Maternal religiosity, adolescent social bonding, and adolescent alcohol use. *Journal of Early Adolescence, 16,* 451–468.

Fowler, J. W., *Stages of faith: The psychology of human development and the quest of meaning.* San Francisco: Harper & Row, 1981.

Franco, H., Galanter, M., Castaneda, R., & Patterson, J. (1995). Combining behavioral and self-help approaches in the inpatient management of dually diagnosed patients. *Journal of Substance Abuse Treatment, 12,* 227–232.

Francis, L. I., & Mullen, K. (1993). Religiosity and attitudes towards drug use among 13–15 year olds in England. *Addiction, 88,* 665–672.

Fry, L. J. (1985). Social thought, social movements, and alcoholism: Some implications of AA's linkages and other entities. *Journal of Drug Issues,* 135–146.

Galanter, M. (1979). Religious conversion: An experimental model for affecting alcoholic denial. *Currents in Alcoholism, 6,* 69–78.

Gelderloos, P., et al. (1991). Effectiveness of the transcendental meditation program in preventing and treatment of substance misuse: A review. *International Journal of the Addictions, 26,* 293–325.

Giannetti, V. J. (1987). Religious dimensions of addiction. *Studies in Formative Spirituality, 8,* 187–197.

Gorsuch, R. L. (1976). Religion as a significant predictor of important human behavior. In W. J. Donaldson, Jr. (Ed). *Research in Mental Health and Religious Behavior.* Psychological Studies Institute.

Gorsuch, R. L. (1995). Religious aspects of substance abuse and recovery. *Journal of Social Issues, 51,* 65–83.

Hanna, F. J. (1992). Reframing spirituality: AA, the 12 steps, and the mental health counselor. *Journal of Mental Health Counseling, 14,* 166–179.

Gottlieb, N. H., & Green, L. W. (1984). Life events, social network, life-style, and health: An analysis of the 1979 national survey of personal health practices and consequences. *Health Education Quarterly, 11,* 91–105.

Hardesty, P. H., & Kirby, K. M. (1995). Relation between family religiousness and drug use within adolescent peer groups. *Journal of Social Behavior and Personality, 10,* 421–430.

Hardy, P. H., & Kirby, K. M. (1995). Relation between family religiousness and drug use within adolescent peer groups. *Journal of Social Behavior and Personality, 10,* 421–430.

Hasin, D., Endicott, J., & Lewis, C. (1985). Alcohol and drug abuse in patients with affective syndromes. *Comprehensive Psychiatry, 26,* 283–295.

Hater, J. J., Singh, K., & Simpson, D. D. (1984). Influence of family and religion on long-term outcomes among opiod addicts. *Advances in Alcohol and Substance Abuse, 4,* 29–40.

Hawks, R. D., & Bahr, S. H. (1992). Religion and drug use. *Journal of Drug Education, 22,* 1–8.

Hoffman, N. G., Harrison, P. A., & Belille, C. A. (1983). Alcoholics Anonymous after treatment: Attendance and abstinence. *International Journal of Addictions, 18,* 311–318.

Jolly, S., & Orford, J. (1983). Religious observance, attitudes towards drinking and knowledge about drinking, among university students. *Alcohol and Alcoholism, 18,* 271–278.

Johnsen, E. (1993). The role of spirituality in recovery from chemical dependency. *Journal of Addictions and Offender Counseling, 13,* 58–61.

Keisler, D. (1966). Some myths of psychotherapy research and the search for a paradigm. *Psychological Bulletin, 65,* 110–136.

Keller, J. E. (1990). *Models of alcoholism from days of old to nowadays.* Pamphlet Series, Center for Alcohol Studies, Rutgers University, New Brunswick, NJ.

Keller, J. E. (1994). Spirituality in treatment and recovery. In G. S. Howard & P. E. Nathan (Eds). *Alcohol use and misuse by young adults.* University of Notre Dame Press, Notre Dame, IN, 109–132.

Khavari, K. A., & Harmon, T. M. (1982). The relationship between the degree of professed religious belief and the use of drugs. *International Journal of Addictions, 17,* 847–857.

Koenig, H. G., et al. (1994). Religious practices and alcoholism in a southern community. *Hospital and Community Psychiatry.*

Istvan, J., & Matarazzo, J. D. (1984). Tobacco, alcohol, and caffeine use: A review of their interrelationships. *Psychological Bulletin, 95,* 301–326.

Kus, R. J. (1995) (Ed). Spirituality and chemical dependency. Harrington Park Press/Haworth Press, Inc; New York, NY.

Larson, D. B., & Wilson, W. P. (1979). Religious life of alcoholics. *Southern Medical Journal, 73,* 723–727.

The influence of religious leaders on smoking cessation in a rural population—Thailand, 1991. (1993, May 21). *Morbidity Weekly Report, 42,* 367.

Levin, J. S., & Vanderpool, H. Y. (1987). Is frequent religious attendance really conducive to better health? Towards an epidemiology of religion. *Social Science and Medicine, 24,* 589–600.

Lorch, B. R., & Hughes, R. H. (1985). Religion and youth substance use. *Journal of Religion and Health, 24,* 197–208.

Mansky, R. A. (1992). Working with functional alcoholics and addicts. *Psychiatric Quarterly,* 86–105.

Mariz, C. L. (1991). Pentecostalism and alcoholism among the Brazilian poor. *Alcoholism Treatment Quarterly, 8,* 75–82.

Mathew, R. J. (1992). Alcoholism in biblical prophecy. *Alcohol and Alcoholism, 27,* 89–90.

Mathew, R. J., Georgi, J., Wilson, W. H., & Mathew, V. G. (1996). A retrospective study of the concept of spirituality as understood by recovering individuals. *Journal of Substance Abuse Treatment, 13,* 67–73.

Midanik, L. T., & Clark, W. B. (1995). Drinking problems in the United States: Description and trends, 1984–1990. *Journal of Studies on Alcohol, 56,* 395–402.

Miller, W. R. (1996). Motivational interviewing: Research, practice, and puzzles. *Addictive Behaviors, 21,* 835–842.

Miller, W. R. (1997). Spiritual aspects of addiction treatment and research. *Mind/Body Medicine, 2,* 37–42.

Miller, W. R., Benefield, R. G., & Tonigan, J. S. (1993). Enhancing motivation for change in problem drinking: A controlled comparison of two therapist styles. *Journal of Consulting and Clinical Psychology, 61,* 455–461.

Miller, W. R., & Rollnick, S. (1991). *Motivational interviewing.* Guilford: New York.

Moore, M., & Weiss, S. (1995). Reasons for non-drinking among Isreali adolescents among four religions. *Drug and Alcohol Dependence, 38,* 45–50.

Muffler, J., Langrod, J., & Larson, D. (1995). There is a balm in Gilead: Religion and substance abuse treatment. In: Lowinson, J. H., Ruiz, P., Millman, R. B., Langrod, J. G., Eds. *Substance abuse: A comprehensive textbook.* 2nd edition. Baltimore, MD: Williams & Wilkins, 584–595.

Pages Larraya, F. (1978). The journal of the Guarayos into the land of the Dead: A transcultural psychiatric study. *Confinia Psychiatrica, 21,* 234–257.

Parfrey, P. S. (1976). The effects of religious factors on intoxicant use. *Scandanavian Journal of Social Medicine, 4,* 135–140.

Peteet, J. R. (1993). A closer look at the role of a spiritual approach in addictions treatment. *Journal of Substance Abuse Treatment, 10,* 263–267.

Project MATCH Research Group. (1997). Matching alcoholism treatments to client heterogeneity: Project MATCH posttreatment drinking outcomes. *Journal of Studies on Alcohol, 58,* 7–29.

Reinert, D. F., Estadt, B. K., Fenzel, L. M., Allen, J. P., & Gilroy, F. D. (1995). Relationship of surrender and narcissism to involvement in alcoholism recovery. *Alcoholism Treatment Quarterly, 12,* 49–58.

Royce, J. E. (1985). Sin or solace? Religious views on alcohol and alcoholism. *Journal of Drug Issues, 14,* 51–62.

Sheeren, M. (1988). The relationship between relapses and involvement in Alcoholics Anonymous. *Journal of Studies on Alcohol,* 104–106.

Shuler, P. A., Gelberg, L., & Brown, M. (1994). The spiritual/religious practices on psychological well-being among inner city homeless women. *Nurse Practitioner Forum, 5,* 106–113.

Skolnick, J. H. (1958). Religious affiliation and drinking behavior. *Quarterly Journal of Studies on Alcohol, 19,* 452–470.

Snyder, C. R. (1958). *Alcohol and the Jews.* Glencoe, IL: Free Press.

Taub, E., Steiner, S. S., Weingarten, E., & Walton, K. G. (1994). Effectiveness of broad spectrum approaches to relapse prevention in severe alcoholism: A long-term randomized, controlled-trial of transcendental meditation, EMG biofeedback, and electronic neurotherapy. *Alcoholism Treatment Quarterly, 11,* 187–220.

Thompson, R. (1994). *In research on the effectiveness of Teen Challenge.* Springfield, MO: Teen Challenge and Resource Center.

Turner, N. H., Ramirez, G. Y., Higginbotham, J. C., Markides, K., Wygant, A. C., & Black, S. (1994). Tri-ethnic alcohol use and religion, family, and gender. *Journal of Religion and Health, 33,* 341–351.

Twerski, A. J. (1990). Is divine intervention really a drawback? *Journal of Substance Abuse, 2,* 485–487.

U.S. Department of Health and Human Services. (1988). *The health consequences of smoking: Nicotine addiction. A report of the Surgeon General* (DDHS Publication No. CDC 88–8406). Washington, DC: U.S. Government Printing Office.

Uva, J. L. (1991). Alcoholics Anonymous: Medical recovery through a higher power. *Journal of the American Medical Association, 266,* 3064–3067.

Vaillant, G. E. (1983). *The natural history of alcoholism: Causes, patterns, and paths to recovery.* Cambridge, MA: Harvard University Press.

Vaillant, G. E., Schnurr, P. P., Barron, J. A., & Gerber, P. D. (1991). A prospective study of the effects of cigarette smoking and alcohol abuse on mortality. *Journal of General Internal Medicine, 6,* 299–304.

Voorhees, C. C., Stillman, F. A., Swank, R. T., Heagerty, P. J., Levine, D. M., & Becker, D. M. (1996). Heart, body and soul: Impact of church-based smoking cessation interventions on readiness to quit. *Preventive Medicine, 25,* 277–285.

Weill, J., & Le Bourhis, B. (1994). Factors predictive of alcohol consumption in a representative sample of French male teenagers: A five year prospective study. *Drug and Alcohol Dependence, 35,* 45–50.

Weiss, S., & Moore, M. (1992). Perception of alcoholism among Jewish, Moslem, and Christian teachers in Isreal. *Journal of Drug Education, 22,* 253–260.

Zucker, R. A., & Hartford, T. C. (1983). National study of the demography of adolescent drinking practices in 1980. *Journal of Studies on Alcohol, 44,* 974–985.

RELIGIOUS PERSPECTIVES ON MENTAL HEALTH

13

RELIGION AND MENTAL HEALTH FROM THE PROTESTANT PERSPECTIVE

H. NEWTON MALONY

Graduate School of Psychology
Fuller Theological Seminary
Pasadena, California 91101

Martin Marty once wrote, "Connecting health/medicine with religion is not difficult. . . . Connecting health/medicine with religious *tradition,* and worse, specific *traditions* is far more problematic" (Marty & Vaux, 1982, p. 3). What Marty contended was true of general health is even more true of *mental health* when it is related to the *Protestant tradition* or, better stated, *traditions.* Many churches are defined as "Protestant," because they are "not Catholic." The range of religious convictions within that spectrum is significantly broad. While churches within Protestantism might be identified along this theological continuum as fundamental, evangelical, orthodox, mainline, or liberal, these self-identifications would not fully encompass the beliefs and practices of the churches. Attendees at services of worship might find remarkable similarities in the words that were used existing alongside great differences in styles and emphases. My students and I have been working for over a decade and a half on a measure of religious maturity that we have claimed encompasses the total Christian tradition, Catholic, Protestant, and Orthodox, but we have become convinced that the effort may be a bit grandiose (Malony, 1988). There may be more differences within Protestant denominations than between them. Nevertheless, there may, indeed, be some Protestant *emphases* that could significantly impact mental health.

DIVERSITY AMONG PROTESTANTS

Consider this: All people do, indeed, live within traditions, as Marty and Vaux (1982) noted, but I have become convinced that some people are more self-con-

---

scious of and committed to their specific traditions than others. In fact, I no longer believe that it can be assumed that applying a label to oneself, such as Protestant, means anything significant unless it implies greater-than-average involvement and commitment. The Israeli psychologist of religion, Benjamin Beit-Hallahmi (1986), concluded that most religious labels do nothing more than provide social identity. Social identity is composed of a variety of labels reflecting multiple roles and associations, religion being only one of them. Although I think that Beit-Hallahmi is overly pessimistic in saying that the only thing that religious identity will predict is frequency of attendance at certain types of religious activities, I do agree that average to less than average involvement will have next to no influence on behavior (Malony, 1995a). Therefore, when thinking about the relationship between Protestantism and mental health, it is best to think of a religious social identity as a conscious *interest,* similar to interest in wood carving or classical music. Considering religion as an *interest* is similar to the manner with which interests of all kinds are dealt in predicting vocational and recreational interests. Only higher than average interests will predict who will choose a given activity over other options when choices are available.

Religious attitudes toward mental health should be no different. The research literature on religion and mental health supports this conclusion. Although higher than average religious maturity has been found to relate to less distress in older Christian women (Atkinson & Malony, 1994), religion in general has not proven to be a uniformly decisive factor in other mental health research (Batson, Schoenrade, & Ventis, 1993, pp. 241–254). In my opinion a given religious tradition will have a significant impact on attitudes of mental health and reactions to counseling only among those whose interest in that religious tradition goes significantly beyond cultural conformity.

However, there may be some significant differences in orientation among the several Protestant groups worth considering that might affect attitudes toward mental health among the very committed. Barkman (1968) detailed these in a format that makes sense but which has never been tested. He contended that the type of religious organization to which a person belonged reflected his or her basic personality styles. Those whose personality style was *verbal,* Barkman contended, were inclined to join Reform and Baptist churches, in which correct statements of belief were emphasized. Those whose personality style was *affective* were inclined to join Wesleyan and Pentecostal churches, in which personal religious experience was emphasized. Those whose personality style was *action oriented* were inclined to join Anabaptist type churches, such as the Quakers, the Brethren, and the Mennonites, in which social action was emphasized. Finally, those whose personality style was more *ethereal* were inclined to join Episcopal or Lutheran churches, in which mystery, ritual, and liturgy were emphasized.

As noted earlier, although this model is suggestive, I am convinced that people initially go to a given church because friends invite them rather than out of a desire to find a group that matches their particular personality styles (Lofland & Stark, 1965). However, long-term satisfaction in a given group may indeed reflect temperamental preferences as persons become acclimated to given churches' specific emphases. Pargament, Johnson, Echemendia, and Silverman (1985) did find some positive relationships between tolerance of ambiguity and group norms among active members of both Protestant and Catholic churches. Thus, while the emphases noted by Barkman (1968) would seem to be present to a certain degree in all Protestant churches, groups do seem to take on dominant characteristics that are worth noting with regard to mental health.

As opposed to Barkman's (1968) typology, I propose a fourfold continuum ranging from fundamentalist to liberal—terms which, while dated, still refer to significant differences in outlook within Protestantism. This continuum reflects two parallel foci: (a) the extent to which a given group looks to the Bible, the tradition, religious experience, or rational thinking as its prime source of authority; and (b) the modal criterion which a given group uses to judge whether a person is religious or not. My typology is as follows:

Fundamentalist Protestant churches in which the Bible is the prime source of authority and obedience to biblical commands is the criterion of judgment as to who is religious or not.

Evangelical Protestant churches in which experience is the prime source of authority and having undergone an event that resulted in emotional assurance of salvation is the criterion of judgment as to who is religious or not.

Traditional Protestant churches in which historical tradition is the prime source of authority and active involvement in a particular religious group is the criterion of judgment as to who is religious or not.

Liberal Protestant churches in which rational thinking is the prime source of authority and ethical behavior is the criterion of judgment as to who is religious or not.

With this model in mind, I now consider the way in which each type of Protestant group might address the following questions:

How shall "mental health" be conceived?
What will be expected in treatment?

In addressing these questions I depend largely on my clinical experience and intuition, although at times I may draw on published material.

HOW SHALL "MENTAL HEALTH" BE CONCEIVED?

Strangely, I believe Fundamentalist and Liberal Protestants would answer this question in the same way but for different reasons. Both would assert that spiritual and mental health were distinct states of mind that should not be confused. However, for Fundamentalist Protestants, those who are spiritually healthy are those who are obeying God's commands, as derived from the Bible, and thus are prepared to go to heaven when they die. The only other type of health worth considering, for this group, is *physical* health, which has nothing to do with spiritual health. There is no such entity as mental *health,* which is not synonymous with spiritual health. Those who are depressed or disturbed are disobedient to God's demands as gleaned from the Bible. There is no nonspiritual *mental health.* The whole mental health movement is a misguided effort to define mental health in secular isolation from the religio/spiritual understanding of life (Bobgan & Bobgan, 1979).[1]

Liberal Protestant Christians understand mental health in a similar manner from a drastically different perspective. They, too, contend that mental health can best be defined by the concept of "obedience." However, the obedience is less a matter of personal ethics and correct belief and more a matter of obeying the scriptural call to love the neighbor and work for justice. Mental health is action in behalf of social and environmental health. Howard Clinebell expressed this point of view taken to its logical extreme in his book *Ecotherapy: Healing Ourselves: Healing the Earth* (1996). John Cobb expressed it well in his endorsement of this volume: "Psychological health and the health of the earth are deeply intertwined. The boundaries between therapy, education, spirituality, and eco-justice melt away in Clinebell's revisioning of our common calling." While Liberal Protestants do not deny the reality of mental health or contend that physical health is entirely separate from spiritual health, they definitely contend that mental health is encircled and engulfed by *spiritual health,* defined as obedience to biblical teachings about creation, justice, and peace.

Evangelical and Traditional Protestants do not combine spiritual and mental health as do Fundamentalists and Liberals. These two groups contend that both are real but are distinctly different. The Evangelicals, for example, distinguish between the two words "joy" and "happiness"—both of which are desirable emotions but refer to different domains. Joy is the goal spiritually healthy persons should seek, whereas happiness is the goal for those who would be mentally healthy. Joy refers to the assurance that one has been "born again" and that God is available for companionship in daily living. Happiness is the experience of being well-adjusted and productive in one's social environment. Johnson, Malony, and Lim (1995) partially confirmed this in a sample of college students in which level of happiness could be predicted only 4% of the time from level of religious maturity. Since the scale they used to measure happiness was composed of the reverse of questions on a depression scale, it was inferred that a high happiness score would imply a somewhat naive giddiness. It was suggested that those who were religiously mature might never look upon life with such an emotion even though they might be very "joyful" in their religious experience.

Traditional Protestants make a similar distinction between spiritual and mental health but for a different reason. They tend to be acculturated in much of their life experience and tend to not question the bifurcation of culture into religion and mental health. Since their religious traditions are well accepted by society, they adjust easily to the distinctions between sacred and secular. They fit comfortably into being church persons and public citizens, and they are comfortable with the separation of church and state. Mental health is a state of mind that refers to overall adjustment to one's environment, whereas spiritual health is a state of mind that refers to one's religious involvement. Both have cultural meaning. They are not in competition with each other; they refer to different domains. Without meaning to disparage this type of Protestantism, it is apparent that this viewpoint tends to be less reflective than the others as to how spiritual and mental health might differ.

THE EFFECT OF THE DIFFERENCES
ON TREATMENT

What effect might the differences among Fundamentalist, Evangelical, Traditional, and Liberal Protestant Christians have on treatment? This is the question to which I turn while reminding the reader that I believe that these differences will have little effect on the average member of any one of the groups. Where members' involvement is significantly greater than average, however, these differences in understandings of mental health may impact the expectations they have when coming to mental health counselors for treatment. [I acknowledge that Marty and Vaux (1986) have included some more specific denomination-based approaches to these matters. These approaches (by Ferngren, Harrell, Klassen, Lindberg, Smylie, Raboteau, Vanderpool, Wacker, and Weber) are included in the references to this essay. I have intentionally chosen a more inclusive grouping in comparing Fundamentalist, Evangelical, Traditional, and Liberal approaches.] In brief, these differences in expectations are as follows.

Fundamentalists might be suspicious of any counsel given; feel guilty about being there; and only trust the advice given by a Christian counselor at their churches who would encourage them to examine their faithfulness to biblical standards.

Evangelicals might be accepting of the counsel they receive but would want to check out the credentials of the counselors in terms of whether they were themselves born again. Furthermore, they might expect the counseling to begin with prayer and that scriptural and religious resources be recommended in the treatment.

Traditionalists would not question the religious background of the counselors but would want to know whether they were well trained in professional skills. They would be surprised if counselors mixed religious and psychological approaches. While they personally might become more regular in their own devotional practices, they would not expect these to be recommended by counselors.

Liberals might eschew the introduction of standard religious resources or practices by counselors and be open to approaches which enable them to get in touch with higher mental processes and meditative practices designed to help them get into a harmonious relationship with their bodies and with the universe.

I have no doubt that such implications for treatment as I have described are real for those who take their specific type of Protestantism seriously. Behind the observations I made about definitions of mental health lie anthropologies about the nature of human beings, cosmologies about the essence of realities, psychopathologies about what can disrupt normal development, theories of healing about what can restore persons to health, and utopian ideas about what life is intended to be (Malony, 1995b). There is consistency in these foundational assumptions only in very involved participants, as I have repeatedly noted, but, where these presumptions are operative, one can assume they will impact treatment expectations.

Among Fundamentalist approaches the writing of Jay Adams is a classic example. His books *Competent to Counsel* (1970) and *More Than Redemption: A Theology of Christian Counseling* (1979) firmly state the biblical criteria for mental health and the means to achieve it. Psychological counseling which analyses cognitions and feelings is of no avail. Change can come only from understanding and obeying the laws of life as contained in the Bible.

Among Evangelical Protestants, the approach of S. Y. Tan (1990) is illustrative. Although he is sensitive to the dangers of imposing religion into treatment, he asserts the values of *explicit integration*—a method of counseling which intentionally introduces religious questions and resources into counseling. Tan concludes that many Christians will expect the counselor to pray with them and to recommend ways in which they can interrelate their faith and their healing.

Among Traditional Protestants, Allen Bergin (1985) is a representative theorist. Although a Mormon, Bergin clearly considers himself to be Christian and his writings affirm the importance of participation in a religious tradition for life adjustment. More important, he asserts the confluence of religious and secular values among psychotherapists as illustrating the lack of conflict in counseling. He contends that the underlying goals of mental health treatment are in accord with the goals of religion and that persons can avail themselves of both resources without feeling any contradictions. Bergin's conclusions would be echoed by such luminaries as Oates (1962) and Oden, Warren, and Schoonhoven (1974).

Finally, as noted earlier, Howard Clinebell (1996) is representative of Liberal Protestants. He recommends appreciating the spiritual core of all efforts to help persons achieve "wholeness" and expands an understanding of treatment to include a sensitivity to the place of human beings in the universe. He criticizes the type of counseling which focuses too much on individual needs and wants. He affirms a type of healing which comes from a concern for others, action in behalf for social justice, a witness to the unity of all creation, and a caring for the natural world. Clinebell's approach is a form of moral therapy seen so vividly in the writing of the late O. Hobart Mowrer, who advocated *integrity therapy*—an approach which suggested that all emotional disturbance was due to real guilt resulting from ethical transgressions that needed readdressing.

In this chapter, I have attempted to relate mental health to the Protestant tradition. After emphasizing that given traditions would impact the definition of mental health and treatment only among those who were significantly involved above the average level, a fourfold model for understanding differences within Protestantism was proposed. Fundamentalist, Evangelical, Traditional, and Liberal Protestant groups were compared on the basis of their understanding of authority and their criteria for religiousness. The implications of these assumptions for understanding counseling and mental health were considered.

EDITOR'S NOTE

[1]There is a considerable range of belief within Fundamentalists on this issue; some would have no problem with the notion of mental health being distinct from spiritual health and would provide Biblical references to back up their view.

REFERENCES

Atkinson, B. E., & Malony, H. N. (1994). Religious maturity and psychological distress among older Christian women. *International Journal for the Psychology of Religion, 4*(3), 165–180.

Batson, C. D., Schoenrade, P., & Ventis, W. L. (1993). *Religion and the individual: A social–psychological perspective.* New York: Oxford University Press.

Beit-Hallahmi, B. (1986). Religion as art and identity. *Religion, 16,* 1–17.

Clinebell, H. (1996). *Ecotherapy: Healing ourselves, healing the earth.* Minneapolis, MN: Fortress Press.

Ferngren, G. B. (1986). The Evangelical–Fundamentalist tradition. In R. L. Numbers & D. W. Amundsen (Eds.), *Caring and curing: Health and medicine in the Western religious tradition* (pp. 486–513). New York: Macmillan.

Harrell, D. E., Jr. (1986). The Disciples of Christ–Church of Christ tradition. In R. L. Numbers & D. W. Amundsen (Eds.), *Caring and curing: Health and medicine in the Western religious tradition* (pp. 376–396). New York: Macmillan.

Johnson, J., Malony, H. N., & Lim, O. B. (1995, July). *Religious maturity and happiness.* Paper presented at the European Congress of Psychology, Athens, Greece.

Klassen, W. (1986). The Anabaptist tradition. In R. L. Numbers & D. W. Amundsen (Eds.), *Caring and curing: Health and medicine in the Western religious tradition* (pp. 271–287). New York: Macmillan.

Lindberg, C. (1986). The Lutheran tradition. In R. L. Numbers & D. W. Amundsen (Eds.), *Caring and curing: Health and medicine in the Western religious tradition* (pp. 173–203). New York: Macmillan.

Lofland, J., & Stark, R. (1965). Becoming a world saver: A theory of conversion to a deviant perspective. *American Sociological Review, 65,* 865–874.

Malony, H. N. (1988). The clinical assessment of optimal religious functioning. *Review of Religious Research, 30*(1), 3–17.

Malony, H. N. (1995a). *Religion as interest rather than instinct: Why religion seems to not predict behavior.* Paper presented at the annual meeting of the Christian Association for Psychological Studies, Virginia Beach, VA.

Malony, H. N. (1995b). A turbo-prop model for integrating mind, body and spirit. In H. N. Malony (Ed.), *Integration musings: Thoughts on being a Christian professional* (pp. 65–70). Pasadena, CA: Integration Press.

Marty, M. E., & Vaux, K. L. (Eds.). (1982). *Health/medicine and the faith traditions: An inquiry into religion and medicine.* Philadelphia: Fortress Press.

Marty, M. E., & Vaux, K. L. (Eds.). (1986). *Caring and curing: Health and medicine in the Western religious traditions.* New York: Macmillan.

Oates, W. (1962). *Protestant pastoral counseling.* Philadelphia: Westminster.

Oden, T. A., Warren, W. C., & Schoonhoven, C. (1974). *After therapy what?* Springfield, IL: Charles C Thomas.

Pargament, K. I., Johnson, S., Echemendia, R., & Silverman, S. (1985). The limits of fit: Examining the implications of person–environment congruence within different religious settings. *Journal of Community Psychology, 13,* 20–30.

Raboteau, A. J. (1986). The Afro-American tradition. In R. L. Numbers & D. W. Amundsen (Eds.), *Caring and curing: Health and medicine in the Western religious tradition* (pp. 539–562). New York: Macmillan.

Smylie, J. H. (1986). The Reformed tradition. In R. L. Numbers & D. W. Amundsen (Eds.), *Caring and curing: Health and medicine in the Western religious tradition* (pp. 204–239). New York: Macmillan.

Southard, S. (1989). *Theology and therapy: The wisdom of God in a context of friendship.* Dallas: Word.

Tan, S. Y. (1990). Explicit integration in Christian counseling. *Christian Journal of Psychology and Counseling, 5*(2), 7–13.

Vanderpool, H. Y. (1986). The Wesleyan-Methodist tradition. In R. L. Numbers & D. W. Amundsen (Eds.), *Caring and curing: Health and medicine in the Western religious tradition* (pp. 317–353). New York: Macmillan.

Wacker, G. (1986). The Pentecostal tradition. In R. L. Numbers & D. W. Amundsen (Eds.), *Caring and curing: Health and medicine in the Western religious tradition* (pp. 514–538). New York: Macmillan.

Weber, T. P. (1986). The Baptist tradition. In R. L. Numbers & D. W. Amundsen (Eds.), *Caring and curing: Health and medicine in the Western religious tradition* (pp. 288–316). New York: Macmillan.

14

RELIGION AND MENTAL HEALTH FROM THE CATHOLIC PERSPECTIVE

NANCY CLARE KEHOE

*Harvard Medical School
Cambridge, Massachusetts 02139*

Denominational affiliation is not the same as a *DSM-IV* diagnosis. A "Catholic" cannot be described by five easily identifiable characteristics. Rather than refer to Catholic patients as "religious patients" as Spero (1985) does or as "the religiously committed patients" as Stern (1985) does, it may foster clinical neutrality to think of people as individuals, couples, and families who are in pain and who seek treatment. They may belong to a particular religious denomination, and their manner of belonging and the way they think about their religious affiliation may add to their distress or it may be an area of comfort and support as they attempt to deal with their pain. "Religious or spiritual issues" cannot be separated from other aspects of the person's history and psychological development. One of the difficulties about the new *DSM-IV* category, "Religious or Spiritual Problem," is that it isolates the religious or spiritual problem from the context of a person's life. The therapist needs to be attentive to the particular ways in which a person's religious tradition affects him or her.

A religious tradition is a complex phenomenon composed of doctrine, community identity, structure, stories, and rituals. A person receives a religious tradition. There is not a Catholic psyche, a Methodist psyche, a Jewish psyche, nor a Muslim psyche—only a person with his or her unique psychological makeup.

By examining religion and mental health from various perspectives, the studies in this book attempt to understand, in a limited way, what are the elements of a particular tradition, and how the person's religious tradition was shaped by various influences that will affect his or her mental life. Even within a particular religious denomination, individuals will differ, despite an apparently similar formation. As we consider religion and mental health from various religious perspectives, it will be important to remember that it is the individual who has internalized the religious formation. Just as an individual's psychic life has been formed, informed, and in some cases "deformed" by his or her family, physical health, and life experiences, so too the person has been formed, informed, and perhaps "deformed" by his or her experience of religious formation that has taken place within a broad context.

Although there may not be a "Catholic perspective," specific Catholic teachings and formation do exist. The Roman Catholic Church is universal; its structure and its head, the Pope, are very visible. His pronouncements are frequently public and, in some instances, even addressed to the world's citizens. Thus, in some ways, Catholicism may be better known than other religions, at least in this country, and there may also be more negative transference because of the authority structure and the public nature of some official statements. As Greeley (1985, p. 7) notes, "No one is without personal biases or opinions when the subject is Catholics." However, the Catholic collectivity or subculture is not the same as the Catholic Church as institution (Greeley, 1977). A failure to make that distinction may have negative clinical effects.

In this chapter, after a review of the literature, I will consider the educational differences among Catholics who were raised before the Second Vatican Council (an international meeting of church officials that took place from 1962 to 1965) and those who received their religious instruction and formation after 1965. The Second Vatican Council was a watershed event for Catholics, one that changed many aspects of the Church's self-understanding. A person born after 1965 may have been raised by parents influenced by the pre-Vatican II Church which can lead to confusion.

It is not only pre-Vatican II Catholics and post-Vatican II Catholics that may differ: There are also ethnic/educational/socioeconomic differences. Some attention will be given to these differences in order to minimize a therapist's risk of generalizing to all Catholics. What we are interested in as clinicians is what the person learned, what was the context in which that learning occurred, how that learning may have influenced an individual's psychological development, and how mental health professionals need to respect and take all these facts into consideration without labeling religious material pathological, defensive, or delusional. The mental health professional should attend to the way a person makes use of his or her experiences, either for good or for ill, either in taking responsibility for his or her life or as an attempt at abdicating responsibility rather than judge these experiences by strictly clinical standards. Attention will be given to the clinical implications of a person's Catholic upbringing and countertransference issues.

REVIEW OF LITERATURE

In reviewing the literature on mental health and Catholicism or on treatment issues and Catholicism, one discovers a paucity of clinical material and research.

References to Catholicism and mental health in the literature, when present, are frequently in the form of observations that supposedly apply to all Catholics. As far back as 1902, James wrote that "Protestantism has been too pessimistic as regards the natural man, Catholicism has been too legalistic and moralistic" (p. 102). According to Bridges and Spilka (1992), Holter reports that Catholic and Jewish women learn roles that their faith states are the lot of the female in life. He found positive correlations between religious commitment among Catholics and Jews and the acceptance of traditional female roles. However, the age, ethnicity, and educational and socioeconomic backgrounds of the women are not factored in.

Jacobs (1992, p. 292) claims that "confession ends the penitent's moral isolation, reducing the effects of alienation on a shamed member of society." However, for some Catholics, depending on the reception they receive from the priest, the experience of confession may increase the sense of shame. Worthen (1974) tries to bridge the gap between psychotherapy and confession but lacks sufficient knowledge of the historical background of the sacrament. She also has unrealistic expectations, especially when she says,

> An even more critical problem is the necessary understanding of those Catholics who choose to use both methods (i.e., psychotherapy and confession), for it requires that the psychotherapist have full knowledge of the Catholic history out of which the client speaks and that the priest have sufficient knowledge of the therapeutic process so that he may guide the client toward the "wholeness" that both Christianity and psychotherapy strive to achieve (p. 276).

It is neither essential nor possible for the therapist to "have full knowledge of the Catholic history out of which the client speaks" nor does the priest need "sufficient knowledge of the therapeutic process." If Worthen was concerned about the patient's splitting, she should have addressed that as an issue. For therapeutic purposes, it may be helpful to understand how the person sees his or her participation in the sacraments and the relationship between a sin and a more diffused sense of guilt which may be more psychological.

The study by Guarnaccia, Patta, Deschamps, Milstein, and Argiles (1992) found that the Roman Catholic Church is the most important social institution in Hispanic communities and that their religious faith is their most important psychological support. Guarnaccia studied the family experience of Hispanics, Afro-Americans and Euro-Americans who were caring for a seriously mentally ill family member. In this group, 62% of the Hispanic families were Catholic and 69% Euro-Americans. The Hispanic families made the greatest use of spiritual help and could use Catholic resources as well as spiritist centers. Based on this study, a therapist treating an Hispanic patient or family could utilize the resources in the community, both those of the church and those of the spiritist centers. Utilizing both is not problematic for Hispanics, whereas it could be in other ethnic groups.

For a clinician, the book which may be the most useful is that by Lovinger (1984). He presents material specific to different religious denominations which is informative but not universalized. Clearly, he studied changes within denominations and uses this knowledge to enrich his understanding of the patient. He addresses central doctrines of the Catholic Church, such as the sacraments, belief in heaven and hell, original sin, and several others from a respectful psychological vantage point and is careful not to generalize.

In a blatant example of inappropriate generalization, Hailparn & Hailparn (1994) treat all Catholics as if they were homogeneous and claim that

> The dynamics of the patient raised in a traditional Catholic mode present a special challenge to the therapist, due to the patient's powerful superego guilt. Thus the Catholic patient can be misunderstood by most therapists for two basic reasons: (1) Much of the training and personal background of therapists is vastly different from that of Catholic patients, and (2) most importantly, the traditional Catholic lives in a very different world from non-Catholics. (p. 271)

The article contains much erroneous information and gives no indication that the author was familiar with any changes in the Church.

As researchers continue their endeavor to study the role of religion and spirituality in relation to mental health, the differences as well as similarities within a particular tradition must be accounted for. Greeley (1977) points to the importance of attending to differences when he says that

> One can be a "devout" Catholic, an "active" Catholic, a "practicing" Catholic, a "marginal" Catholic, or a "disaffiliated" Catholic and one can move back and forth among the various positions along the affiliation continuum. One can be angry at one's Catholic past, ignore it, be militant about it, be fascinated by it or endeavor to forget it completely (although Catholic as a worldview and Catholic as a means of ethnic identity are both acquired very early in the childhood experience and hence, both are very difficult to dispose of). (p. 28)

He goes on to say that "American Catholics are an ethnic group in the general sense of the term, as well as being a group of ethnic groups, in the special use of the work 'ethnic' as meaning descendants of European immigrants" (p. 9).

What follows is based on thousands of hours of clinical experience in working with Catholic patients and on my own personal experience as a Catholic. Both of these have made it evident that there are important differences among Catholics based on age, family, religious formation, education, ethnic background, and socioeconomic level.

EDUCATION AND RELIGIOUS FORMATION

THE ROMAN CATHOLIC EXPERIENCE BEFORE
THE SECOND VATICAN COUNCIL

Education of Children

In 1962, Pope John XXIII convened the Second Vatican Council. This meeting of the highest Church officials was a response to worldwide pressure for change; the results of the Council effected radical changes within the Catholic Church. It was a watershed event whose effects are still being felt within the Church. In particular, Catholics who received all their religious formation before 1965 may continue to live out of their earlier learned experience. What was that experience? As noted previously, it is impossible to generalize. However, some common experiences can be given.

The Catholic Church in the United States has been an immigrant church. What that has meant is that when each new wave of immigrants arrived and settled in neighborhoods with others from their homeland, they set up parochial schools. Because the tuition was minimal, even the poorest children were not excluded. Furthermore, the Church frowned on children going to public schools, so parents and priests made every effort to send their children to a Catholic school.

The minimal tuition in the schools was possible because the schools were staffed by nuns who wore religious habits and who were not paid a salary. Rather, they were supported by the parish; this support varied greatly depending on the financial state of the parish. The educational level of the nuns also varied considerably. Some nuns were only high school graduates with some college preparation, whereas others had college degrees or advanced degrees. Psychological sensitivity was not a characteristic either of the formation of the nuns or of their educational systems. Prior to the 1960s, no required psychological batteries of tests were administered to candidates for religious orders or the priesthood. Consequently, one could find priests and nuns who were not really suited psychologically for religious life or the priesthood. The children in the classroom or parishioners may have experienced the negative effects of adults who were in a vocation for which they were ill suited.

Religious formation especially in grammar school or in Sunday school classes (for those who attended public school) consisted of memorizing the Baltimore Catechism with its question and answer format: "Who made you?: God made me. Why did God make you: God made me to know Him, to love Him, to serve Him in this world and to be happy with Him in the next." There was a certain obsessive–compulsive quality about the educational process, with the teachings presented as lists that one was to memorize—the commandments, the laws of the church, the holy days of obligation, the seven deadly sins, the criteria for venial sins, and the criteria for mortal sins. Exploration, investigation, and questioning of these truths was not the educational mode. The sacraments of the church were foundational to Catholic membership: Baptism, Penance, Eucharist, Confirmation, Matrimony, Ordination, and Extreme Unction. Mass was in Latin and hence incomprehensible to most of the congregation. Catholics were forbidden to attend religious ceremonies of other denominations. Catholic teaching about sexuality was very clear and explicit: Masturbation was a mortal sin, as was sex outside of marriage; artificial birth control was not allowed; and couples could only practice the rhythm method.

The religious content of Catholic education may have been consistent, but the affective quality of a child's experience varied according to the individual instructors who were mostly nuns and a few lay teachers. There are hundreds of Catholic religious orders, and each had its distinctive characteristics. Even within particular orders, differences were possible. Some students could experience rigidity and harshness on the part of some of their teachers, whereas others may have experienced nurturance and understanding (Kehoe & Gutheil, 1993). The same was true of parish priests. Some were rigid and controlling, whereas others were pastoral and compassionate.

Education of Adults

The religious formation of Catholics who did not attend Catholic secondary school or Catholic college ended with elementary school. Any further instruction came principally from the sermons preached at mass on Sundays, which, as a rule, focused on Catholic doctrine and reinforced what had been learned in grammar school. As a result, the religious formation of these Catholics essentially did not develop much beyond an elementary level.

Although Catholics who attended Catholic secondary school and Catholic college had the opportunity to develop their Catholic formation along with their intellectual formation, the process was still within the Catholic context. Some priests discouraged students from attending non-Catholic colleges, suggesting it was sinful. Educational formation that took place solely in Catholic schools resulted in a certain insularity of thought, and fostered stereotypes, because of the lack of interaction with other faiths. When an interfaith marriage occurred, the non-Catholic had to promise that he or she would raise the children within the Catholic faith. A religious education that essentially ended in grammar school or one that may have included high school or college could still be more underdeveloped than other aspects of a person's life. There was, however, a well-articulated and agreed upon paradigm of what it was to be a Catholic. This provided a foundation for life and a solid framework within which to make decisions.

Theological Language, Beliefs, and Assumptions

In this section, I examine some language, beliefs, and possible assumptions that individuals raised in the Catholic tradition would have learned as a matter of course. Later, I consider some clinical implications. I intend only to cite some examples that I have encountered frequently enough in my work to know that they can be problematic.

A pamphlet titled, "Outlines of the Catholic Faith: Teachings, Beliefs, Practices and Prayers" (1978), is readily available in many parishes. Although it was published after the Second Vatican Council, the contents reflect a pre-Vatican II mentality. It is the kind of pamphlet that members of a parish might purchase or that might be used by people under instruction. It claims to provide a summary of the principal teachings of the Church. When describing the first article of the Creed which says, "I believe in God the Father Almighty, Creator of Heaven and Earth," the author expands this by saying that God can accomplish all things: In Him nothing is impossible, and He is all knowing and sees all things. God created all things—the first human beings, the good angels who are in Heaven, and the fallen angels, devils, that are in Hell. Further on there is the statement that when Jesus comes to judge the living and the dead, the evil will be sent to Hell and the just will be taken to Heaven.

The faithful are encouraged to honor the saints in heaven and pray for the faithful who have died. Sin is described as an offense against God in thought, word, desire, deed, or neglect. Sins are divided into two categories, venial and mortal, the former a less serious violation and the latter a serious offense that merits eternal damnation if not repented and forgiven before death. However, mortal sins were not easy to commit; a person had to be in his or her right mind, fully conscious of the seriousness of what was intended, and the deed had to be of a serious nature, such as murder.

Though not mentioned specifically in this pamphlet, other expressions that are frequently used in instruction, by families, or in sermons are the following: "God will provide," "this is the will of God," "God fits the back to the burden," "each person has a guardian angel who protects and guides them," and "God never asks more of us than we can handle."

How, in what circumstances, and at what stage of development an individual hears these messages and learns these truths can have a very different impact (Ventis, 1995). To discover how these affect a person's mental health is the work of the clinician in the context of therapy.

THE ROMAN CATHOLIC EXPERIENCE AFTER
THE SECOND VATICAN COUNCIL

Education of Children

The Second Vatican Council is a convenient reference point for change, though it runs the risk of simplification and fails to recognize the larger sociological changes that were at work in the world during the 1960s. This was an era of dramatic changes on several fronts and the changes within the Catholic Church took place in that context. However, for the purposes of this chapter, I will only focus on how the Second Vatican Council affected Catholics. It was the first Council of the Church in which non-Catholics, as well as lay- and religious people, were present in addition to the Catholic hierarchy. The ordinary Catholic, to this day, probably has never read the original documents from the Council and thinks of it as the event that changed the mass from Latin to the vernacular, that encouraged Church members to see engagement with the world and social justice issues as constitutive elements, that led to major changes for nuns (such as the change from religious habit to regular dress), that made abstinence from meat on Friday no longer an obligation, that made interdenominational marriages easier, and that encouraged dialogue with other religious denominations.

In a period of dramatic change, the consequences of those changes are not immediately perceptible. This was true in regard to Catholic education. Women religious, for a variety of reasons, moved away from teaching in Catholic schools and into new ministries or left religious life. Parochial schools were administered by laymen and women. The Baltimore Catechism was no longer the main tool for communicating Catholic doctrine. Instead, for a while at least, there was very little content in religion classes. The clear paradigm of religious instruction was lost. There was a "culture" of sorts, but it was more a culture of confusion as new modes and meanings concerning a Catholic's self-definition evolved. The mass was in the vernacular. Scripture, human interest stories, and multimedia approaches were used in the classroom. Much of the past was rejected without a clear sense of what should be put in its place. Consequently, Catholics who were children in the years after Vatican II had a very uneven religious formation.

Education of Adults

Greeley (1985) explores various factors that have influenced Catholics since 1964 and suggests that some of these include the Council but also the level of education among Catholics, the change in their economic status, the encyclical on birth control that was written soon after Vatican II, and their identification or lack of identification with a particular parish and particular priest. All these affect how an adult is a Catholic today. While the education of children has been less structured, there have been more possibilities for adult religious formation through courses, retreats, spiritual direction, and renewal programs in parishes.

FAMILY AND ETHNIC CONTEXT

Since Catholic education has been so central to the development of Catholics, I have elaborated on it. However, it is not the sole influence. How Catholicism was practiced, talked about, and lived within a family also affects the person's religious formation. Within the same family or with different families, there may be great variation concerning such things as church attendance, the celebration of certain religious holidays, familiarity with saints, and relationships with members of the clergy. Furthermore, it is not just the nuclear family that shapes the transmission of a religious identity; a generational influence, such as an intermarriage in a prior generation, may have a great impact on how a family thinks about being Catholic. The family's level of education and its socioeconomic status and changes in both areas over the years also play a part in how a person internalizes his or her religious tradition.

Not only the family but also the ethnic context and the neighborhood shape what is learned. It is not possible to talk about being an "American Catholic" without realizing that there are Irish Catholics, German Catholics, Italian Catholics, Slavic Catholics, Polish Catholics, Puerto Rican Catholics, Mexican Catholics, etc. Each ethnic group nuances "Catholicity" in a way that is particular to itself, and even within similar ethnic groups there may be regional differences. The regional differences may be related to the country of origin or the region in the United States in which the family originally settled. There are also generational differences within ethnic groups.

Not all ethnic groups live in tightly formed communities. An Irish Catholic who grew up in a predominantly Jewish neighborhood may be different from an Irish Catholic who grew up in an Irish neighborhood. A Polish Catholic who grew up in a predominantly German Lutheran area may be different from a Polish Catholic who is third generation and lived in a Polish neighborhood all his or her life. There are numerous ways in which family/ethnicity/Catholicism nuance the way in which a person "is" Catholic. The clinician needs to be aware of the possibility of these subtle differences.

CLINICAL IMPLICATIONS

TREATMENT MODALITY

Reference has been made to the Baltimore Catechism and to the question and answer process whereby children were educated prior to 1965. This educational method neither invited exploration nor fostered an inquisitive approach. When a Catholic person begins therapy, the therapist might benefit from learning from the patient the kind of religious instruction he or she received. The therapist can then distinguish for the patient between questions in therapy that are used to invite self-reflection and questions that have "correct answers." A failure to do so might result in unnecessary frustration for both therapist and patient. Kehoe and Gutheil (1984) illustrate the problems that may result when the therapist does not consider how the patient may be hearing his or her questions.

AUTHORITY FIGURES, CHURCH TEACHING, AND INDIVIDUAL RESPONSIBILITY

"Every living soul has to come to terms with authority, power, and responsibility. These three categories are charged with affect; they are integral to religion and conversely religions have a good deal to say about them" (Pruyser, 1968, p. 262). Pruyser refers to religion in general, not any particular denomination. It is not just Catholics who have issues with authority figures and personal responsibility. However, given the very explicit and clear doctrines and the pronouncements of Catholic Church leaders, Catholics may struggle with authority and personal responsibility in ways that have been shaped by their experience of being Catholic. Yet, Vatican Council II, the birth control issue, the increased role of the laity in the local parish, and the opportunities for higher education all have potentially altered the way adult men and women in the Church view authority figures who were raised after the 1960s. Therefore, the age of the person in therapy and his or her religious formation may affect the way he or she views the therapist and the issue of personal responsibility. As with all patients, this needs to be explored.

The therapist does the patient a disservice by assuming anything. That is a major problem in the Hailparn and Hailparn (1994, p. 277) article. The authors, in exploring the implications for psychotherapy with a Catholic patient, state, "Foremost is the unique role of the therapist. Unlike usual analysis which focuses on projected transference, here a direct attack on the superego is vital. The old superego must be minimized and a new, accepting one put in its place." They proceed to state that "we, as therapists must 'exorcise' the punitive superego and replace it with a loving, accepting one" (p. 279). That is a powerful authoritarian position and is not seen as a possible reenactment.

FANTASIES AND SINS

Another area to explore that has implications for treatment with a person with a Catholic formation is that of fantasy. The "Confiteor," a prayer which is frequently said at the beginning of the mass, contains the phrase "I have sinned exceedingly in thought, word, and deed." That is a problematic expression because it includes a person's inner world as well as his or her actions, words, and deeds. As it is frequently said, many people undoubtedly do not attend to the words they are saying or may not even mean them. However, for a scrupulous person or for an obsessive–compulsive person, those words can have damaging effects.

In preparing young children for their first confession and in the review one is to make before each subsequent confession, one considers whether he or she has sinned in thought, word, or deed. A distinction between spontaneous thoughts, desires, or fantasies and willful thoughts, desires, or fantasies that were entertained with the concomitant desire to carry them out was not made. A murderous wish that is a response to being hurt is different from a carefully thought out, intentionally willed desire to kill someone or to seriously harm a person. Rather than exploring the significance of certain thoughts, religious formation often suggested a judgment about them and then a sense of guilt for having them. Hence, many individuals experience both pain and confusion about the meaning of "sinning in thought, word, and deed."

When the therapist asks the person about his or her fantasies, the patient might understand it as "tell me what you have done wrong" or "tell me your sins." Sexual fantasies, angry feelings, envious feelings, etc., may be perceived by the patient as sins. Resistance then may ensue based on a sense of shame and guilt, but the resistance may be misinterpreted by the therapist who is ignorant of the patient's Catholic formation. Some further exploration may be useful, thus enabling a person to distinguish how he or she decides what is harmful/sinful and what is not.

RELIGIOUS MESSAGES AND LANGUAGE

Earlier, I referred to some religious messages that were taught in schools, in families, or preached from the altar. When a patient talks about hell or the fear of being punished in hell, or angels that protect him or her, that does not mean the person is psychotic. It also does not rule it out. However, it is crucial for the therapist to know that Catholic teaching includes the concept of hell and the devil as well as heaven and angels. What a person associates with these beliefs and how they see themselves in relation to them need to be investigated but they do not necessarily mean that the person is delusional.

When a child hears at the age of 4 and later that God can do all things, that in Him nothing is impossible, and that He is all knowing and all seeing, the child's imagination can conjure up all sorts of fantasies and desires about what this Being can do. The meaning of that concept or others like it was not always reframed and rethought at other developmental stages. Since religious education and formation for many people ended with grammar school, high school, or possibly college, many earlier messages were not reexamined.

An example of these conflictual messages is the following: A young girl is abused by her father but has been told by the nuns that she has a guardian angel who protects her. This child then might wonder if perhaps she does not have a guardian angel. Did she do something to lose her angel? Were the nuns lying? What does "protect" mean?

When children in an alcoholic family who are told or hear at church that "God provides" or "that everything that happens to us is God's will" or "that God is all powerful," what are they to conclude? What does God provide? What kind of a God would will such pain? If God is all powerful, why doesn't God change the alcoholic parent? If God is all powerful, why doesn't He cure my mother who is dying? Individuals can live many years with the inner conflicts that relate to these messages. By exploring both a person's religious formation and the wishes and fantasies attached to what they have learned, the clinician can help the person to rethink them from a different developmental perspective.

In this section, I have focused more on issues that relate to a person's religious formation before the mid-1960s. The absence of such a clear paradigm after the 1960s may have its own problems but makes it more difficult to point to specific formation that may impact treatment.

COUNTERTRANSFERENCE ISSUES

If Greeley (1985, p. 7) is correct in saying that "no one is without personal biases or opinions when the subject is Catholicism," then therapists need to be attentive to their countertransference issues. These will differ for the therapist who may have been raised in a Catholic tradition, either before or after the 1960s, in contrast to the therapist who was not and whose knowledge of Catholicism comes either from the media or from people he has known.

Whether the therapist is or is not still affiliated with his or her Catholic tradition, what prompted the disaffiliation, the religious formation of the therapist, the ethnic background, and the person's family experience all may contribute to possible countertransference difficulties. Because of the wide divergence within the Catholic Church today, a therapist who continues to be affiliated with the Church may react very strongly to a person whose interpretation of certain beliefs or attitudes toward authority figures differs from that of the therapist. The assumption that the therapist will understand the patient if he or she shares the same religious background may also be problematic because it inhibits the exploration of what the patient's experience has been.

As noted in my earlier review of literature, not much has been written about patients who are Catholic and issues for their treatment. In the absence of such material, the article by Hailparn and Hailparn (1994) is potentially more detrimental. The article does highlight, however, the fact that such perceptions exist and may influence uninformed therapists. Supervision and consultation may be useful in order to address any countertransference issues that a therapist might have in working with patients who are Catholic.

CONSULTATION AND REFERRALS

Therapists cannot and need not have extensive knowledge about various ethnic groups or various religious denominations. In order to understand what is a norm within the community, a consultation with someone from the ethnic group may be useful. This prevents the therapist from making erroneous diagnostic judgments. Except in the case of cults, the community is usually the norm for what may be deemed healthy or not. Also, in working with someone from a particular religious denomination, at times it may be useful to consult with someone within the same religious community.

For Catholics who value the sacrament of Reconciliation, formerly referred to as Penance, a therapist might raise the question whether a person would benefit from talking to a priest, particularly in cases in which the person has been estranged from the Church. Knowing that there have been changes in the Church in the past 25 years may help someone who is burdened by guilt but who has not been connected with the Church due to a "sin" that may have occurred years ago.

CONCLUSION

Rizzuto (1993) states that,

> The undeniable fact that all people have their own sacred landscapes as explicit or implicit context for their lives has been ignored by clinicians. Many patients undergo lengthy psychotherapeutic treatments without ever attending to the beliefs coloring the background of their experiences. (p. 16)

As we have seen, a person raised with a Catholic formation may possess many beliefs that are supportive to him or her or that are a source of pain and conflict. Although I have attended to those beliefs and messages which in my experience have caused individuals the most difficulty as they work toward their own healing, there are other beliefs and messages that are a source of enormous comfort for people.

A growing body of research indicates that there is evidence that religion has positive effects on mental health. However, this relationship will only be known in the context of treatment as therapists become more at ease with the respectful exploration of religious material. Information, such as that provided in this chapter, is only one resource needed for this exploration. More important is the attitude of respect and curiosity for all that has shaped an individual life.

REFERENCES

Anonymous. (1978). *Outlines of the Catholic faith: Teachings, beliefs, practices, prayers.* MN: Leaflet Missal.

Bhugra, D. (Ed.). (1996). *Psychiatry and religion: Context, consensus and controversies.* London: Routledge.

Bridges, R., & Spilka, B. (1992). Religion and the mental health of women. In J. F. Schumaker (Ed.), *Religion and mental health* (pp. 43–53). New York: Oxford University Press.

Greeley, A. M. (1977). *The American Catholic: A social portrait.* New York: Basic Books.

Greeley, A. M. (1985). *American Catholics since the council: An unauthorized report.* Chicago: Thomas More.

Guarnaccia, P. J., & Parra, P. (1996). Ethnicity, social status and families' experiences of caring for a mentally ill family member. *Community Mental Health Journal, 32*(3), 243–260.

Guarnaccia, P. J., Parra, P., Deschamps, A., Milstein, G., & Argiles, N. (1992). Si Dios quiere: Hispanic families' experiences of caring for a seriously mentally ill family member. *Culture, Medicine and Psychiatry, 16*(2), 187–215.

Jacobs, J. (1992). Religious ritual and mental health. In J. F. Schumaker (Ed.), *Religion and mental health* (pp. 291–299). New York: Oxford University Press.

James, W. (1958). *The varieties of religious experience.* NJ: New American Library.

Kehoe, N., & Gutheil, T. (1984). Shared religious belief as resistance in psychotherapy. *American Journal of Psychotherapy, 38*(4), 579–585.

Kehoe, N., & Gutheil, T. (1993). Ministry or therapy: The role of transference and countertransference in a religious therapist. In M. L. Randour (Ed.), *Exploring sacred landscapes* (pp. 55–80). New York: Columbia University Press.

Koenig, H. G. (1995). *Research on religion and aging.* Westport, CT: Greenwood.

Koenig, H. G. (1997). *Is religion good for your health: The effects of religion on physical and mental health.* New York: Haworth.

Lovinger, R. (1984). *Working with religious issues in therapy.* New York: Jason Aronson.

Pruyser, P. W. (1968). *A dynamic psychology of religion.* New York: Harper & Row.

Rack, P. (1982). *Race, culture, and mental disorder.* London: Tavistock.

Rizzuto, A. (1993). Exploring sacred landscapes. In M. L. Randour (Ed.), *Exploring sacred landscapes* (pp. 16–33). New York: Columbia University Press.

Spero, M. H. (Ed.). (1985). *Psychotherapy of the religious patient.* Charles C Thomas: Springfield, IL.

Stern, M. (Ed.). (1985). *Psychotherapy and the religiously committed patient.* New York: Haworth.

Ventis, W. L. (1995). The relationships between religion and mental health. *Journal of Social Issues, 51*(2), 33–48.

Walsh, J. (1995). The impact of schizophrenia on clients' religious beliefs: Implications for families. *Families in Society: The Journal of Contemporary Human Services, 76*(9), 551–558.

Worthen, V. (1974). Psychotherapy and Catholic confession. *Journal of Religion and Health, 13*(4), 275–284.

15

RELIGION AND MENTAL HEALTH FROM THE MORMON PERSPECTIVE

SALLY H. BARLOW AND ALLEN E. BERGIN

Department of Psychology
Brigham Young University
Provo, Utah 84602

THE CHURCH OF JESUS CHRIST OF LATTER-DAY SAINTS

In 1997, members of the Church of Jesus Christ of Latter-Day Saints (LDS or Mormons) celebrated the sesquicentennial of the arrival of their pioneer predecessors in the valley of the Great Salt Lake in 1847, then part of Mexico. While this celebration received favorable worldwide publicity and reflected, generally, the successful settlement of the west by LDS pioneers, it had been preceded by persistent persecution that forced the newly formed church, officially established in April 6, 1830, to relocate from New York to Ohio, Missouri, Illinois, and to the barren lands of what eventually became the state of Utah. These intense persecutions included an extermination order by Missouri Governor Boggs, routine looting, property confiscation, and the eventual assassination of their prophet, Joseph Smith, in June 1844, at the age of 38. Smith had offended many by (i) his insistence that he had witnessed a vision of God the Father and Jesus Christ, in which extant religions were declared to be apostate; (ii) his claim to have received from an angel the *Book of Mormon,* which contained a record of Israelites in the Americas, including a visitation to them by the resurrected Christ; (iii) his communal church organization headed by a restored apostolic priesthood which differed from traditional church organizations by claiming direct modern authority from God; (iv) his emphasis on a patriarchal family model including Old Testament-style plural marriage for some; (v) his declaration that Zion, or the Kingdom of God, was being reestablished through him in preparation for the second coming of Jesus Christ; (vi) his success in gathering converts from America and Europe and establishing a major new city in Illinois (Nauvoo, population 12000–15000, 1845, about the same as Chicago at that time) with a growing political power and its own militia; and (vii) his declaring himself a candidate for the President of the United States in the election of 1844. This boldness eventually cost him his life. His followers were faced with giving up their faith or being murdered. They chose a third alternative: migration into the wilderness under the leadership of their successor prophet, Brigham Young (for a more complete history, see Allen & Leonard, 1976; Arrington & Bitton, 1979).

This Mormon diaspora was fraught with difficulties including continued hardship, disease, and death over a period of years as refugees and new converts from eastern states and Europe made their way west in covered wagons and handcarts from 1847 to 1869, when the transcontinental railroad made the arduous western trails obsolete. About 80,000 pioneers made the trek, but 6000 died in route to their "promised land" in the valleys of the Wasatch Mountains, the westward front of the Rockies. From their capital in Salt Lake City under the leadership of Brigham Young, they were organized into new waves of pioneers who established nearly 400 communities in a vast territory that is now divided into eight states. In the words of the Pulitzer prize winning author, Wallace Stegner, a Western chronicler (1964),

> The Mormon migration was . . . the permanent hegira of a whole people—grandparents, parents, children, flocks, herds, household goods and gods. . . . They were literally villages on the march, villages of sobriety, solidarity and discipline unheard of anywhere else on the western trails. (p. 11)

> They were the most . . . successful pioneers in our history. . . . The Mormons moved like the Host of Israel. (p. 6)

After this region became part of the United States in 1848, the United States organized the Territory of Utah and sent agents of the government to monitor affairs therein. Conflicts between Washington and Utah ensued over many issues for the next 48 years. For instance, the federal government confiscated lands and incarcerated many of the males involved in polygamy, even sending an army to quell the "Mormon rebellion" in 1857. This governmental campaign did not abate until the church rescinded the policy of plural marriage and Utah was able to apply for statehood, which was granted in 1896.

The pioneers and their progeny eventually became a prosperous, well-educated people, no longer driven by persecution toward separatism. With 5 million members in the United States, the LDS church is one of America's largest and increasingly influential denominations. An additional 5 million members distributed in 159 nations and territories make its growth a phenomenon of note. Rodney Stark, Professor of Sociology and Religion at the University of Washington, has predicted, based on a demographic and statistical profile, that Mormonism will emerge during the twenty-first century as the next major world religion. Stark (1994) notes, "After a hiatus of fourteen hundred years [since Mohammed], in our

TABLE 15.1   Geographic Distribution of LDS Church Membership in North America

State/province	No. of members	State/province	No. of members
Utah	1,484,000	Tennessee	27,000
Mexico	728,000	British Columbia	26,000
California	726,000	Alabama	25,000
Idaho	327,000	Alaska	24,000
Arizona	271,000	Louisiana	24,000
Washington	211,000	South Carolina	24,000
Texas	182,000	Kansas	22,000
Oregon	126,000	Kentucky	21,000
Nevada	124,000	Minnesota	20,000
Colorado	101,000	New Jersey	19,000
Florida	98,000	Arkansas	17,000
Virginia	61,000	Massachusetts	16,000
Alberta	60,000	Wisconsin	16,000
Hawaii	55,000	Nebraska	15,000
Wyoming	54,000	Mississippi	15,000
New Mexico	54,000	Iowa	14,000
Georgia	51,000	Connecticut	11,000
North Carolina	51,000	West Virginia	11,000
New York	49,000	<10,000: DC, DE, MB, ME, NB, ND, NH, NS, PQ, RI,	
Ohio	43,000	SD, SK, VT	
Illinois	43,000		
Missouri	43,000	Approximate USA membership by regions	
Montana	39,000	(in millions)	
Ontario	34,000	West (15 states in Mountain, Pacific,	4.0
Pennsylvania	33,000	and Southwest areas)	
Michigan	33,000	South (14 southeastern states)	0.5
Oklahoma	31,000	Midwest (11 Midwest & plains states)	0.3
Maryland	30,000	East (10 mid-Atlantic & New England states)	0.2
Indiana	30,000	Total	5.0

Note. Statistics in rounded number from *Deseret News 1997–1998 Church Almanac,* Deseret News, Salt Lake City (1998).

time a new world faith seems to be stirring" (p. 22). It may be helpful for clinicians to be aware of how the Mormon population is distributed in North America (Table 15.1).

DOCTRINE, CULTURE, AND HEALTH STATUS

While Mormons, or Latter-Day Saints as they prefer to be called, are generally viewed positively by outsiders, there is still some residual apprehension on the part of both parties as members have moved from minority status to the mainstream. Outsiders base this on a perception of Mormons as unorthodox in several doctrines and practices that place them outside the traditional Christian community. Though Mormons are no longer considered a people with horns and many wives, they do evoke curiosity about the ceremonies conducted in "members-only" temples, their strict moral code, their seeming insular self-sufficiency, and their aggressive missionary program with its 60,000 missionaries in more than 150 countries who include other Christians among their proselytes. Latter-Day Saints are also known for their specific health code titled the "Word of Wisdom," which prohibits tobacco, alcohol, tea, and coffee and encourages good nutrition and other health habits.

Aside from the beliefs already noted, other views set Latter-Day Saints apart from Protestants and Catholics, including the doctrine of eternal progression (humans have the potential to become Godlike), revelation (a modern-day prophet), the repudiation of the doctrine of original sin (humans are responsible for their own sins and not for Adam and Eve's transgression), and the Godhead as three distinct personages who are one in purpose but not in substance. Mormons believe that humans were born in a premortal existence as spirit offspring of a Mother and Father in Heaven and that they are on an eternal journey that includes (i) preexistence, where a war in heaven had been fought to support God's plan of agency; (ii) mortal existence, the purpose of which is to gain a physical body and learn obedience to God's laws through trials and tribulations; and (iii) exaltation, once the mortal test has been passed successfully, one may live with God. Mormon scripture depicts this afterlife as divided into three levels of glory depending on the extent of ones faithfulness as well as a region of outer darkness where Satan, a literal spiritual being, and his followers are cast off forever.

Another distinction is the Mormon Temple, which is not used for weekly church services but is considered a holy place where only LDS members who have been certified worthy by their local bishops may enter. There, priesthood sealings occur of couples and families for "time and all eternity" in a "new and everlasting covenant" as do endowment ceremonies, which, through ordinances and covenants, guide one toward eternal life and exaltation. Such rites, including baptisms, are also performed vicariously for deceased persons who had no opportunity during mortal life to participate in these "savings" ordinances. The work for the dead is a unique, and some say "peculiar" Mormon practice which is based on the world's most extensive collection of genealogical records of the human family.

Some of these notions are foreign to other religions, even Christianity. In fact, one criticism of Mormonism made by other Christian denominations is that Mormons are not Christians. However, major doctrines do parallel other Christian faiths, central of which is that Jesus Christ is the savior of humankind, as do other doctrines, such as the importance of repentance, salvation by the grace of God and our own works, baptism (this occurs at the age of 8 and includes complete immersion), free will or agency, and some liturgy, though this is limited to two specific sacramental prayers during Sunday church service as well as specific ceremonies that take place in temples. A complete review of doctrinal issues is beyond

TABLE 15.2   The Articles of Faith of the Church of Jesus Christ of Latter-Day Saints

---

We believe in God, the Eternal Father, and in His Son, Jesus Christ, and in the Holy Ghost.

We believe that men will be punished for their own sins, and not for Adam's transgression.

We believe that through the Atonement of Christ, all mankind may be saved, by obedience to the laws and ordinances of the Gospel.

We believe that the first principles and ordinances of the Gospel are: first, Faith in the Lord Jesus Christ; second, Repentance; third, Baptism by immersion for the remission of sins; fourth, Laying on of hands for the gift of the Holy Ghost.

We believe that a man must be called of God, by prophecy, and by the laying on of hands, by those who are in authority to preach the Gospel and administer in the ordinances thereof.

We believe in the same organization that existed in the Primitive Church, viz., apostles, prophets, pastors, teachers, evangelists, etc.

We believe in the gift of tongues, prophecy, revelation, visions, healing, interpretation of tongues, etc.

We believe the Bible to be the word of God as far as it is translated correctly; we also believe the Book of Mormon to be the word of God.

We believe all that God has revealed, all that He does now reveal, and we believe that He will yet reveal many great and important things pertaining to the Kingdom of God.

We believe in the literal gathering of Israel and in the restoration of the Ten Tribes; that Zion will be built upon this [the American] continent; that Christ will reign personally upon the earth; and, that the earth will be renewed and receive its paradisiacal glory.

We claim the privilege of worshiping Almighty God according to the dictates of our own conscience, and allow all men the same privilege, let them worship how, where, or what they may.

We believe in being subject to kings, presidents, rulers, and magistrates, in obeying, honoring, and sustaining the law.

We believe in being honest, true, chaste, benevolent, virtuous, and in doing good to all men; indeed, we may say that we follow the admonition of Paul—We believe all things, we hope all things, we have endured many things, and hope to be able to endure all things. If there is anything virtuous, lovely, or of good report or praiseworthy, we seek after these things.

—Joseph Smith

---

the scope of this chapter. A succinct description of LDS belief can be found in the Articles of Faith (see Table 15.2). An in-depth coverage of LDS belief can be found in Talmage's *Articles of Faith* (1984) and in LDS scriptures (the Bible, King James Version, with inspired emendations by Joseph Smith; *The Book of Mormon: Another Testament of Jesus Christ; The Doctrine and Covenants*—revelations to Joseph Smith and his prophetic successors; and *The Pearl of Great Price*—inspired addition to the Old Testament writings and prophesies of Moses, Abraham, and Enoch (all available from the church-owned Deseret Book Co., P.O. Box 30178, Salt Lake City, UT 84130).

A general overview of statistics suggests that the Mormon health codes do tend to benefit the Mormon population both emotionally (Bergin, Payne, Jenkins, & Cornwall, 1994) and physically (Bahr, 1994; Lyon & Nelson, 1979). Mormons have strikingly lower rates of cancer (Lyon & Nelson, 1979), including predictable ones (those related to smoking and sexual promiscuity) and those not predictable (liver and kidney). A comprehensive description of the entire subculture is available in the definitive *Encyclopedia of Mormonism* (Ludlow, 1992).

While most researchers note the limited sample size, most data on Utahns (Utah is 70% Mormon) suggest, when compared with national base rates, "real" rates of mental illness are lower, suicide rates are just slightly above the national average and just below the average for the mountain states, alcohol and drug use is significantly below national averages, and divorce statistics are near the national average (Bergin et al., 1994, p. 141). When active LDS are separated out from these broad statewide statistics, the physical and mental health benefits are more striking. Bergin and colleagues also note that on standard personality measures, Mormons do not differ significantly from normative groups or other mainstream religious samples and suggest that variables other than religious preference may be better predictors of negative or positive traits. However, as Bergin cautions, ambiguities remain in a comprehensive understanding of the Mormon experience. In addition, he acknowledges that Mormonism, like other religious cultures that are strict, orthodox, and demanding of high expectations, can set the stage for disturbances in certain kinds of vulnerable individuals. His in-depth case studies may shed light on this in the future. Most notable about this research is the attention to how people are religious rather than whether they are religious.

Certainly, apparent differences do exist between the Mormon and non-Mormon community. Some of these are a result of the previously discussed doctrinal beliefs. A strong doctrinal emphasis on eternal progression appears to influence Mormons' beliefs about education. In comparison to national survey data, Mormon samples show a strong positive correlation between level of education and religiosity, which is quite different from the general trend in America which suggests that the more education one has, the less likely he or she might be to practice religion. Other differences may be a result of practices that are an outgrowth of local cultural phenomena that occurred during the church's initial expansion along the Wasatch Front (a concentration of members in and around Salt Lake City) and are applicable mostly to that geographic area (Cornwall, Heaton, & Young, 1994).

A study comparing Utah Catholics, Protestants, Mormons, and nonaffiliates showed Utah Mormons to be highest on all indicators of religiosity (self-definition, church attendance, tithing paid, and private family prayer). Parenthetically, non-Utah Mormons have been known to eschew this "hyperreligiosity" and occasionally denigrate Utah Mormons as a group, saying it is better to be a practicing Mormon in the "mission field" (anywhere outside of Utah). Overall, however, active Mormons (in Utah and outside of Utah) are similar to each other in behaviors and attitudes, and recent sociological data, collected nationally, suggest that on a number of indicators Mormon families are generally like other mainstream religious families (cohesive and relatively egalitarian in structure).

MINORITY PSYCHOLOGY
AND CULTURAL CONFLICT

Despite successes as an institution, wealth, representation in congress, and growing diversity in race, ethnicity, and national origin, a strong residue of "outsider" feeling continues to exist within the main core of the LDS population in the United States. There is a degree of suspicion between Mormon adherents and their neighbors. This has been reinforced by a small but constant and vocal anti-Mormon sentiment, especially among the more fundamentalist Protestant groups who continue to publish inaccurate, sometimes bizarre, caricatures of Mormon doctrine, practice, and people. As a consequence, there is a degree of guardedness and anticipated rejection that is also common among all minority groups in America. Clinically this is manifested in the care with which mental health providers are selected by church members: "Can they be trusted to understand?" "Is my conservative lifestyle going to be threatened?" and "Will my beliefs be respected?" Although there is no corroborating evidence, it is our impression that Mormons prefer counselors of their own religion or others known to be supportive. In the intermountain west, where there is a strong concentration of LDS people, mental health services appear to be utilized at the usual rate. According to limited research, these therapists use a wide variety of spiritual interventions in their professional therapeutic work consistent with that of therapists from other Christian denominations (Richards & Potts, 1995), but in many urban areas where Mormons are a distinct minority and fewer LDS therapists are available, psychological services appear to be underutilized by Mormons, similar to other minorities (Sue, Zane, & Young, 1994), for fear that their faith will be undermined. This is not altogether based in fiction because many religious people, not just LDS, who were seeking mental health services in the 1970s and 1980s were sometimes encouraged, for instance, to solve sexual inhibition by "having an affair" or anxiousness by "having a glass of wine." These therapeutic "solutions," perceived as coming from an agnostic or amoral profession, further galvanized the church leadership as well as its members against non-LDS mental health professionals.

FOCUS ON THE FAMILY

Christian psychologist James Dobson's famous "Focus on the Family" endorses values and commitments that are virtually identical with those central to Mormon theology and practice. Mormons perhaps go even a step further than Dobson and other religions in asserting that righteous families will be bound together eternally. In Mormon temples, couples are "sealed together for time and all eternity."

This strong family focus can be therapeutic in its supportive, loving network that spreads out to other extended family as well as congregation families. Within these families there is a strong inculcation of morals (including prohibition against sex outside of the marriage covenant, abortion, same-gender sexual relationships, and drugs; and an instillation of values of self-control, hard work, service, and self-sacrifice). Understandably, this strength can have unintended consequences as the inculcation occasionally turns to an unhealthy indoctrination that isolates family members who do not believe or who do not participate fully in the carefully prescribed levels of activity. These activities include lifetime commitments that move from the youth organization, Primary, to priesthood for males and comparable organizations for females.

There has also been an emphasis on having large families, and the Utah birthrate is the highest in the nation. This results in extensive kinship networks, huge family reunions, and extensive genealogical studies, all of which can enhance cohesion, belonging, sense of community, and secure social identity. Thus, generally, this family focus appears to create healthy networks for most. The counterpart to this is that large families and complex social networks can also create interpersonal stresses and difficulties in managing the care of children, especially as more couples feel the need to work outside of the home. Such problems as divorce, drug use, teen delinquency and pregnancy, and domestic abuse, once low, are on the rise. The family has become a target for social distress, and marriage and family problems are the number one reason for self and bishop referral to LDS Social Services, the Mormon social service agency.

THE SOCIAL SYSTEM

The LDS church is organized exclusively as a lay church, and there is no paid ministry. Participation by males and females at all ages throughout the lifetime is built into daily life through a number of organizations and programs. In addition to the priesthood ordination at predictable stages if worthy (beginning at age 12), males generally become involved in scouting and other youth programs; girls are involved in a young women's program that includes moral instruction, personal growth, camping, and sports; and both are often involved in seminary (religion classes often attended before regular school) and in regular family home evening (Monday night events generally held within families for the purpose of instruction and fun). These are in addition to weekly sunday school and sacrament meetings (communion service). Adult males and females routinely visit each other and families monthly as home teachers and visiting teachers, respectively. Under the instruction of this particular program, ideally, every ward (congregation) member is visited monthly. This highly structured, daily practice of their religion leaves many adults socially and emotionally fulfilled via a strong sense of order, cohesion, and stability in what might appear to be a transitory world. However, the problems inherent in such organization also cause some concern. These include those members who do not like such daily activity or experience the expectation to serve their "brothers and sisters" as a burden. In addition, given the strong sense of community that attends such routine activities, isolation (self-imposed or other imposed for a number of reasons, such as lifestyle deviations, morality infractions, or excommunication) leads to many of the problems for which members seek help from therapists.

While the ethic to participate and serve dominates the cultural system of Mormons and is represented in a number of successful programs worldwide, including the church's welfare system, humanitarian aid, service missions, and Deseret Industries (jobs for the poor and disabled), the overall focus on service also has its drawback if a person is unable to mobilize himself or herself to help through depression, introversion, or aversion to such activity.

HUMAN DEVELOPMENT ANCHORED IN THE SPIRITUAL DIMENSION

With all the previously discussed programs, service aims, lifetime involvement, moral standards, family ties, and theologically based aspirations, an individual's identity is considered to be both socially linked and eternal. All these programs and activities are aimed at human development that aspires eventually to nothing less than becoming more Godlike inwardly and in conduct, for "Who shall ascend into the hill of the Lord, or who shall stand in his holy place? He that hath clean hands and a pure heart." (Psalms 24:3–4). The ideal process involves the interplay of individual and group identity, instilling such attributes as faith, unselfishness, love, patience, and humility. Problematic by-products of this include isolation for those who feel disenfranchised or the opposite—an oversubscription to activity by those who robotically step through each rite of passage (e.g., advancement to the priesthood, mission, and marriage in the temple) without genuine reflection on and consequent development of intrinsic religiosity.

THE SPECIAL ISSUES OF WOMEN AND UNMARRIED MEMBERS

LDS females are not ordained to the priesthood, in contrast to a number of Christian organizations starting with the Methodists in the 1950s. The priesthood authority is considered the most important key restored through Joseph Smith. Women participate in the blessings of the priesthood through marriage, and within the church many women are puzzled by outsiders' claims that they are second-class citizens. Their specific organization, The Relief Society, one of the oldest and largest women's organizations in the world, is a strong auxiliary arm of the church that focuses on service to a number of groups both within and outside the church. However, some women may feel disenfranchised if they view priesthood ordination as the only route to God or if they feel badly that they must "go through my husband" (or father, etc.) to enjoy the benefits of the priesthood. Single women may be particularly at risk for feelings of isolation. Criticisms of dogmatic patriarchy (leveled at other Christian religions as well; see Ruether, 1983) certainly exist in the LDS church, even though there is a strong injunction against such "unrighteous dominion."

LDS and other religions are struggling to free themselves from a historical patriarchy that evoked an exclusively male language and consequently implied and often enforced a notion of lopsided redemption. These practices have been embedded in thousands of years of male-dominated society. However, the LDS belief that Joseph Smith restored the fullness of the Gospel, including Christ's unmatched and exquisite sense of equity, encourages LDS females and males to view ordination to the priesthood as an issue of division of labor and order rather than exclusivity. A vast network of priesthood availability from a father's blessing to home teacher visits and other ward and stake leaders ideally create for all members the "Priesthood of all believers" written of by John (Revelations 20:6) in the New Testament that is for the purpose of blessing the lives of all members. Indeed, the current LDS male priesthood ethic is to serve rather than to dominate as in Mark 10:44–45: "And whosoever of you will be the chiefest, shall be servant of all. For even the Son of man came not to be ministered unto, but to minister, and to give his life a ransom for many."

The role of women is valued and consistently supported by church leaders (Hinckley, 1996) who remind LDS women that the role of mother is essential and eternal. As Stegner (1964) states, "That I do not accept the faith that possessed them does not mean I doubt their frequent devotion and heroism in its service, especially their women. Their women were incredible" (p. 13). LDS church leaders have also consciously increased their support of childless women by reminding them that if they are unable to have children in this life, they may be entitled to do so in the next one.

Another area of concern involves what has been referred to by some as being "unmarried in a married church." Certainly not all adults are married, but the strong emphasis on family and marriage creates a potential for isolation in those members who have never married or are divorced or widowed. Many ward and "stake" (several wards) activities are organized for couples. As the church grows larger and the possible number of unmarried members increases, LDS leaders are paying particular attention to the programs that unwittingly promote such disenfranchisement by developing activities for all members that emphasize participation around principles of the Gospel of Christ and not narrow particularities of stereotyped membership.

PARTICULAR PSYCHOPATHOLOGIES POSSIBLY INFLUENCED BY MORMON CULTURE

As Carbo and Gartner (1994) point out, certain pathologies of religious culture can maintain individual psychopathologies, though as Moench (1985) suggests, "Mormon religion does not predispose one to psychopathology . . . but just as one's personality traits become exaggerated under stress and illness, what is already important to one may become the focus or matrix upon which one's symptoms become evident" (p. 64). Moench states that the following factors in the Mormon orientation may contribute to this matrix:

1. Evangelism: The active missionary effort often appeals to the dissatisfied seeking a better life, which may include "passive-dependent personalities, people ostracized from their social group, or those with a narcissistic bent for the limelight" (p. 64).

2. Trust in miracles, mistrust in medicine: Members who have genuine emotional or physical illnesses may needlessly bypass medical care in lieu of priesthood blessings.

3. Spirituality or supernaturalism: These can lead to superstition, wishful or even magical thinking rather than the mature development of faith.

4. Authoritarianism: The expectations of obedience that accompany authority can sometimes induce a number of unhealthy responses in the membership, including passive-aggressiveness, obsessive-compulsiveness, and inappropriate guilt.

5. Inflexibility: Mormon doctrine answers a number of questions about life left unanswered by the majority of religions. This sometimes leads some members to develop an inability to deal with the "mysteries of the kingdom," insisting on a black-and-white problem-solving style that inhibits healthy flexibility and tolerance for ambiguity. Richards and Bergin (1997) have published an outline of seven possible ways of being religiously unhealthy contrasted with seven healthy counterparts. These guidelines, presented in Table 15.3, expand upon the commentary by Moench and are intended to aid clinicians who work with religious clients, Mormon or otherwise. They can be used as a guide for both diagnostic and psychotherapy interviews.

In addition to challenging the inappropriate appropriation of certain religious beliefs, therapists must also challenge the creed of such religious subcultures which may be reinforcing, directly or indirectly, a resistance to mental healthiness. For instance, busyness is often instigated and maintained by a ward or stake or churchwide ethic that has built up over the years to show who is most "anxiously engaged in a good cause." Over the years, through General Conference talks (held semiannually in the Tabernacle on Temple Square and broadcast internationally) Mormons have been admonished to participate in a number of activities above and beyond their regular church callings and weekly attendance at several hours of meetings. These include but are not limited to food storage, gardening, parenting (often large families), community service, scripture reading, exercising, genealogy, keeping a journal, family home evening, and developing individual talents. Excessive subscriptions to keeping busy can preclude the development of an emotional, contemplative inner life necessary to the maintenance of good mental health and intrinsic religiosity.

Therapists also need to examine their own countertransference reactions to certain "tight" religious communities that can, at times, parallel the dynamics of incestuous families: Rigid distinctions between insiders/outsiders reinforce the idea

TABLE 15.3   Religious–Spiritual Values, Lifestyles, and Mental Health:
An Interview and Assessment Guide

Adaptive—healthy values and lifestyles	Maladaptive—unhealthy values and lifestyles
1.A. Intrinsic	1.B. Extrinsic
● Sincere	● Role-playing
● Congruent	● Incongruent
● Lives religion	● Uses religion
● Personal faith	● Normative faith
2.A. Actualizing	2.B. Perfectionistic
● Growth-oriented	● Righteous performances
● Self-regulated agency	● Overcontrolled inefficacy
● Experiential–creative	● Ritualistic–stagnant
● Self-renewing–repentant	● Self-punitive–depressed
● Integrates ambiguity and paradox	● Anxious about the unanticipated
3.A. Reforming–renewing	3.B. Authoritarian
● Change-oriented	● Rigid
● Benevolent–reforming power	● Dogmatic–absolutistic
● Tolerant	● Intolerant–prejudiced
● Egalitarian	● Controlling–dominating
4.A. Interpersonal–social orientation	4.B. Narcissistic
● Networking–familial–kinship	● Self-aggrandizing
● Cooperative	● Competitive
● Open–authentic–integrity	● Manipulation–deception
● Self-sacrificing	● Self-gratifying
5.A. Nurturing	5.B. Aggressive
● Tender–protective	● Angry–abusive–violent
● Warm–faithful–intimate	● Antisocial–unfaithful
● Caring	● Sadistic
● Facilitating growth	● Power-seeking
● Empathic	● Insensitive
6.A. Reconciling	6.B. Dependent
● Forgiving	● Pleasing–submissive
● Humble	● Compliant–masochistic
● Appropriately direct	● Passive-aggressive
● Problem-solving	● Conflict-avoidant
7.A. Inspiring	7.B. Hyperspiritual
● Attunement to spirit of truth	● God-controlled–externalizing
● Prophetic	● Occult–evil inspired
● Mystical–good reality testing	● Mystical–poor reality testing

Note. This schema shows how personality and lifestyle dimensions can be intertwined with values, religion, and spiritual themes. This table may be used by clinicians as an interview and assessment guide for evaluating the health and adaptiveness of clients' religious and spiritual values and lifestyles at the beginning and throughout therapy. It also is a helpful outline for setting therapeutic goals. Reprinted from Richards and Bergin (1997, p. 189). Copyright 1997. Used by permission of the American Psychological Association.

of getting too many needs met within the community. Therapists need to resist simply "rescuing" such clients from these communities and help develop instead understanding and raised awareness of persons in such communities as well as strengthening their ego boundaries which encourages appropriate choices. As the analyst Alice Miller (1984) reminds us, the issue is not freeing ourselves from representations but rather becoming enlightened witnesses when we watch or participate somehow in those representations.

Unquestioning reliance on patriarchy has the impact for some of unhealthy dependency. As Durham (1985) points out, those members of the LDS religion who rely blindly on priesthood leaders are also at risk for blind reliance on the helping professions. Thus, therapists must beware not to substitute one blind system for another and must confront overreliance on authority. At risk are some Mormon women who, according to some writers (Bennion, 1985; Cornwall, 1994; Iannaccone & Miles, 1994) can be caught up in prescribed roles that may preclude the development of their own personhood; that is, they become involved in "place-taking" in which their identities are based only on their roles (i.e., mother). This notion of role playing, often constructed of ideals, can be a problem for both genders as men and women seek to fulfill their callings in their church jobs (the lay leadership of the LDS church requires this; Shepherd & Shepherd, 1994), their roles as fathers and mothers, and various community and professional positions.

Conceptualization of pathology itself can be influenced by certain religious beliefs. Some Mormons view emotional and mental illness as manifestations of sin. If taught from an early age that one can overcome anything (apparently including genetic predisposition), a person with bipolar disorder, for instance, may not be adequately diagnosed or treated, given the stigma of the erratic, supposedly sin-induced behavior. Some mental health professionals, in an attempt to give circumspect credence to the sin and mental illness connection (Narramore, 1994), suggest that the depth and dynamics of sin is rooted in character pathology. This may hold for some disorders and not others. This debate will not yield to solution anytime soon. In the interim, therapists must attempt some understanding of the client's pathology by separating out (i) long-standing problems of the person or family of origin from the mission of the religious community, (ii) possible genetic predisposition, and (iii) environmental influences including the tensions within and outside of the religious community.

Regardless of the origin (sin, genetic predisposition, unhealthy family dynamics, etc.), pathology impairs or confuses a client's contact with and conception of God. It is hoped that therapy frees such impairments. It is our belief that God can help client and therapist penetrate pathologies and directly bless those who have been deprived, neglected, abused, or caused to suffer from inherited or socialized intergenerational dysfunctions. This can ultimately lead to hope, insight, and healing. Enabling a Mormon client to untangle his or her encumbered relationship to Deity by, for instance, uncovering self-punitive, perfectionistic introjects associated with God allows the client to relate to both God and self more tenderly as well as to draw on the surrounding religious community for support. Therapists who are aware of the Mormon doctrine, history, traditions, and culture are more likely to serve such clients (Koltko, 1990). This will aid the therapist in making distinctions between cultural representations (how the daily practice of religion has become inaccurately codified) versus the client's sincere attempts to live his or her religion from day to day. The following example illustrates this point.

Mormons are industrious. As stated previously, one of the largest concentrations of Mormons is in Utah, whose state symbol is the beehive. Many Mormons have internalized this value for action as a devotion to busyness. Psychiatrist Louis Moench (1985) suggests that the struggles of one of his clients, an overly anxious middle-aged white woman, were directly related to her internalization of this creed, never leaving time for her own self-reflection. When a major depression finally stopped her, she was forced to take time to introspect about her own life, its meaning, and what really mattered: Was it fulfilling all the roles (mother, wife, Relief Society President) perfectly? Or was it caring for herself more lovingly and in turn finding time to lovingly relate to others? Though recovery from the depression and the consequent hospitalization were painful for her, she emerged with a new sense of worth no longer based on busyness and was also able to develop a quality relationship with the Divine, based on more mature object relatedness (i.e., she no longer saw God as the one who would punish her relentlessly were she to fail at her church jobs).

Bergin et al. (1994) remind us of the restorative aspects of all religions and the healthy interchange between psychology and religion when they write about Mormons:

> A positive relationship between mental health and Mormonism seems to depend on the level of commitment and the degree of involvement . . . the healthy features of intrinsic religiousness will be better actualized when the institutional and familial environments allow for honest recognition and acceptance of moral imperfections, thus emphasizing growth relative to moral principles rather than an outward perfectionism that reinforces rigidity and ensures lowered adaptability. (p. 155)

PREDICTING RESISTANCE IN THE MORMON CLIENT

Managing resistance in LDS clients can be a daunting task. As most therapists know, clients seek treatment and engage in the process with an odd ambivalence—working hard to change and yet resisting those efforts to face their pain, thus causing a stalemate. Resistance in the religious client can often take on religious overlays such as an unwillingness to consider indepth feelings of anger, given a superficial interpretation of the injunction to forgive. A number of issues from the Mormon culture can create resistance, including the busyness ethic mentioned previously (clients will not make time for treatment) as well as several other areas which include resistance to (i) analyzing spiritual beliefs, (ii) exploring negative feelings, and (iii) disagreeing with perceived opinions of authorities. Generally, these resistances must be dealt with by utilizing strategies that decrease resistance and encourage working through, although a few caveats exist for this population.

LDS clients may not have clearly articulated all spiritual aspects of their lives. This may create a reluctance to discuss spiritual issues, fearing that speaking them aloud will strip them of their sacredness. This becomes troubling for some therapists because it is not simply an exercise to uncover unhealthy encoding of doctrinal practices. Such dialog may also uncover the entire issue of "religion as illusion" which casts its shadow equally upon Mormons and other believers. Therapists will have to tolerate their own countertransference reactions. McDargh (as quoted in Randour, 1994) states, "Does it make a difference if and how the clinician admits, if only to himself or herself, the possibility that a client's religious convictions do in some way resonate with a reality that is not simply the client's creation?" (p. 176). This debate is best addressed in other sources (Jacobs & Capps, 1997). The advantage of clarifying a client's object relation to God is the development of a clarity of focus and function. As Rizzuto (1996) suggests, God representations influence self and other object relations and they must be explored to uncover the vast array of relationships other than God as well as with God.

LDS clients may not wish to acknowledge "negative" feelings, such as envy, rage, and hatred, as well as examine private issues or personal temptations, such as those concerning sex, dishonesty, and abuse. Dealing with resistance issues in this category includes healthy exploration of those affects considered unfamiliar or negative, especially anger, because Mormons have been known to be conflict-avoidant. However, with respect to deviant sexual thoughts, Mormons have been cautioned on a number of occasions to not yield to temptation even in imagery. "Since Jesus spoke of the wrongness of mental adultery—are we free to sanction salacious imagery in therapy?" (Maxwell, 1976). Given this, the therapist must proceed with caution by avoiding "flooding" the client with images he or she cannot tolerate.

LDS clients may feel reluctant to discuss openly their disagreement with doctrines, practices, or "the brethren," those priesthood leaders in charge of the ward (bishop), stake (stake president), or church (leaders at the highest level of organization are called "general authorities" including the First Presidency and Twelve Apostles). Dealing with resistance issues in this category includes a careful examination of relations both to the social peer group and to authority, as well as an affirmation from the therapist that confidentiality is in place (i.e., the therapist does not intend to repeat anything, including a client's anger toward a particular authority). Resolving authority issues often includes an honest appraisal of overly positive (dependent) or overly negative (hostile) feelings, and an integration of previously split-off part objects that might have been conveniently projected onto such authorities, accompanied by subsequent acknowledgment that authorities may have made mistakes because they are human too as it is generally understood that "almost all men misuse authority and power" (Maxwell, 1976). Alienation from the religious peer community is an equally difficult problem to resolve, especially if one's attitudes or behaviors deviate from norms or alienate people who would ordinarily be sources of support. Group tendencies to judge or to press for conformity without trying to understand can impede the client's progress. This can sometimes be overcome only by assistance from sympathetic local church leaders who have been enlisted with client permission.

LEAVING THE FOLD

A clear doctrinal/cultural/historical by-product of being a practicing Mormon is that one is taught from an early age (and it is emphasized during discussions with potential converts) that the LDS church is the one true religion on the earth. While this exclusiveness is by no means unique to Mormonism, much distress can accrue to those members who doubt or dispute. In addition, once having been part of the fold, should one decide to leave, the exit can be very painful because of doubt, hostility, or fears and because of the perceived or actual loss of multiple and often deep attachments.

Mormons who have become disengaged or disaffiliated with the church have been studied by several researchers (Albrecht, 1989; Albrecht & Cornwall, 1989; Albrecht, Cornwall, & Cunningham, 1988). Those who became inactive (disengagement) or left altogether (disaffiliation) reported difficulties with an emotional sense of marginality, conflicts over spouse or family religiosity, and questions regarding one's future, whereas issues of doctrine played a less significant role. Over an individual's lifetime, religious activity changes depending on a number of circumstances. The importance of a person's beliefs and the importance of belonging to a church generally increases with positive life events, whereas the opposite appears to accompany negative life events (though there is anecdotal evidence that faith may increase during crises). Albrecht and Cornwall (1989), who classified Mormons in their sample into nine types along a continuum from fervent followers to apostates, suggest that this holds for events that are distinctly religious in nature and other events that may not be perceived as being related to religion (employment changes, illness, death, injury, and divorce). They note the following at-risk categories as well: 15- to 28-year olds, women ages 17–25, and recent converts. In addition, the therapist must attend to issues of suicide risk because the value system and the social connectedness that may have precluded this previously are no longer in place.

SUMMARY

Freud called religion "the universal obsessional neurosis of humanity . . . a system of wishful illusions together with a disavowal of reality." (1964, p. 71) He also believed, however, that the most insidious by-products of religion (expecting God to make us safe and free from pain—astutely referred to as Christian narcissistic entitlement by Alter, 1994) were the biggest problem with religion and not the deep religious feeling. Unlike Freud, we do believe in the saving grace of religion, in particular the salvation offered to us by Jesus Christ, as restored through his prophet Joseph Smith. We do agree with Freud, however, that certain insidious by-products of religion can and do exist. Among Mormon communities, those are part of a cultural overlay that has some distinctions and some similarities to the potentially pathogenic features shared by other religions.

The hope is to create a community of true charity in which we help each other. However, the building of communities can be a slow process, and the beauty of each religion is sometimes accompanied by the inculcation of a cultural encoding of doctrine that interferes with the individual's or community's ability to engage in this mutually uplifting endeavor. Sometimes the appropriate aid of a psychotherapist restores the individual to his or her community with a new sense of self and an increased ability to relate to others and to God. This is especially true if therapists (i) respect religious concerns by finding out about the particular religious system and carefully discern constructive cultural belief from manifestations of psychopathology; (ii) acknowledge boundary issues by adhering not only to ethical guidelines regarding dual roles etc. but also, when appropriate, enlisting the support of religious leaders in the client's community when permission is given; (iii) promote therapeutic interventions that encourage client skill-building without contradicting their own sense of morals; (iv) develop ways to understand client spiritual experiences, including accounts of personal revelation that are not automatically attributed to thought disorder; and (v) encourage the development of individuation and appropriate ego skills, including altruism. Such steps will ensure the adequate care of and appropriate service to LDS clients and, it is hoped, the larger religious community.

REFERENCES

Albrecht, S. (1989). The Consequential dimension of Mormon religiosity. *BYU Studies, 29*(2), 57–108.

Albrecht, S., & Cornwall, M. (1989). Life events and religious change. *Review of Religious Research, 31*(1), 23–38.

Albrecht, S., Cornwall, M., & Cunningham, P. (1988). Religious leave-taking: Disengagement and disaffiliation among Mormons. In D. Bromley (Ed.), *Falling from the faith: Causes and consequences of religious apostasy* (pp. 62–80). Newbury Park, CA: Sage.

Allen, J. B., & Leonard, G. M. (1976). *The story of the Latter-Day Saints.* Salt Lake City: Deseret Book.

Alter, M. (1994). *Resurrection psychology: An understanding of human personality based on the life and teachings of Jesus.* Chicago: Loyola University Press.

Arrington, L. J., & Bitton, D. (1979). *The Mormon experience.* New York: Knopf. (This review and critique of Mormon practices and beliefs by two esteemed LDS historians invites the reader to enter the past as well as the present-day world of the Latter-Day Saint. Chapters 15 and 16 are particularly relevant.)

Bahr, S. (1994). Religion and adolescent drug use: A comparison of Mormons and other religions. In M. Cornwall, T. Heaton, & L. Young (Eds.), *Contemporary Mormonism: Social science perspectives* (pp. 118–137). Chicago: University of Illinois Press.

Bennion, F. (1985). Women and roles: Transcending definitions. *Journal of the Association of Mormon Counselors and Psychotherapists 11*(1), 48–51.

Bergin, A. (1994). Religious life-styles and mental health. In L. B. Brown (Ed.), *Religion, personality and mental health* (pp. 70–93). New York: Springer-Verlag.

Bergin, A. (1996). Life and testimony of an academic clinical psychologist. In S. Black (Ed.), *Scholars testify* (pp. 3–16). Salt Lake City: Deseret Book.

Bergin, A., Masters, K., & Richards, P. (1987). Religiousness and mental health reconsidered: A study of an intrinsically religious sample. *Journal of Counseling Psychology, 34*(2), 197–204.

Bergin, A., Payne, R., Jenkins, P., & Cornwall, M. (1994). Religion and mental health. In M. Cornwall, T. Heaton, & L. Young (Eds.), *Contemporary Mormonism: Social science perspectives* (pp. 138–158). Chicago: University of Illinois Press.

Carbo, R., & Gartner, J. (1994). Can religious communities become dysfunctional families? Sources of countertransference for the religiously committed psychotherapist. *Journal of Psychology and Theology, 22*(4), 264–271.

Cornwall, M. (1994). The institutional role of Mormon women. In M. Cornwall, T. Heaton, & L. Young (Eds.), *Contemporary Mormonism: Social science perspectives* (pp. 239–264). Chicago: University of Illinois Press.

Cornwall, M., Heaton, T., & Young, L. (Eds). (1994). *Contemporary Mormonism: Social science perspectives.* Chicago: University of Illinois Press. (Recent explorations of issues in a variety of religions have been augmented by these LDS sociologist who focus on Mormons. They lend credence to the effort that to view oneself from the "outsider's" perspective of science allows for clearer insight. Chapters include such topics as the African American male's admission into the Priesthood, Mormon mental health, and the struggles apparent in becoming a global church.)

Durham, C. (1985). Women and the helping professions: A Judicial view. *Journal of the Association of Mormon Counselors and Psychotherapists 11*(1), 40–47.

Finn, M., & Gartner, J. (1992). *Object relations theory and religion: Clinical applications.* Westport, CT: Praeger.

Freud, S. (1964). *Future of an illusion.* New York: Anchor. (Original work published 1927)

Gallup, G. (1985). *Religion in America* (p. 387). Princeton, NJ: Gallup Report.

Hinckley, G. B. (1996, November). Women of the church. *The Ensign,* 67–70.

Iannaccone, L., & Miles, C. (1994). Dealing with social change: The Mormon church's response to the change in women's roles. In M. Cornwall, T. Heaton, & L. Young (Eds.), *Contemporary Mormonism: Social science perspectives* (pp. 265–286). Chicago: University of Illinois Press.

Jacobs, J. L., & Capps, D. (1997). *Religion, society and psychoanalysis: Readings in contemporary theory.* Boulder, CO: Westview.

Koltko, M. (1990). How religious beliefs affect psychotherapy: The example of Mormonism. *Psychotherapy, 27*(1), 132–141.

Ludlow, D. H. (Ed.). (1992). *Encyclopedia of Mormonism. Vols. 1–5.* New York: Macmillan.

Lyon, J., & Nelson, S. (1979). Mormon health. *Dialogue: A Journal of Mormon Thought, 12*(3), 87–92.

Masters, K., Bergin, A., Reynolds, E., & Sullivan, C. (1991). Religious life-styles and mental health: A follow-up study. *Counseling and Values, 35,* 211–224.

Maxwell, N. (1976, July). Some thoughts on the Gospel and the behavioral sciences. *The Ensign,* 70–75.

Miller, A. (1984). *Thou shalt not be aware: Society's betrayal of the child.* New York: Farrar, Straus & Giroux.

Moench, L. (1985). Mormon forms of psychopathology. *Journal of the Association of Mormon Counselors and Psychotherapists 11*(1), 61–73.

Narramore, B. (1994). Religious resistance. *Journal of Psychology and Theology, 22*(4), 249–258.

O'Dea, T. (1957). *The Mormons.* Chicago: University of Chicago Press. (Though over 40 years old, this classic text by the distinguished Catholic sociologist from Columbia University represents an insightful look at a number of issues in the Mormon church, including his analysis of the intense in-group/out-group tension between Mormon and non-Mormon communities that some would suggest still exists today.)

Randour, M. (1994). *Exploring sacred landscapes: Religious and spiritual experiences in psychotherapy.* New York: Columbia University Press.

Richards, P. S., & Bergin, A. E. (1997). *A spiritual strategy for counseling and psychotherapy.* Washington, DC: American Psychological Association.

Richards, P. S., & Potts, R. (1995). Using spiritual interventions in psychotherapy: Practices, successes, failures, and ethical concerns of Mormon psychotherapists. *Professional Psychology: Research and Practice, 26*(2), 163–170.

Rizzuto, A. (1996). Psychoanalytic treatment and the religious person. In E. Shafranske (Ed.), *Religion and the clinical practice of psychology* (pp. 409–431). Washington, DC: American Psychological Association.

Ruether, R. R. (1983). *Sexism and God-talk: Toward a feminist theology.* Boston: Beacon.

Shafranske, E., & Malony, N. (1996). Religion and the clinical practice of psychology: A case for inclusion. In E. Shafranske (Ed.), *Religion and the clinical practice of psychology* (pp. 561–586). Washington, DC: American Psychological Association.

Shepherd, G., & Shepherd, G. (1994). Sustaining a lay religion. In M. Cornwall, T. Heaton, & L. Young (Eds.), *Contemporary Mormonism: Social science perspectives* (pp. 161–181). Chicago: University of Illinois Press.

Stark, R. (1994). Modernization and Mormon growth. In M. Cornwall, T. Heaton, & L. Young (Eds.), *Contemporary Mormonism: Social science perspectives* (pp. 13–23). Chicago: University of Illinois Press.

Stegner, W. (1964). *The gathering of Zion. The story of the Mormon trail.* New York.

Sue, S., Zane, N., & Young, K. (1994). Research on psychotherapy with culturally diverse populations. In A. E. Bergin & S. L. Garfield (Eds.), *Handbook of psychotherapy and behavior change* (pp. 783–817). New York: John Wiley.

Talmage, J. T. (1984). *Articles of faith.* Salt Lake City: Deseret Book. (This book is the best official digest of Mormon doctrine, teachings, organization, and practice. Published in 1899 and last revised in 1924 by the author, a scientist who became one of the Twelve Apostles of the Church, the *Articles of Faith* is used routinely by teachers and missionaries throughout the world.)

Vande Kemp, H. (1966). Historical perspective: Religion and clinical psychology in America. In E. Shafranske (Ed.), *Religion and the clinical practice of psychology* (pp. 71–112). Washington, DC: American Psychological Association.

16

RELIGION AND MENTAL HEALTH FROM THE UNITY PERSPECTIVE

GLENN R. MOSLEY

*Association of Unity Churches
Lee's Summit, Missouri 64081*

TREATING PATIENTS WITH A UNITY BACKGROUND

Unity people are eclectic in their pursuit of spirituality as well as in their pursuit of other complex interests. While no two Unity students necessarily describe their spiritual experiences or beliefs in exact, and at times not even in similar terms, what academic and clinical psychiatrists, psychologists, and other mental health professionals need to know about treating mental health problems in persons with a Unity background is that nearly all hold one belief in common: That all persons are triune beings (spirit, mind, body).

In addressing the mental health problems of a Unity student (as most prefer to be called), a mental health care professional needs to address all three areas of the student's being. Most Unity students increasingly consider it a "given" that a therapist will explore the effects their distress is having on the three phases of their person—spirit, mind, body (Grof & Grof, 1989, p. 52). (Unity students do not use "and" before the third word in the series precisely because they do not believe one can effectively separate the three; they are "one.")

Because of Unity students' belief that they are one—spirit, mind, body—they feel a pervasive sense that even their "chaotic" experiences will ultimately be resolved. Increasingly, those with mental/emotional problems recognize that they are in the midst of personal change and transition which may even take on the guise of an overwhelming turbulence. At times they express the feeling that their world

    245

as they have known it is coming to an end—an awe-inspiring and a fearsome experience. They may experience terrible anxiety and at the same time feel hopeful, believing they have come to an important crossroad in their ongoing spiritual development. They see, sometimes in a painful way and at other times with simple, painless clarity, that their present turmoil is part of their evolution into the next phase of personal and spiritual growth which may well include an expanded awareness that they are a spirit, mind, body. This sense of an ultimately optimistic outcome and the desire to experience it substantially guides the Unity person in the selection of a mental health professional.

MEDICATION AND TREATMENT(S)
IN THE CONTEXT OF BELIEFS

Whatever the phase of being requiring specific attention (i.e., spirit, mind, body), a majority of Unity students tend not to take over-the-counter or prescription medication. Exceptions might include short-term use of analgesics for pain relief or antibiotics to treat infection. There are three basic reasons for this consistent behavior among Unity people:

1. They have an inherent belief, underscored by their spiritual studies, that spontaneous healing is possible and have a vested interest in not overproviding external help.

2. They are inclined to look to other modalities of treatment besides, or in addition to, medication.

3. They wish to play an active role in their treatment.

A Harvard Medical School (1993) survey indicated that 20% of the general population with depression turns to alternative therapies, suggesting that these persons wanted to play an active role in their treatment. In a similar survey of Unity students (Unity ministers, licensed teachers, and laity), 87% reported that they actively participated in their own treatment whether working with a spiritual counselor, a physical, or a mental health care professional (Association of Unity Churches, 1997). Furthermore, 81% sought alternative therapies either instead of or concurrent with traditional mental health care.

The 87% of students reported previously indicated that two major roles they played in their own mental, physical, or spiritual health care were (a) the category of health care professional they choose and (b) who they choose to work with as a health care professional. Eighty percent reported they prayed for guidance about both (a) and (b). They hold sacred their individual right to such selection, much as advocated by psychiatrist Dorsey (1965):

> I cannot imagine what it would be like to be unable to choose my own physician, but I cherish that freedom of choice quite as I cherish my civic right to choose the religious living which I prefer. I consider "taking a physician" to be almost as private and personal a matter as is "taking a mate." Where my health is concerned I need as much harmony of spirit,

consent of will, and unification of self-consciousness as I can mobilize, in order to recover and maintain my clear sense of the wholeness–allness–unity of my human being. Thus, I might not choose you, on account of your extreme subjectivist theories, but if anyone else wished to choose you, I hold that he should not be denied that possibility. (pp. 445–446)

Having made the choice of health care professional(s), Unity students also report that they actively take part in the decision-making regarding the type of treatment they will participate in, whether mental, physical, or spiritual. These people have an expressed interest in moving from disease management to promotion of both their own and others' health by incorporating the principles of integrative medical treatment.

EVOLUTION OF MEDICAL TERMS IN THE UNITY STUDENT'S THINKING

The use of the term "integrative medical treatment" is evidence of evolution in the thinking of the Unity student. Unity people were among the first to adopt the use of the term "alternative medicine," some as long ago as the late 1950s. Typically, all modalities of treatment which were not allopathic medicine were placed in the "alternative" category, with other modalities in their own groupings, e.g., chiropractors, nutritionists, and herbalists. Some students began to recognize that the word alternative connoted an "either/or" rather than a "both/and" range of options, which seemed to be a threat to both the patient and physicians, and began using the term "complementary medicine" during the mid-1980s, as did some members of the allopathic medical profession.

Later, in the early 1990s, Unity people began adopting the term "integrative medicine" and recently have begun using the terms "integrative modalities of treatment" or "integrative medical treatment" interchangeably with integrative medicine.

A FUNDAMENTAL UNITY BELIEF

Unity students believe that God indwells humankind and all creation and that prayer and meditation are the direct access routes to an awareness of that indwelling Presence. We shall pursue the subject of prayer and meditation and its relationship to therapist(s) in more detail later. Over 80% of Unity people do not think of treatments by chiropractors, use of nutritional supplements for physical and emotional problems, precautionary dieting, acupuncture, prayer and meditation, therapeutic touch, healing hover touch, osteopathy, vitamin and mineral therapy, breathing exercises, etc., as peripheral to allopathy but rather as a part of the core of integrative modalities of treatment. The Unity student sees the various disciplines of health care as being part of the entree with allopathy and not as incidental side dishes.

PHYSICAL EXERCISE, NUTRITION,
BREATHING EXERCISES, AND PRAYER
AND MEDITATION

As noted earlier, Unity students are eclectic in many ways, including their pursuit of mental and physical health and well-being. They tend to read, study, and experiment with myriad ways to maintain health and to regain health for any of the three phases of being—spirit, mind, body—once it has broken down. Eighty percent of those who responded to the survey (Association of Unity Churches, 1997) exercise from one to six times a week, from 15 to 45 min each time. Even those who do not exercise regularly know of the benefits of exercise.

Exercises and spiritual practices with a physical component that are most often engaged in by adult Unity students are tai chi, hatha yoga, martial arts, stair climbing, golf, brisk walking, swimming, dance, low-impact aerobics, hiking, bicycling, and stretching. They generally practice, or at least have read about or studied, relaxation techniques, meditation, nutrition, breathing exercises, etc. Many of these studies are included in the adult education programs of the ministry they attend (Mosley, 1980). The study and practice of *pranayama,* a part of the ancient East Indian breath control associated with yoga, is a popular class in the Unity adult education classroom. Pranayama is both authentic spiritual practice and one of the pathways to regaining and maintaining mental and physical health. A mental health practitioner who would work well with a Unity patient/client might prescribe a varying combination of the previously discussed practices.

THE NEED TO TREAT THE WHOLE PERSON:
SPIRIT, MIND, BODY

In order to treat mental health problems in a person with a Unity background, the mental health caregiver needs to treat the whole person—spirit, mind, body. In their eclectic pursuit of complex interests, Unity students are likely to have learned of the side effects of the three types of prescription antidepressants, tricyclics, monamine oxidase inhibitors, and serotonin reuptake inhibitors (especially Prozac). If depression is only mild to moderate in severity, the therapist might wish to avoid these drugs and consider with the patient important lifestyle choices and/or herbal medication alternatives, such as St. John's wort extract. Weil (1997) observes,

> St. John's wort . . . used in Europe for 15 years (prescriptions in Germany now outnumber those for Prozac 25 to 1), . . . was until recently largely dismissed by our own medical community. . . . Meanwhile, a major multicenter trial of the herb is finally in the works here, involving the National Institute of Mental Health (NIMH) and the National Institutes of Health's Office of Alternative Medicine. (p. 8)

Unity students might also choose other natural products, including passion flower, kava extract, oat straw, valerian, amino acid therapy, or ginkgo biloba extract, which are purported to offer antidepressant effects.

Seasonal affective disorder (commonly known as "cabin fever" in northeastern Ohio and southeastern Michigan (locations of my last two churches before becoming CEO in our international offices) has a number of useful home remedies known to many Unity students who live in those somewhat damp and cloudy climates. These home remedies might also be prescribed by a mental health care professional. In addition to taking nutritional and herbal antidepressants instead of, or in addition to, seeking assistance from a mental health care professional, Unity students may include in their regimen of self-care—or respond well to the health care professional's suggestions—to plan a winter vacation in a sunny climate if at all possible; remove or trim from around windows vegetation and/or open shades and blinds which prevent sunlight from entering through windows; receive a massage from a professional masso-therapist if possible or from a friend or family member if necessary; and exercise outdoors at midday, every day if possible. Finally, a popular home remedy in treatment of seasonal affective disorder which is also used by both alternative and conventional medicine is to sit in front of a fluorescent light that is 10–12 times brighter than average indoor light for 2 hrs daily.

The "Talking Cure" and Nutritional Therapy

The Unity student may be willing to continue talking with the trained therapist but would welcome other treatment programs that address the needs of spirit, mind, body. For example, as an option to drugs to correct the brain's chemical imbalances, which may trigger clinical depression, the Unity person generally prefers nutritional therapy which may reestablish a healthy balance of brain chemicals through less powerful medicines. As suggested in the work of Althoff, Williams, Molvig, and Schuster (1997, p. 68), "The amino acid tryptophan is needed for the synthesis of serotonin, a mood-regulating chemical in the brain, and the amino acid tyrosine is needed for the brain chemical norepinephrine." If they are lacking, adding these amino acids is one way that will help to regain balance of brain chemicals.

Before pursuing these subjects further, I must state for the benefit of the nonprofessional reader/prospective Unity patient who has not already studied and discovered options to psychoactive drugs with possible undesired side effects that one needs to exercise caution regarding self-diagnosis. While it is useful to "listen" to your body, mind, spirit and to determine needs and courses of action, it cannot be overemphasized that it is also good to work with a health care professional regarding the use of nutritional products. If you are already using a prescribed medicine such as either one of the benzodiazepines (Valium and Xanax are two of the better known versions) or Prozac, mentioned previously, you must work closely with your physician before discontinuing any drug (Murray, 1996). One should also not mix herbal extracts with other psychoactive drugs. If you wish to consider more natural methods, be certain to discuss it with your therapist. Should the physician need more information about the integrative modalities of treatment, this can be found in the studies I have referenced in this chapter (studies published in medical journals and other health care publications).

The Way Unity Students Eat

Unity people generally attempt to be well informed about nutrition. They consider their diet as important to mental health as it is to physical health; their four basic diets are (a) a vegetarian diet (no animal foods or animal by-products), (b) a lactoovo vegetarian diet (dairy products as the only animal foods), (c) a general diet that includes as meats only fish with scales and poultry (skinned), and (d) a general diet that includes moderate amounts of red meat. Of those Unity students responding to our survey (Association of Unity Churches, 1997), 47% report following one of the first three diets.

There are also specific diets for persons with different blood types (e.g., type A and O) (D'Adamo, 1996). With regard to the effects of diet on my own health in relationship to my blood type (type A), I relate the following experience. Some time ago, I was diagnosed with borderline diabetes. I had this problem for several years until I made a small shift in diet. Within 3 weeks, my glucose level dropped from 163 to 71; it is now consistently 85–90 with a simple diet for those with type A blood. Diets of Unity students are often rounded out with nutritional supplements, easily available from health food stores, for both physical and mental problems.

A number of researchers suggest a relationship between blood sugar and human behavior. For example, a well-dressed woman visited internist Dr. Marc Siegel (Bonnie View Productions, 1997) without an appointment. She said that she was diabetic. Upon checking, Dr. Siegel determined that the diabetes was controlled. Over several weeks, Dr. Siegel recognized that there seemed to be a relationship between radically different glucose levels and radical changes among the various emerging personalities of the woman who now appeared to have dissociative identity disorder. Dr. Marc Siegel referred the woman to psychiatrist Dr. Greg Alsip. Concerned for her safety, Dr. Alsip placed her in a New York City hospital.

The nurses quickly noticed that the glucose level of each personality was different from each of the other personalities. At a glucose level of 80, the patient expressed a male personality who wondered why he had been referred to a psychiatrist. One of the female personalities with extremely erratic behavior had a glucose level of 250. Some of the personalities tended to be diabetic. Others clearly were not diabetic. While Dr. Alsip was able to draw this patient back to the most stable personality, that of the woman with controlled diabetes, he appropriately did not draw conclusions based on this one case.

It would be most difficult to determine whether a dangerously high blood sugar level caused extraordinarily erratic behavior or whether the extraordinarily erratic behavior prompted the dangerously high blood sugar level. The causative relationship probably would not be possible to determine with a single case study, although it is suggestive.

A Unity student who was aware of the possible correlation of blood sugar to behavior might well feel comforted if a psychiatrist or other mental health care professional ordered a blood sugar test and then took the results into consideration while planning and providing a treatment program.

THE DESIRE FOR AND PRACTICE OF PRAYER
AND MEDITATION

Researcher, psychiatrist, and president of the National Institute for Healthcare Research, David Larson (as cited in Versau, 1997, p. E1), says that "Not only is religious commitment associated with improved coping and recovery from both physical and mental illness, but a number of recent studies have suggested that religious commitment could also have a prophylactic or preventative effect on physical and mental health."

The previous statement follows Larson's (as cited in Reynolds, 1996) previous observation concerning research into the factors of faith and prayer:

> Of 300 studies on spirituality in scientific journals, the National Institute for Healthcare Research found nearly three-fourths showed that religion had a positive effect on health. Research also shows four out of five patients want doctors to ask them about their faith, and one in two want their doctors to pray with them. (p. 10A)

Despite this, according to a *USA Today* survey, only 10% of people indicated that their doctors had "talked to them about their faith as a factor in their healing."

The Association of Unity Churches (1997) survey supports Larson's position, and in the case of Unity people, the data goes slightly beyond his conclusions regarding the desire to discuss their faith and considerably beyond regarding their desire for prayer. Eighty-two percent said that it was "important" to "very important" that their health care professional have an understanding of the impact of the spiritual realm on their health, mental and physical.

Regarding their choice of mental health care professional, the Association of Unity Churches (1997) survey asked respondents to check as many as applied to them (totaling more than 100%) and to indicate whom they would go to first for assistance. Of the three considered to be mental health professionals by Unity people, 78% of Unity students (all three categories, i.e., ministers, licensed teachers, and laity shared this percentage almost exactly) would go first to a spiritual counselor, 41% would either go first to a psychologist or to a psychologist in addition to a spiritual counselor, and 17% would either go first to a psychiatrist or to a psychiatrist in addition to a spiritual counselor.

The first choice, to seek help from a spiritual counselor, is made specifically because the Unity student knows that he or she will be prayed with during the course of a consultation. Among the same survey respondents, 53% would agree to the use of herbal/natural medicines, 25% would agree to prescription medicine, 9% would agree to over-the-counter medications, and the balance would not take medicine. According to David Larson (as cited in Cohen, 1997),

> Most doctors ignore the fact that their patients are fans of God and . . . that 60 percent of the population would like to discuss spiritual issues with their doctors and 40 percent would like their doctors to pray with them. . . . Neither doctors nor psychotherapists are taught to deal with or even bring up religious issues. (p. 70)

Using the American Academy of Family Physicians as their source, Carey and Visgaitis (1997) reported that 42% of family doctors have not been introduced to using spirituality in healing through professional training. Nevertheless, 75% of female doctors and 63% of male doctors "have used prayer or meditation in treating themselves." It would be interesting to know what percentage of psychiatrists and other psychotherapists use prayer when they have healing needs. As evidenced in Larson's statements and from the Association of Unity Churches' survey (1997), 40–50% of the general population and 78% of Unity students would like for their health care professional to pray with them about mental or physical health problems. Therefore, one might ask, "Why do psychiatrists, psychologists, and other mental health professionals not pray with their patients/clients more often?"

Four possible reasons for this come quickly to mind: (a) that a given patient/client may be one in the population who would not want the mental health professional to pray with him or her; (b) in the therapist's mind, to offer prayer might raise questions in the patient/client's mind regarding competence; (c) that the therapist and patient/client are of different religious backgrounds; and (d) that therapists do not know patient/clients would like prayer.

In response to the four scenarios noted previously, I suggest that for the Unity patient (a) the mental health professional ask either on the intake questionnaire or during the first consultation whether the patient/client would want the therapist to pray with her/him; (b) the Unity patient/client will only have more confidence in the therapist's skills as the result of such an inquiry; and (c) since Unity students attempt to honor diversity, patient/client and therapist being of different religious backgrounds would tend to heighten the prayer experience together (the Unity student who had selected a therapist who was Catholic, Jewish, Muslim, or of any other religious background would consider praying with that therapist an added bonus).

It is not suggested that a physician or mental health professional proselytize or in any way apply pressure regarding religious views, but simply allow for the positive effects of coping, restoring hope and peace that are brought about through prayer. At the very least, the psychiatrist, psychologist, or other mental health professional might ask if the Unity patient/client would like a few minutes of silence to close the consultation.

ACKNOWLEDGMENTS

I offer thanks to those who helped with this chapter, colleagues and friends all: Lisa Wittman and Cary Herold for assistance with the Association survey; Carl Osier for his suggestions and assistance with editing; Shirley Hopper for wording processing; and Bets Kirby for her suggestions, editing, and production wizardry. I appreciate the help, and feedback, from the thousands who have participated in my healing workshops. Each has been both student and teacher to me. Finally, thanks to my wife, Martha, also a friend and colleague, for her support in presenting those hundreds of workshops which have taught me so much.

REFERENCES

Althoff, S., Williams, P., Molvig, D., & Schuster, L. (1997). *A guide to alternative medicine.* Lincolnwood, IL: Publications International.

Association of Unity Churches. (1997). *Survey of 781 (of 1960) Unity ministers, licensed teachers, and congregants.* Lee's Summit, MO: Author.

Benson, H. (1996). *Timeless healing: The power and biology of belief.* New York: Scribner.

Bonnie View Productions. (1997, June 26). Television transcript, "Vital Signs," New York.

Carey, A., & Visgaitis, G. (1997, March 27). Doctors pray for selves. *USA Today,* p. 2A.

Cohen, J. (1997, March/April). The greatest story never told. *Utne Reader,* p. 70.

D'Adamo, P. J. (1996). *Eat right for your type.* New York: Putnam.

Dorsey, J. M. (1965). *Illness or allness: Conversations of a psychiatrist.* Detroit, MI: Wayne State University Press.

Grof, S., & Grof, C. (Eds.). (1989). *Spiritual emergency: When personal transformation becomes a crisis.* Los Angeles: Tarcher.

Harvard Medical School. (1993). *Survey on use of alternative medicine.* Cambridge, MA. Harvard Medical School.

Mosley, G. R. (1980). *A comparison of secular and religious experiential education activities in the adult religious education classroom.* Columbus: ERIC, Ohio State University.

Murray, M. T. (1996). *Natural alternatives to Prozac.* New York: Morrow.

Reynolds, B. (1996, May 3). Prayer the medicine patients are seeking. *USA Today,* p. 10A.

Versau, J. (1997, March 29). Religion is beneficial to your health. *The Chicago Times,* p. E1.

Weil, A. (1995). *Spontaneous healing.* New York: Fawcett Columbine.

Weil, A. (1997, July). Can St. John's wort ease depression? *Self Healing.*

17

RELIGION AND MENTAL HEALTH FROM THE JEWISH PERSPECTIVE

MICHAEL R. ZEDEK

The Temple, Congregation B'nai Jehudah
Kansas City, Missouri 64131

Any effort to summarize a 4000-year-old history and tradition cannot help but prove inadequate. However, it is possible to suggest key concepts which are emphasized within Judaism, even as those ideas have been conveyed to much of the world by way of the Jewish people's odyssey.

GOD, TORAH, ISRAEL

Such discussions often focus on three themes: God, Torah, and Israel. This study begins with the third element, Israel. Along with the terms Jews and Jewish, Israel has been used to designate Jewish people even long before the establishment of the modern state with that name because Israel connects Jews to a specific group, one that understands itself to be the spiritual heir of Abraham and Sarah, Isaac and Rebecca, Jacob (as the patronymic for the community, he is also called Israel), Leah, and Rachel.

Also, while almost all Jews feel a connection to a unique history, community, and, perhaps, destiny, there is a complication; no one has offered a sufficiently inclusive definition of what Judaism or Jews are precisely.

Religion, nationality, civilization, and a kinship group all have merit, but no one is sufficient in itself. For instance, there are persons who identify themselves as serious Jews, yet they would object to any suggestion that they are religious. What about a nationality? Consider, can one convert to Italian? While the first instinct may be to respond negatively, the answer is definitely yes. Among nations the process is called citizenship. Within a religious context, the term is conversion. In a family, the preferred word is adoption.

In fact I find the most inclusive suggestion in the notion that "more than being a small group, we are a large family."[1] The comment conveys the understanding that Jews believe themselves to be connected in an intimate way to other "family members" around the world. At its best that means a special concern for the fate of Jews anywhere,[2] even as Jews express a universal concern to establish justice for all people everywhere.

An essential concept that Judaism introduces to the world is a moral passion that we must be concerned for all and a strong conviction, even an urgency, that we bridge some of the distance between what is and what should be.

With such declarations as "Justice, justice you shall pursue" (Deut. 16:20), "You know the heart of the stranger for you were strangers in the land of Egypt" (Exodus 23:9), and "You shall be holy, for I, the Lord your God, am holy" (Lev. 19:2), Judaism introduces ethical monotheism to the world. The concept suggests that there is a unity, a singular force, the cause behind all appearances, that at the heart of the universe there is an ultimate reality which makes for meaning. An essential implication of the Jewish teaching about deity, then, is that our lives are more than "a tale told by an idiot full of sound and fury signifying nothing."

Rather, Judaism makes a bold and what may seem to some not only an unfamiliar but also a puzzling assertion because many are accustomed to consider religion (especially in Western tradition) to be about ensuring a place in God's world when they die. However, instead of a focus on salvation or eternal life, Judaism explores how we might get some "godness" or, to use a less religious orientation, some goodness into the world.

As the prophet Isaiah expresses, "You shall be a light to the nations." In Exodus we are instructed, "You shall be to Me a kingdom of priests and a holy people." In such ways does Judaism articulate an agreement, a covenant with God to make the world better. This concept includes an often misunderstood and maligned idea of Jews as God's Chosen People. While some may view this suggestion as the height of ethnocentric arrogance, the concept does not mean singled out for priority or privilege. Rather, it means that those who tie their fate to the people of Israel have a responsibility to witness through concrete deeds (mitzvot)[3] of God's presence in the world and in our lives. There is never a suggestion that others are excluded from that work, only that Jews are called to do it.

[1] I first heard this offering in a presentation by Rabbi Harold Kushner, the author of *When Bad Things Happen to Good People.*

[2] This suggestion is made explicit in the Talmudic dictum (the Talmud is the essential compendium of Jewish tradition. Its teachings date from approximately 300 BCE to 200 CE), "All Israel bears a responsibility one for the other." Jewish tradition dates years of the civil calendar with a religiously neutral "before the common era" (BCE) and "common era" (CE).

[3] The word *mitzvah* (plural, *mitzvot*) literally means commandment, as in the notion of requirement or obligation. It also suggests good deeds, actions, or restraints from activity that express caring.

Regarding notions of life after death, Jewish tradition certainly includes speculation about a survival of some kind,[4] but it also is possible to suggest that there is no continuing of the individual—that death is the end of the "I." Whatever one's faith or fear, Judaism's bottom line is that we trust God. If there be conscience survival of personality, that will take care of itself. If not, the critical task still remains to live a life that makes a difference. Judaism describes a partnership in which not only do we need God but also, in some mysterious fashion, God needs all of us.

A corollary to this prescription means that Judaism does not embrace a mission to convert the world. While converts are welcomed, there is no conviction that there is only one way to serve God and that the way is Judaism's alone. Even when the sages speculate about afterlife, they insist, "All the righteous [notice all people, not just Jews] have a share in the world to come."[5]

The principle documents of Jewish thought and practice are part of a vast body of literature which begins with the Torah (more fully, Tanach)[6] and Talmud.

Torah in Hebrew means instruction, and it is often used to include a world of law, history, teaching, legend, and story. Therefore, in addition to being the title of the first five books of the Hebrew Bible, Torah by extension also may indicate all of Jewish learning.

ORTHODOX, CONSERVATIVE, AND REFORM JEWS

Halachah means the path or way. The halachah plays a role similar to the *sh'riya* in Islam or to the significant body of church teaching in Roman Catholicism. That means some Jews view the *halachah* as binding. What it describes is what they should or must do. To fail to observe those teachings is to engage in what religions label as sin. For Orthodox Judaism this means that what appropriate (read Orthodox) authorities describe as the authentic halachah is obligatory.

Conservative Judaism views the halachah as an obligation for the observant person, but it also suggests that a more flexible approach may be determined, but again only by the appropriate rabbinic leadership.[7] That means the Conservative

---

[4]Orthodox Judaism is more likely to assert that as a certainty.

[5]The statement is from the introduction of a tractate or section of the Talmud called *Pirkei Avot* (*Ethics of the Sages*).

[6]An acronym in the Hebrew language which indicates the parts of the Bible, Tanach is a more accurate description for Judaism than the Christian title of Old Testament.

[7]The word rabbi means teacher. A rabbi is presumed to be neither more nor less holy than any other member of the community. However, the rabbi derives authority by virtue of knowledge of the tradition and, often, interpersonal skills to maximize influence. Rabbis were not intended to be the Jewish version of a minister or priest. Nonetheless, in the American setting they are often and sometimes appropriately viewed as the equivalent because many Jews view the rabbi as a provider of spiritual guidance and teaching.

movement generally demonstrates a degree of flexibility with regard to the halachah that would be considered inauthentic for Orthodoxy.

Reform Judaism views historic Jewish practice as having a claim on its members; however, Reform embraces a commitment to personal autonomy. That means
the tradition has a voice, a vote, but not a veto.

No doubt there are at least two other groupings, namely, those who view the
tradition as little more than historical curiosity and those who are blissfully ignorant of the material altogether.

However, the halachah is meant to be (depending on one's philosophical commitment within Judaism) either the or a path for a Jew to serve God with "all one's
heart, soul, and might." It intends to transform every aspect of life, not only the
exceptional experiences but also the everyday and common, so that one may recognize the sacred dimension available at all times, in all places, and with every
person.

JUDAISM IN HISTORICAL PERSPECTIVE

As to a brief history, the story of the Jews traces back some 4000 years to the
biblical Abraham and Sarah and to a divine call for Abraham to leave his ances-
tral home and journey to the land of Canaan.

Abraham is the first person called a Hebrew (*Ivri* in the biblical language). The
word means "on the side," and while it may originate as a geographical designation, as on or from the other side of the Jordan River (i.e., from the east), it also
describes an often commented upon characteristic of many Jewish people, namely, to see things distinctly not, per se, in the accepted or majority fashion. Just as
Abraham and Sarah initiated a radical break from the inherited tradition around
them, their spiritual descendants often played the role of iconoclasts. Therefore,
for example, scholars have suggested that Freud's Jewishness gave him a perspective to see things differently and a willingness to dissent from the accepted
wisdom of his time.

The journey continues with Isaac and Rebecca, Jacob, Leah, Rachel, and their
children. Joseph and his brothers bring the then small group to Egypt. There the
initial experience is one of welcome as they grow and prosper into 12 tribes. However, acceptance is soon followed by centuries of enslavement. Then Moses responds to a divine command and leads the Israelites from slavery to freedom, out
of Egypt toward the Promised Land.

The experience in the wilderness culminates in the revelation of God's law at
Mt. Sinai. After 40 years of wandering, Moses dies at the very entrance to the land.
Then Joshua, his chosen successor, leads the tribes in the conquest of Canaan. A
period of instability follows in which the people are led by charismatic leaders
called judges who seem to arise just in time to avert disaster. At the people's urg-
ing, Samuel, the last of these leaders, appoints Saul as the first king.

However, Saul quickly loses divine favor, and authority passes to the remarkable David. Poet, musician, warrior, statesman, and hero, David establishes Jerusalem as an eternal focal point of Jewish yearning. There, his son and successor, Solomon, builds the first great Temple. After Solomon's death, a civil war splits the nation in two. This period of kings and prophets is described as an era of turmoil and testing. Ultimately, the northern kingdom, sometimes called Israel, is destroyed by the Assyrians and its capital sacked in the eighth century BCE. The exiled people disappear from history and come to be known as the Ten Lost Tribes. The southern kingdom called Judah, with its capital of Jerusalem, continued to enjoy a degree of autonomy until 586/5 BCE when the Babylonians destroyed the city and Temple shrine and exiled all leadership.

However, in this circumstance, something unprecedented occurred. For peoples in the ancient near east such a catastrophe meant the end of national identity. Since their deity was presumed defeated, so too were the people finished. However, the Jews understood that God, who demands justice, still could and must be served. With the leadership of Ezra and Nehemiah, they maintained a distinct community and returned to the land about 535 BCE.

The subsequent centuries included encounters with ancient Persia and Greece, especially under the Hellenistic influence of Alexander the Great and his successors.

Roman legions put an end to the second independent Jewish commonwealth. That conquest, with the exception of a brief period of rebellion, put an end to Jewish national authority until 1948.

THE JEWISH PEOPLE IN MODERN TIMES

From the time of the Babylonian exile to the present day, a substantial portion of the Jewish people have lived in diaspora. That means for more than 2000 years Jewish history was written in many locations and in encounters with other communities. Sometimes, the Jewish people were welcomed additions to their new homes. Too often there followed bitter periods of oppression and violence. However, always the circumstance of life in diaspora meant a requirement to live in some creative tension between the attractions and pressures of the world around Jews and the desire to maintain Jewish life.

In that context, the stirrings of modernity, most evident with the American and French revolutions, brought extraordinary opportunity. The previously denied privileges and obligations of citizenship provided an invitation for Jews to participate in the public life of many countries. That new circumstance created a variety of responses. The different branches of Jewish religious life self-consciously defined themselves because of the challenge of modernity. Even as Jews were confronted with an unprecedented climate of accommodation, that welcome produced the necessity of dealing with issues of acculturation and assimilation.

Nonetheless, modernity did not eliminate the specter of anti-Semitism. In fact, at the end of the nineteenth century, the unjust imprisonment for treason of Captain Alfred Dreyfus and the subsequent anti-Semitic violence in supposedly modern France inspired a totally secular Theodore Herzl to revive Zionism, the Jewish movement for a national home. Today, for reasons of theology, history, and family, what happens in Israel matters to Jews no matter where they may reside.

ISSUES IN THE PSYCHIATRIC TREATMENT OF JEWS

As to issues related to psychiatric treatment, Jews frequently may suggest about themselves some variation of "Jews are like everybody else, only more so." Namely, it is entirely possible, in fact likely, that Judaism or Jewishness may be incidental to the clinical evaluation of a patient. However, with some Jewish persons there likely could be several factors that may assist in treatment evaluation.

Especially with someone from the Orthodox community, an authority figure, usually a rabbi, may be able to intervene to attain information, cooperation, and/or compliance from a resistant patient or family member(s). Orthodox Judaism assigns exceptional authority to its leaders, so a rabbi's decisions, at least theoretically, are binding on his congregants.

Another area of concern is the nature of the family constellation. For some time sociologists wrote of a supposedly distinct character to Jewish family life, from the intensity of caregiving to the statistically low occurrence of alcoholism, drug and spousal abuse, as well other notions of exceptionality. If such analyses ever were correct, they seem less so today with the heavy influence on all persons of our highly secular and materialistic culture.

However, the clinician may encounter Jewish persons who subscribe to the possible reality or myth of such distinctiveness. Such persons may evidence a considerable element of denial, guilt, or shame with regard to emotional fragileness on their part. To need a mental health professional and, especially, to be emotionally ill may be viewed as a horrendous embarrassment for the individual, the family network, and, in rare circumstance, the extended community.

Furthermore, Jewish persons are often high achievers, persons who "shouldn't" require assistance from mental health professionals. At the same time, paradoxically, Jews in America (an overwhelming number of whom have undergraduate and advanced degrees) are frequent users of the medical establishment. There is also a long tradition of respect for the medical profession in all expressions of Judaism. A doctor is likely still to be viewed not only as a person of wisdom and prestige but also as an individual who pursues a noble calling. The healer may be viewed as a partner with God in "perfecting the world."[8]

One additional factor which impacts Jewish persons in treatment is the long history as a minority community. At times, non-Jews have ascribed considerable

---

[8]*Tikkun Olam.* The Hebrew denotes an important Jewish value. It literally means to "repair the world," even though that work may need to be done one person at a time.

worth to Jews because of that status. Too often, the position of outsider has subjected Jews to discrimination and violence. As a result, a few Jewish persons may suspect the motives of gentiles. Do good intentions mask an effort to convert or marginalize Jews? Does the non-Jew harbor anti-Semitic attitudes? Does the person view Judaism as somehow inferior to his/her own commitment? Such attitudes may appear irrational, but the time-worn suggestion that even a paranoid may have real enemies is a not altogether unreasonable conclusion in a century that saw fully one third of the Jewish people annihilated.

A sensitive clinician, however, is more likely to confront Jewish persons with unrealistically high expectations about the skills of the practitioner. Jews genuinely trust good medical practice and people who care, of whatever background, are viewed overwhelmingly positively.

An additional aid in ensuring treatment compliance is a significant conviction in Judaism that a person can change. Judaism asserts that what we have been or done does not eliminate a capacity for improvement, transformation, and change.

Jewish theology conveys this conception in its distinction from Christian thought with regard to the doctrine of original sin. Unlike Christianity, Judaism does not consider sin a state of being into which we are born. Rather, sin means individual acts of omission or commission. Therefore, rather than the idea that human beings are by nature corrupt or the naive suggestion that we are in essence fundamentally good, Judaism teaches that we have responsibility for our behavior and that we can change that behavior too. That may prove especially helpful in the effort to return a patient to health.

Regarding any preferences for a specific treatment theory or technique, a pharmacological repertoire, family systems theory, and psychotherapeutic models are all potential therapies that may be recommended. Trust between the patient and caregiver is far more essential than a particular prejudice favoring one theory of intervention over another.

REFERENCES

Donin, H. (1972). *To be a Jew: A guide to Jewish observance in contemporary life.* New York: Basic Books.

Grayzel, S. (1968). *A history of the Jews.* New York: New American Library.

Jacobs, L. (1983). *The book of Jewish values.* London: Ballentine Mitchell.

Jacobs, L. (1984). *The book of Jewish belief.* New York: Behrman House.

Johnson, P. (1984). *A history of the Jews.* New York: Harper & Row.

Seltzer, R. (1980). *Jewish people, Jewish thought.* New York: MacMillan.

Siegel, R., Strassfeld, M., & Strassfeld, S. (1973). *The Jewish catalog.* Philadelphia: Jewish Publication Society.

Strassfeld, M. (1985). *The Jewish holidays: A guide and commentary.* New York: Harper & Row.

Strassfeld, S. (1976). *The second Jewish catalog.* Philadelphia: Jewish Publication Society.

Trepp, L. (1980). *The complete book of Jewish observance: A practical manual for the modern Jew.* New York: Summit Books/Behrman House.

18

TREATING BUDDHIST
PATIENTS

BRUCE W. SCOTTON

Department of Psychiatry
University of California, San Francisco
San Francisco, California 94140

Two sociological trends contribute to the increasing presentation of Buddhist patients to American psychiatrists. The first is the continuing immigration of Asians and their ensuing, although gradual, acceptance of Western psychiatric treatment. The second is the conversion of many native-born Americans to Buddhism. This chapter will examine the similarities and differences of the two groups and suggest an appropriate clinical approach for both. I will begin with a discussion of basic beliefs shared by all Buddhists and then proceed to survey the worldview and psychology which result from those beliefs. Then, the two groups of American Buddhists are examined more closely.

BASIC TENETS OF BUDDHIST BELIEF

Buddhism arose as the report of the results of one man's (Siddhartha Gautama, a prince living on the Indian–Nepalese border about 500 BC) attempt to find a pragmatic system to alleviate the suffering he noted in the world. As a result, the teachings are often descriptive and phenomenological and "nosological" lists abound, describing the pathological operations of our consciousness and the world it creates. Thus, there are "four seals" of belief which were derived from observations of consciousness. The first seal is that *dukkha,* or suffering, is a universal aspect of the human condition. The second seal, *anatta,* or no-self, states that there is no separately existing self to be found in the phenomenal world. Buddha's analysis of consciousness concluded that a separate self could not be found in any of the parts of awareness nor in the sum of the parts of awareness. All that could be found to exist was a set of connected events, objects, emotions, and thoughts. Adopting that understanding—that "reality" and "self" are only a constantly changing play of different events, physical and mental—is an essential step toward release from suffering. The third seal, *annicca,* or impermanence, states that nothing lasts. Possessions, emotional states, relationships, even planets are all created and then pass from existence. The only thing that varies is the rate of change. Staking one's happiness to such transitory phenomena produces inevitable disappointment. The fourth seal is that nirvana or release from suffering exists—release through surrendering attachment to the false sense of a separate self and all that it produces (Sopa & Hopkins, 1976).

Gautama Buddha (which means Gautama the enlightened one) observed that there were four "noble truths" about the nature of existence. First, *dukkha* or suffering is universal. Suffering can be divided into physical and psychological, and is essential to the nature of human beings, but in all cases it is based on the operation of the second truth. The second truth is *samudaya:* Suffering arises from our clinging to things in the form of attraction and repulsion for objects, beings, ideas, and events. Often we are repelled by our current experience and seek to end or avoid it. If we are attracted to our experience, we worry it may soon end and we seek to hold on to it. In both cases we suffer. Such clinging leads to a cycle of "dependent origination," or rebirth. In this case rebirth means both reincarnation and rebirth of the same ego attachments from moment to moment (Buott, 1955). Third, *nirodha,* or cessation of suffering, is possible by breaking the cycle of dependent origination. If we quit re-creating our attached ego we can stop suffering. Fourth, *marga,* a way or a "noble eightfold path," exists which is the way to the cessation of suffering. The eight components are correct views, correct intention, correct speech, correct action, correct livelihood, correct effort, correct mindfulness, and correct concentration.

RESULTING WORLDVIEW AND PSYCHOLOGY

Buddhism differs significantly from the dominant Western philosophic paradigm of rational positivism. While it is nearly a cliche to note that ours is a materialistic society, Buddhism posits a spiritualistic world in which physical reality is ultimately a delusion which seems to exist only because it is constructed by our consciousness. What sort of reality do we then construct? Matter is seen as arising from consciousness of repeated sensory impressions. As the result of repeated sensory impressions, the individual takes bodily form. Materiality is the physical manifestation of previous experience. Such an understanding of the world has obvious implications for healing, both physical and psychological, through the changing of consciousness (Govinda, 1969).

Even within the manifest world, the quality of emptiness or *shunyata* predominates and underlies all phenomena (Govinda, 1969, p. 224). Shunyata forms a yin/yang set of opposites with *thathata,* suchness, the quality of experienced existence in the now. Emptiness and suchness are ultimately polar aspects of the same truth (p. 116).

Buddhism incorporates a sophisticated psychology/philosophy called *abhidharma* which will only be touched upon in this chapter (Scotton, 1996). Although it may seem esoteric to the Western observer, abhidharma is grounded in the shared and mutually monitored experience of thousands of mediators who have spent hundreds of thousands of hours watching their own mental experiences over the course of two and one-half millennia. Again, the emphasis is on developing pragmatic knowledge which will lead the individual to release from the woes of the world. Therefore, abhidharma excels at description of states, enlightened and benighted. In noting such things as the realm of consciousness (the world of physical form, the world of pure form, the world of nonform, or the world beyond the differentiation of the three), the level of consciousness in that realm, the positive and negative emotions present, the current goal of consciousness, and the automaticity or volitionality involved in the consciousness, the Buddhists construct a complex map of awareness (Govinda, 1974, p. 115).

One traditional analysis of the human condition is that of the five *skandhas,* meaning heaps or aggregates. What we think of as a human being consists of the gathering of experiences of five categories. *Rupa skandha,* or corporeality, includes sense organs with their sense objects, the relationships between them, and their psychological products. *Vedana skandha,* feelings, includes emotional responses to sensation and from within. Issuing from both reflection and intuition, *samjna skandha,* or discriminating perception, helps us differentiate experiences. Arising from the karmic consequences of our choices, *samskara skandha* consists of mental formations which produce the illusion of an individual character, e.g., "I've always been the sort of person who. . . ." *Vinjnana* (knowing) *skandha* consists of the collection of awareness of the other skandhas. It coordinates the others and contains the possibility of pure consciousness. Using such a schema the student of Buddhism can analyze the mental contents at any moment, note their category, and disidentify from them: For example, "This is an event from the x skandha which will soon be replaced by another mental event. I can observe it but I am not that event."

PSYCHOLOGICAL AND BEHAVIORAL TENDENCIES OF THE BUDDHIST PATIENT

Obviously, adherence to a worldview so different from that of Western society may result in a very different set of priorities and behaviors. To the degree that the patient remains a practicing Buddhist, behavioral differences may not be just cultural patterns that will gradually be replaced; instead, they may be evidence of basic decisions about values that the patient has no desire to alter. For instance, what may look to the Western psychiatrist like a naive and passive acceptance of a painful state may be the external manifestation of the Buddhist patient's diligent work on altering his or her consciousness and thus the illness at hand (since, in Buddhism, physical reality emerges from patterns of mind).

Several common factors will influence both assessment and treatment of Buddhist patients. Often the same characteristic may pose both a problem in initial understanding and, once learned by the physician, an aid to his or her treatment of the patient. A list of such factors, common to all Buddhist patients, includes the following:

1. A strong valuation of the role of consciousness as a causative and curative agent in dysfunction and illness. At odds with the prevalent perception of Asians as just wishing to be "fixed" by an authority figure/doctor, this factor should be addressed to maximize the working alliance and patient compliance. The diligent Buddhist patient will be seeking to understand both the meaning of the problem and what failed in his or her consciousness that led to that difficulty. The magnitude of this assumption should not be underestimated. The principle of the primacy of consciousness over matter is assumed to be constantly operant for all of us, and the effects of that primacy are seen as profound. Not only can consciousness in ignorance cause disease but also enlightened consciousness can bring about functioning that is better than normal. Each Buddhist tradition has living adepts who demonstrate supernormal functioning, both mental and physical. Called "siddhis" (and also found in other spiritual traditions), such powers were dismissed for centuries as fancy by the Western scientific establishment but were demonstrated in laboratory conditions and became an impetus for the current interest in biofeedback, relaxation training, etc. (Scotton, Chinen, & Battista, 1996, p. 263). Once understood, this factor can greatly aid treatment because the doctor can enlist the patient in applying his or her diligence to further understand and manage the problem. From their experience with Buddhist practice, many Buddhist patients will already be familiar with the psychodynamic concept that focusing attention on a difficulty can cause it to unravel and eventually disappear.

2. An emphasis on the psychological–interpersonal–spiritual context for the current problem. Closely related to the first, this factor can also affect compliance and outcome. The psychiatrist should ask the patient what he or she thinks caused the problem, ask for clarification of foreign concepts as necessary, and listen to the description symbolically as well as literally. Failure to do so can result in dismissal of the treatment (and of the psychiatrist) as simplistic and ineffectual. Once comprehended, this factor actually makes Buddhist patients unusually open to intervention in an up to date, multifactorial, biopsychosocial–spiritual model (Scotton et al., 1996, pp. 409–415).

3. A tendency to present illness and dysfunction as a Kraepelin-like list of symptoms rather than as a disease entity. In my experience, Buddhist patients are

more likely to describe their presenting problem as, for instance, "My sleep has been disturbed and I'm not eating well," whereas other patients, even other Asian patients, are more likely to say, for instance, "I've been down lately," or "I've been a little depressed." This tendency seems related to the repeated training in Buddhist practice to watch mental and emotional events as they pass and to disidentify from them. This factor, when coupled with factor 2, can present as an "all or nothing" experience in history taking for the doctor. As he or she evidences interest in the context, the initial sparse list of symptoms often mushrooms into a long description of the patient's world. Once again, when understood, this tendency proves useful in management in that the Buddhist patient may prove particularly adept at watching the progress of target symptoms and at being vigilant for the appearance of symptoms warning of decompensation.

4. A patience with dysfunction that may seem like pathological passivity to the psychiatrist. Related to the basic tenet of annicca, or impermanence, which was discussed previously, this factor may result in the Buddhist patient calmly relating a painful situation whose depth and duration would have a typical Western patient presenting at the emergency room. Part of the patience is due to a trust that "this too shall pass" (annicca is true here too) and part may be due to a willingness to tolerate painful states as a natural part of life (the assumption of dukkha). Rather than seeing this Buddhist trait as pathological, the doctor may come to see our Western society's intolerance of suffering ("Take Maskurpane now and get fast relief!") as the abnormal position. The understanding psychiatrist can use this patience to gradually build a lasting cure for the condition at hand.

5. An assumption that the patient's Buddhist teacher, the patient's best guide to the ultimate nature of reality, will be an appropriate consultant on the progress of the psychiatric treatment. The psychiatrist should remember that the study of the mind and the study of spiritual issues are not treated separately in Buddhism but rather seen as inextricably linked. In my experience, practicing Buddhists (as opposed to Buddhists who were born into the religion but do not practice regularly) have invariably discussed their psychiatric treatment with their teachers, although in some cases I was not informed of these discussions for months. Furthermore, the teachers' comments have usually been taken with the weight of important teachings for the patient's spiritual and physical well-being. At times these interventions by the teacher have caused significant changes in the course of the therapy, usually for the better.

Not surprisingly, such patient–teacher consultations reinforce the treatment best when the psychiatrist is perceived as open to, and at least somewhat understanding of, Buddhist teachings. I have established collegial working relationships with several teachers who have been most helpful in keeping treatment of their students on course. Almost all my contacts with the teachers have been indirect: The patient tells me what the teacher says and I comment; the patient tells the teacher what I say and the teacher comments. Through such an arrangement I have found that the teacher can often be used to constellate a superego/higher Self inner figure for the patient who can be consulted when the patient feels the need for guidance. Such work in therapy is seen as quite consonant with spiritual practice in which the guru becomes internalized.

EXAMINING AND TREATING THE TWO MAIN GROUPS OF AMERICAN BUDDHISTS

THE ASIAN AMERICAN BUDDHIST

Although so far concentrated on the coasts and in university communities, Asian American Buddhists are becoming increasingly common throughout the United States. It is important for the clinician to remember that the Asian American may have multiple religious affiliations. Due to the nature of Asian society (Joseph Campbell once remarked that the idea of heresy seemed confined to the religions springing from Jerusalem and the Kremlin), the clinician may encounter (as I have) a Korean family which is both Christian and Buddhist; a Japanese patient who is Shintoist and Buddhist; a Chinese patient who is Taoist, Confucian, and Buddhist; or an Indian patient who resides in and consults with the board of directors of a Hindu ashram but is Buddhist. The clinician should inform himself or herself about all parts of the patient's background.

Much of the patient's presenting picture will be affected by his or her culture of origin, apart from his or her religious beliefs. Dr. Juthani has done an excellent job of summarizing those cultural qualities for Hindus in her chapter in this book and much of what she says can be applied to Asians in general. Asians will tend to attribute much status and respect to doctors and will, in turn, expect the doctor to act as an active leader in responding to the presenting situation. They will tend to be confused and disappointed by an open-ended, nondirective approach. Therefore, the clinician hoping to do psychotherapy from a traditional "neutral" stance must do a careful job of assessing the patient's understanding of such an approach and must not assume that difficulty in participating in such treatment constitutes pathological defensiveness.

Asian patients will appear acquiescent to treatment recommendations but the psychiatrist must not assume that treatment will be followed to the letter. Particularly early in treatment, and particularly when the patient is unsure that the clinician understands him or her and his or her culture, treatment recommendations will be tempered, adjusted, and combined with other traditional responses as the patient attempts to find treatment appropriate for an Asian person like himself or herself in these Western circumstances. The treating psychiatrist, wishing to maximize treatment, must therefore learn about the culture at hand and the interventions the patient may be mixing in or wondering about the absence of. Armed with such knowledge, the psychiatrist can adjust treatments appropriately. As the treatment progresses the psychiatrist will find that, having established himself or herself as informed and sensitive, his or her recommendations are followed more completely.

As a measure of how biased our discipline has been in the area of tolerance of other cultures' spiritual experiences, the clinician should remember that, until the groundbreaking work of Lu, Lukoff, and Turner that resulted in the inclusion of a "V code" for nonpathological religious experience in the *DSM-IV*, even spiritual experience that was validated by entire cultures was forced to be labeled psychotic (American Psychiatric Association, 1994; Lukoff, Lu, & Turner, 1996).

THE AMERICAN CONVERT TO BUDDHISM

American converts are becoming increasingly prevalent, a fact that the clinician may overlook if he or she does not routinely take a spiritual–religious history. Many Buddhist converts continue to think of themselves as being simultaneously part of their religion of origin. The psychiatrist may therefore think he or she works with "a typical American" when in fact he or she is faced with a Catholic–Buddhist, Protestant–Buddhist, or atheist–Buddhist patient, each of whom may have his or her own particular twist on Buddhism. Jewish–Buddhists seem particularly prominent and include a number of popular Buddhist teachers (Boorstein, 1996). Again, the clinician is behooved to learn about all the formative influences if he or she is not already familiar with them.

Practices differ widely among Buddhists. Tibetan Buddhists often practice detailed prescribed visualizations of figures who personify spiritual attributes. These practices often require hours to follow through once. Theravadan Buddhist practice from Southeast Asia may prescribe sweeping inch by inch over the body with the consciousness or watching thoughts and feelings arise and then pass away. Zen Buddhists are often instructed to "just sit." In all cases the practice can produce states of altered consciousness and mental experiences which the clinician could mistakenly label as pathological in a Westerner. For instance, a visualized figure may move or speak, a mediator may experience his or her body as dissolving, and a "sitter" may experience the world as a delightful fabrication of vibrating energy. The doctor must inquire about the meaning of such experiences in the context of the spiritual tradition. Most important, even if the experience seems novel to the tradition, the doctor must examine it from a pragmatic point of view for the patient. Is the atypical experience at hand part of a context of spiritual experience that produces growth and insight for the patient, is it part of a context of other pathological symptoms that inhibit good functioning, or is it a mixture of the two (Scotton, 1985)? Given that a basic part of the Buddhist approach is to alter one's perception of the world, the psychiatrist must not assume that any atypical perception is automatically pathological.

SUMMARY AND CONCLUSION

The evaluation and treatment of Buddhist patients has been seen to include the practice of sound clinical principles such as taking a good spiritual–religious history, learning about the patient's cultural background and understanding its influence on the treatment, and adopting a pragmatic, rather than rigid, standard for evaluating unusual mental events. Specific information about basic Buddhist beliefs and about the numerous cultures of origin of Buddhist patients have been given to aid the clinician's understanding. Once the psychiatrist has demonstrated a sensitivity to these issues, the Buddhist emphasis on the individual's use of consciousness often works to produce an unusually diligent and cooperative patient.

REFERENCES

American Psychiatric Association. (1994). *Diagnostic and Statistical Manual IV.* Washington, DC: Author.

Boorstein, S. (1996). *That's funny, you don't look Buddhist.* San Francisco: Harper.

Buott, E. (Ed.). (1955). *Teachings of the compassionate Buddha.* New York: Penguin.

Govinda, A. (1969). *Foundations of Tibetan mysticism.* New York: Weiser.

Govinda, A. (1974). *The psychological attitude of early Buddhist philosophy.* New York: Weiser.

Lukoff, D., Lu, F., & Turner, R. (1996). Diagnosis: A transpersonal clinical approach to religious and spiritual problems. In B. Scotton, A. Chinen, & J. Battista, (Eds.), *Textbook of transpersonal psychiatry and psychology.* New York: Basic Books.

Scotton, B. (1985). Observations on the teaching and supervision of transpersonal psychotherapy. *Journal of Transpersonal Psychology, 17*(1), 57–75.

Scotton, B. (1996). The contribution of Buddhism to transpersonal psychiatry. In B. Scotton, A. Chinen, & J. Battista (Eds.), *Textbook of transpersonal psychiatry and psychology.* New York: Basic Books.

Scotton, B., Chinen, A., & Battista, J. (Eds.). (1996). *Textbook of transpersonal psychiatry and psychology.* New York: Basic Books.

Sopa, L., & Hopkins, J. (1976). *Practice and theory of Tibetan Buddhism.* New York: Grove Press.

19

UNDERSTANDING AND TREATING HINDU PATIENTS

NALINI V. JUTHANI

Albert Einstein College of Medicine
New York, New York 10461

There is an emerging consensus among mental health professionals studying religion that understanding patients' religious beliefs/faith and practices is extremely important in diagnosis and treatment. Just as one cannot treat the body without closely examining the mind, one cannot treat the disorders of the mind without understanding its spiritual dimension.

Religious beliefs and faith have helped many people understand the meaning of life, cope with struggles, and provide social support. All the world's religions are alike in this respect; however, they differ in their cultural expression.

Psychiatric patients may have a conscious or unconscious fear that clinical probing of their religious values may lead to undermining of a cherished belief or exposure to ridicule (Presser, 1971). Patients who are culturally different, such as Hindus, may feel this more strongly, creating an additional barrier in communicating such beliefs to their mental health providers.

This chapter attempts to guide mental health clinicians in the understanding and treatment of Hindu patients. It is based on the author's understanding of Hindu religion and Hindu culture. It is estimated that over 800 million people in the world adhere to Hinduism. The majority of these people are from the Indian subcontinent, North America, Europe, and Africa. Surprisingly to many Americans, North America has three numerically large generations of Hindus as native-born or naturalized citizens.

INTRODUCTION TO HINDUISM

Hinduism is one of the world's oldest religions. It has no known beginning, no human founder, and predates recorded history. It is an integral part of many human lives and is well integrated with the cultural practices of its followers. The major scriptures of Hinduism are the Vedas, the Upnishads, and the Bhagwad Gita. The Vedas are considered the oldest; therefore, Hinduism has been called the "Vedic" religion as well.

Hinduism has involved itself in a continuous exchange of thoughts and beliefs with the Jain, Buddhist, and Sikh religions. This interaction has benefitted the evolution, reformation, and progress of Hindu Society, traditions, and rituals. The rules of society and the ways of conduct (Dharma) are laid down in Smriti by the Rrisis or Saints.

The most important of Smriti text is The Laws of Manu. The Smriti can make adaptation to time, place, and circumstances. The Upnishad reformed some of the Vedic rituals. The two epics, Ramayana and Mahabharata, played an important role in understanding of Vedic system of thoughts. The Bhagwad Gita, which was recited by Krishna in the epic Mahabharata, played a very important role in understanding the concept of God, devotion, reincarnation, etc. Hinduism sees no conflict between science and religion, notably in the doctrines of creation, evolution, and causality. Hindu tradition considers Rrisis as scientists and the Hindu way of life encourages both outer and inner pursuit of truth. The ultimate goal is God realization or self-realization. The state does not legislate Dharma.

Since Hinduism prevailed in India predating recorded history, it can be viewed as an ethnic religion. However, in understanding Hinduism, one identifies a universalizing core. This concept of universality implies plurality rather than uniformity or isomorphic equality (Sharma, 1993). Hinduism, therefore, is a system of philosophy rooted in the experience of many Rrisis or Saints. The Hindu "believes in one creator and a supreme reality which is the ground of one's divinity." The Upnishad calls this divine simply Atman, Brahma, or Self. This Self is seen to be one, the same in everyone. The Self is in all creatures and is not different from the Ultimate Reality called God (Easwaran, 1987a). This reality is said to be beyond description, but it is a "pure consciousness" which makes the eye see and the mind think. This divine power is changeless, holds everything together, creates, dissolves, and re-creates.

This informing power or spirit is God, who is recognized by many names. These names are both male and female. In Bhagwad Gita there is a great verse which states, "Whenever righteousness declines and the purpose of life is forgotten, I manifest myself on earth. I am born in every age to protect the good, destroy the evil and re-establish the truth." This is how Hindus look upon Krishna, Rama, Buddha, Vishnu, and others as divine incarnations of God (Easwaran, 1987b). Based on individuals' faith in these reincarnated beings, several sects of Hinduism developed.

Hinduism considers the concept of God as ever-loving and purely benevolent.

It is in all lives and manifests as love, truth, and light. All life is therefore sacred, to be loved, respected, and revered. Hindus believe in nonviolence or *ahimsa* and Universal Love for all creatures.

BASIC COMPONENTS

Hindu philosophy is based on the following major elements:

1. Law of Karma: All deeds or actions of a human being are called Karma. The law of Karma states that every event is both a cause and an effect. "As you sow, so shall you reap." Every action will have its reaction, and every cause will have its destiny determined in due course of time (Thakkar, 1988). Therefore, the law of Karma is the law of (a) action and reaction, (b) cause and effect, and (c) effort and destiny. The law of Karma states unequivocally that though we cannot see the connections, we can be sure that everything that happens to us, good or bad, originated once in something we did or thought about doing. We ourselves are responsible for what happens to us. It follows that we can change what happens to us by our efforts to change ourselves. We can take destiny into our own hands. This Karma is committed not only physically but also by our thoughts. Hindu philosophy compares a thought to a seed: very tiny, but it can grow into a huge, deep-rooted, wide-spreading tree. Similarly, it is believed that thoughts, although as small as a seed, lead to actions. It is also believed that good Karma is rewarded and sinful Karma is punished. Superficially the Law of Karma may be considered punitive, but it is much more illuminating to consider Karma an educative force whose purpose is to teach an individual to pursue life selflessly toward the welfare of the whole. In this sense, life is considered a school in which one learns, skips a grade, stays behind, or can graduate. As long as a debt of Karma remains, a person has to keep coming back for further education and self-realization. This is the basis of the cycle of birth and death (Easwaran, 1987b).

2. Reincarnation: Soul is eternal and immortal. It undergoes endless cycles of creation, preservation, and destruction. It takes a different body in each birth until it is completely self-realized. All souls, therefore, evolve toward union with creator, ultimately find spiritual knowledge, and are liberated from the cycles of rebirth, thereby reaching "Nirvana."

3. Dharma: Dharma is rules of society and the ways of conduct. Therefore, Dharma is the essential order of things which brings an integrity and harmony to the universe. It means rightness, justice, goodness, and purpose through selflessness. Underlying this concept of Dharma is the oneness of life. The Upnishad discovered that lives are interconnected because at its deepest level creation is indivisible. This oneness bestows a basic balance on the whole of nature such that disturbance in one place sends ripples everywhere until balance is restored. The highest Dharma of a Hindu is ahimsa or nonviolence through Universal Love for all creatures (Easwaran, 1987b).

4. Guru: Hindus believe that a spiritually awakened teacher or "Guru" is es-

sential in one's life. Guru shows a path to righteous life through understanding of *jnan* (real knowledge), Karma (deeds), and *bhakti* (devotional worship).

5. Idol worship: Images are very important in Hindu religion. Many Hindus have idols in their homes and in temples which serve as objects of devotion. Philosophically, it is important to note that the idol itself is not worshipped but rather is representation of an aspect of the divine. However, to many Hindus the idol itself is of significance. Human mind is very powerful. It can re-create anything it concentrates on. Concentration cannot exist without bhakti or devotion. In the first stage of idol worship the devotee will concentrate his or her mind on the physical image of the God he or she loves. Once fixed on God's physical image with faith, the mind gradually turns to God's nonphysical qualities. These qualities gradually manifest in the worshipper's life. Ultimately, the devotee progresses beyond these manifest qualities and attains the realization that "God is with me, indwelling" and "I am the spiritual joy." Thus, Gita says that the idol worship plays a very important role in making the mind sensitive, powerful, and progressive (Athavale, 1988). It sublimates libido into spiritual love. It is the nature of the mind to worry about the past, dream about the future, and to be discontent with the present. The only way the mind can be purified and made stable is by engaging it in worship. The form of God we choose to worship depends on our inclination and our faith. Gita merely instructs "Fix your mind on me." Idol worship is considered a perfect science and a psychological necessity. It is believed that concentration on a form of God (an idol) gives peace to the conscious mind and purifies the unconscious mind by regulating it. Full concentration during idol worship takes the mind into a complete state of meditation. It is during this state of meditation that the conscious mind and the unconscious mind unify in the worship of God. The unconscious instincts and libidinous desires sublimate into spiritual love and fullness (Athavale, 1992).

6. Ayurveda: In understanding a Hindu patient, one needs to become familiar with the ancient Indian science of life called *Ayurveda*. The purpose of Ayurveda is to tell us how our lives can be influenced, shaped, extended, and ultimately controlled without interferences from sickness or old age. The guiding principle of Ayurveda is that the mind exerts influence on the body and freedom from sickness depends on contacting one's awareness, bringing it into balance, and then extending that balance to the body. The state of balanced awareness, more than any kind of physical immunity, creates a higher state of health. Ayurveda embodies the collected wisdom of sages who began their tradition many centuries ago and it has been carried forward generation after generation. According to ayurvedic understanding, every human has a body type which is like a blueprint outlining the innate tendencies that have been built into his or her system. By knowing one's body type an Ayurvedic practitioner can tell which diet, physical activities, and therapies can help treat a person (Chopra, 1991).

The classification of mental illness conforms to the Ayurvedic categories of *nija* (endogenous, arising out of the imbalance of doshas) and *agantu* (exogenous, mostly possession states) (Desai, 1989). The endogenous category consists of symptoms such as inappropriate smiling or laughing, dancing or singing (flighty), anger, excitement, and violence. These symptoms are considered curable by corrective dietary regimen, emesis, massage, enemas, reassurance, and a variety of Ayurvedic drugs.

The exogenous type of insanity is caused by the wrath of gods or ancestors or possession by various categories of spirits. It is usually regarded as incurable. Some think this insanity is caused by bad Karma of the previous life.

COMMON PRACTICES OF HINDU FOLLOWERS

In most concrete terms a Hindu strives to evolve from a material human to a spiritual one and considers God as an inspirer. The following practices are used in the day to day life of a Hindu; some carry out these practices as a tradition with or without understanding:

1. Express gratitude to God by praying in the morning, at meal times, and at bed time. One also bows in gratitude to one's Guru, parents, and elders.

2. Obtain knowledge and good thoughts from a Guru and by reading scriptures directed at living a righteous life. This is also accomplished by attending regular discourses given by saints.

3. Do Karma to evolve from a selfish materialistic life to a more selfless life. Examine one's deeds on a daily basis, with a hope that such an introspection will lead to a higher stage of spiritual development.

4. Worship an idol of a deity of one's choice and learn to concentrate one's mind on the deity's virtues and absorb its values and philosophy of living. Idol worship leading to meditation is used to purify one's mind and become free of evil forces created by materialistic desires. The words "OM," "Shanti," or "Peace," are often recited during meditation.

5. Fast on a regular monthly or bimonthly schedule to control and regulate desires.

6. Work in harmony with the cosmos. Many Hindus believe in astrology whereby it is believed that the movement of the planets and the stars in the universe have an effect on all creatures including humans. Therefore, major life events are planned according to the astrological predictions. Certain days and times are considered more desirable than others in the lunar calendar. Therefore, major life events are planned on such desirable days and times. Horoscope matching of a man and a woman is a common element in arranging a marriage. If the horoscopes do not match, it is believed that the marriage will have many problems and may end up in divorce or death of a spouse.

7. Share the good thoughts from Hindu scriptures with others out of love and Dharma or responsibility. Making such visits to people is considered God's work.

8. Offer a portion of one's energy, physical, emotional, intellectual, or economical, toward the selfless work.

9. Provide warmth and support to all human beings, build a community, and develop a social network.

10. Bathe in holy rivers like the Ganges when on a pilgrimage. Hindus desire to have their bodies cremated after death and the ashes carried to the River Ganges. It means an eventual merger with nature. Many of these practices are carried out by generation after generation of Hindus. For some, these practices have become traditions that are carried out as rituals without full understanding.

11. Revere and worship one's ancestors. Hindus have great reverence for one's ancestors, who often serve as inspirational images. Therefore, many rituals and customs are based on what ancestors have done.

CLINICAL EVALUATION AND TREATMENT OF HINDU PATIENTS

Religion and culture are integral parts of life for Hindu patients. Patients are rarely self-referred Most of them are referred by a friend, a wise man of the society, or a priest. Prior to seeing a psychiatric clinician, a patient may often consult a folk healer or a priest and get treated with herbal medication.

A recent study published in the *New England Journal of Medicine* stated that fully one-fourth of Americans who seek help from a physician for a serious medical condition may also be using spiritual healing, herbal medicines, folk remedies, or other forms of nonconventional treatment (Sharp, 1995). This is certainly true for Hindu patients. It is only when symptoms persist that a psychiatrist is consulted. These patients usually have the following expectations:

1. The psychiatrist will be an advisor, teacher, and a guidance counsellor—almost like a Guru.

2. The psychiatrist will listen to all members of the family and involve them in treatment.

3. The psychiatrist will prescribe some medications.

4. The psychiatrist will provide symptom relief.

Therefore, in initial assessment it is recommended that the clinician listen to family members describe the patient's symptoms. The physician should identify the spokesperson and decision maker of the family. This spokesperson is usually educated and a good communicator. Compliance from the patient may depend on the rapport with the family.

During evaluation, the clinician should

1. Be interactive and abandon a nonjudgmental, passive, neutral stance.

2. Be focused at the very beginning. Exploratory talk therapy does not work in early phases of treatment.

3. Identify the problems. Cognitive and behavioral psychotherapy may be useful, but Hindu patients tend to conceal pathology and suffer quietly. Therefore, the clinician must probe vigorously.

4. Be authoritative. Expect that the patient will agree with the prescribed treatment plan but do not expect compliance automatically. Patients tend to agree as part of showing respect toward the psychiatrist but may continue to modify medications and mix them with herbal medications—without consulting the psychiatrist.

5. Use medical model of treatment. Somatic symptoms are frequently described by the patient. Listen for the larger or perhaps symbolic meaning of these symptoms.

6. Target for symptom relief through medications in the initial phase of treatment. Self-improvement and character change are desired only by a very few highly motivated patients. Such patients will respond to traditional exploratory insight-oriented psychotherapy.

7. Involve the family at every stage of treatment and make special efforts to get those family members who do not show up for sessions involved.

8. Identify the social network and utilize it to help patients connect within the sociocultural network.

9. Do not dismiss the patient's beliefs but listen empathically and provide support. Patients may explain inexplicable illnesses and untimely death similarly to accidents and misfortune that are often explained as the unseen workings of Karma.

10. At times a clinician may support a family decision to see only faith healers since in many instances traditional healing ceremonies may work similarly to psychotherapy for that patient. Patients with possession states, for example, respond to drug, recitation of mantras, offerings to deities, vows, performance of rituals, and worship of Gods. Underneath such possession states, some patients may have unconscious desires to bring the behavior of family members into compliance with their own wishes.

11. Do not interpret a patient's expectation of the psychiatrist to be a Guru as transference but understand it as part of the culture.

12. Do not interfere in patients' beliefs, rituals, and practices, but instead offer advice to prevent illness and improve health. Such an attitude of acceptance goes a long way in easing cross-cultural tensions.

ISSUES IN EVALUATING AND DIAGNOSING HINDU PATIENTS

Having understood the cultural and religious ways of approaching a Hindu patient, a clinician should remember to distinguish between healthy and unhealthy religious factors in a patient's adaptation to life situations. Healthy spirituality involves courage, prudence, love for oneself, love for others, as well as knowledge and open-mindedness. These factors work together to make a person well integrated. True knowledge and open-mindedness constitute wisdom. Effective psychological integration and wisdom go hand in hand.

From a Hindu viewpoint, unhealthy religiosity involves excessive fear, lack of prudence, selfishness, self-hate, hate of others, ignorance and close-mindedness, as well as more extreme symptoms such as delusions and hallucinations of a religious nature. The former factors lead to conflicts and result in stunted emotional and spiritual growth and destructiveness (Xavier, 1987). Psychiatrists may encounter Hindu patients who are at various stages of spiritual development and cultural adaptation. In many cases spiritual issues may be related to psychological issues, e.g., a constantly angry person may perceive God as punitive and sadistic. Psychological treatment may then free the patient to move to a higher level of spirituality. It should be noted, however, that psychiatric treatments may not lead to the greatest level of spirituality and that patients' faith and cultural practices may continue where the psychiatrist has left off.

REFERENCES

Athavale, P. (1988). *The call of duty.* IL: Devotional Associates of Yogeshwar.
Athavale, P. *(1992). The system.* Bombay: Sat Vichar Darshan Trust.
Chopra, D. (1991). *Perfect health: The complete mind/body guide.* New York: Harmony Books.
Desai, P. C. (1989). *Health and medicine in the Hindu tradition.* New York: Crossroad.
Easwaran, E. (1987a). *The Upnishads.* CA: Nilgiri Press.
Easwaran, E. (1987b). *The Bhagwad Gita.* CA: Nilgiri Press.
Presser, P. C. (1971). Assessment of the patients' religious attitudes in the psychiatric case study. *Bulletin of Menninger Clinic, 35,* 272–291.
Sharma, A. (1993). *Our religions.* New York: Harper Collins.
Sharp, D. (1995). Culture clash. *Hippocrates, 2,* 37–41.
Thakkar, H. (1988). *Theory of Karma.* Ahmadabad: Navajivan Mudranalaya.
Xavier, N. C. (1987). *The two faces of religion: A psychiatrists' view.* AL: Portals Press.

20

RELIGION AND MENTAL HEALTH FROM THE MUSLIM PERSPECTIVE

SYED ARSHAD HUSAIN

University of Missouri at Columbia
Columbia, Missouri 65212

Islam is the most rapidly growing religion in the United States, and if this trend continues, Islam will become the second largest religion in this country. There are over 1.5 billion Muslims in the world and Islam is the majority religion in 48 countries. For these reasons, it is relevant for health care providers to become familiar with the basic tenets of Islam.

Each major religion of the world has its own quest for spirituality and wellness. The religious quest in general tells us about the basic human makeup, its inner weaknesses, potential qualities, and the need for a set of guiding principles for leading a meaningful life and attaining a healthy state of mind. In this chapter, I will attempt to illustrate the spiritual and moral systems of Islamic faith and the value Islam attaches to the spiritual, mental, and physical health of mankind. Before we embark upon this discussion, it will be helpful to review briefly the history and general principles of Islam.

HISTORICAL BACKGROUND OF ISLAM

Islam is the last of the great Semitic religions. The word Islam means "Peace" and "to submit to the will or law of God." The Islamic laws were revealed to prophet Mohammed over a period of 23 years beginning in the year 610 AD and are preserved in the holy book Qur'an.

Muhammad was born in 570 AD in Mecca. His father died before his birth, and his mother died when he was 6 years old. Mohammad was first raised by his grandfather and, after his grandfather's death, by his uncle Abu Talib. As a young boy he traveled with his uncle to Syria, and some years later he made similar trips in the service of a wealthy widow named Khadijah. He transacted the widow's business honestly and with great expertise. Khadijah was very impressed by young Mohammad's character, loyalty, and steadfastness, the attributes which earned him the title "Al-Amin" (the trustworthy). She soon asked his hand in marriage. He agreed even though she was 15 years older than he.

Mohammed belonged to the clan Banu Hashim, a subsect of the powerful and prosperous tribe Al-Quresh. The Quresh were the descendants of Abraham through Ishmael. The Ka'bah was erected in Mecca by Abraham for the worship of One God, but over time the objective changed to idol worship. There were few who still longed for the religion of Abraham and were known as *Hunafa* ("by nature upright"), Muhammad being one of them. Every year Mohammad used to retire with his family to cave Hira on the top of Jabal-Alnoor ("the mountain of light"), not far from Mecca, for meditation. It was there one night at the age of 40 that the first revelation came to him. He heard a voice say: "Read!"

> "Read: In the name of thy Lord who Createth.
> "Createth man from a clot.
> "Read: And it is thy Lord the Most Bountiful
> "Who teacheth by the pen,
> "Teacheth man that which he knew not."

He saw an angel who said: "O Muhammad! Thou art Allah's messenger, and I am Gabriel." At first he was frightened and ignored the angel, thinking that his imagination or a spirit was playing a trick on him. Muhammad, frightened and confused, reported this experience to his wife Khadijah. He was very distressed and perturbed about the whole experience but Khadijah reassured him and took him to an old man, Waraqa Bin Nawfal, who was familiar with "the Scriptures of the Jews and Christians." Waraqa told Khadijah and Mohammed that the heavenly messenger who previously came to Moses had come to Muhammad, and that Mohammad was chosen as the prophet of his people. Mohammad was still very perturbed. The angel Gabriel appeared before him several times and finally assured him that what he was experiencing was not a figment of his imagination. Once convinced of his prophethood, Mohammed accepted the overwhelming task assigned to him by his creator. From then on, he became filled with an enthusiasm of obedience to his lord which justifies his proudest title of "The Slave of Allah."

The verses revealed to Mohammad when in a state of a trance for the following 23 years are held sacred by the Muslims as the words of God. Also, because the angel on Jabal-Alnoor, the mountain of light, bade him to "Read!" and insisted on his "Reading" though he was illiterate, the sacred book is known as *Al-Qur'an,* ("The Reading:" the reading of the man who knew not how to read).

For the first 3 years of his Mission, the Prophet preached only to his family. His wife Khadijah was the first to accept Islam, followed by his first cousin Ali, whom he had adopted, then his servant Zeyd, a former slave. His old friend Abu Bakr also was among those who accepted Islam early along with some of his slaves and dependents.

At the end of the third year, the Prophet received the command from Allah to "Arise and warn," whereupon he began to preach in public and began to speak against their idol worshiping. The Quresh responded with severe hostility, persecuting his poorer disciples and mocking and insulting him. So cruel was the persecution that the Prophet advised some Muslims to emigrate to Abyssinia (present-day Ethiopia), then a Christian country. Despite persecution and emigration, the Muslim community continued to grow in number. The Quresh, in an effort to stop this steady growth of Muslim community, tried a compromise and offered to accept his religion and make him their chieftain if he would give up attacking idolatry. When this effort failed, they went to his uncle Abu Talib, asking his permission to kill Mohammad and promising to give him all that he desired. Abu Talib refused.

The opposition to Mohammad's preaching grew tougher and he had little success among the Meccans. His mission was becoming a failure when, during the season of the yearly pilgrimage, a small group of men from Yathrib, since known as *Madinah,* approached him. At Yathrib, Jewish rabbis had often spoken of a Prophet soon to come among the Arabs who would help Jews to destroy the pagans. The men from Yathrib saw Muhammad and recognized him as the prophet the rabbis had described. At the following season of pilgrimage, a deputation from Yathrib came to meet the Prophet. They swore allegiance to him in the first pact of Al-'Aqabah. They returned to Yathrib with a Muslim teacher who spread the message of the prophet in that city.

During the following pilgrimage, 73 Muslims from Yathrib came to Mecca and vowed allegiance to the Prophet. At this time Mohammed decided to immigrate to Yathrib. When Meccans learned of this plan, they conspired to kill him.

The Hijrah, the flight from Mecca to Yathrib, marks the beginning of the Muslim era. The 10 years which followed Hijrah represent the years of success, the fullest that has ever crowned one man's endeavor. The Hijrah establishes a clear distinction in the story of the Prophet's mission, which is evident in the Qur'an. Until then he had been a preacher only. Henceforth, he became the absolute spiritual and political leader of a state which grew in 10 years into the empire of Arabia. He instituted a series of reforms and laid the foundations of the nascent Islamic state. At the time of Muhammad's death in June 632 AD the whole of Arabia had embraced Islam. His successors, the caliphs, who were elected by the people, were designated as the heads of the state and the religious community but had no power to enunciate laws or define dogma. The entire fabric of Islamic life, both private and public, was governed by the laws of Islam. They spread the domain of Islam within a century from the shores of North Africa to deep into central Asia up to India.

THE MEANING OF ISLAM

The word Islam means submission to the Will of God and obedience to His Law. Only through submission to the Will of God and by obedience to His Law can one achieve true peace and enjoy lasting purity. Allah is one and has no partners. He is the creator of the heavens and the earth. He is the Absolute Transcendent Creator, the Lord and Master of all. Allah is the one who Adam, Noah, Abraham, Isaac, Ishmael, the Tribes Moses, Jesus, and Muhammad all worshiped. Allah alone is infinite and original being, all else is created by him and suffer finitude. The Qur'an (59: 22–24) mentions many attributes of Allah:

> He is Allah, than whom there is no other God, the knower of the invisible and visible. He is the beneficent, the Merciful, the Sovereign Lord, the Holy One, peace, the keeper of faith, the guardian, the Majestic, the Compeller, the Superb. Glorified by Allah from all that they ascribe as partners (to Him). He is Allah, the Creator, the Shaper out of nothing, the Fashioner. His are the most beautiful names. All that is in the Heaven and the Earth glorifies him and He is the Mighty the Wise.

The Muslims believe that Muhammad was the last, not the only, prophet who reinforced and immortalized the eternal message of God to mankind. This message was revealed by God to many prophets of different nations at different times, including Abraham, Ishmael, Isaac, David, Moses, Jesus, and Muhammad. A Muslim accepts all the prophets previous to Muhammad without discrimination. He or she believes that all those prophets of God and their faithful followers were Muslims, and that their religion was Islam. The Qur'an (3: 83) states,

> Say: We believe in Allah and that which was revealed to us, and that which was revealed to Abraham and Ishmael and Isaac and Jacob and the tribes and that which was given to Moses and Jesus and to the Prophets from their Lord; we make no distinction between any of them, and to Him we submit.

QUR'AN

The definitive sources of Islamic Law are Qur'an, Sunnah, and Hadith. The Qur'an consists of 114 Suras or chapters containing 6616 ayahs (verses). The Qur'an has been preserved in original Arabic both in writing and memory for the past 1400 years. The Qur'an has been the source from which Muslims have derived not only their law and theology but also the principles and institutions of their public life. The Qur'an assigns the prophet four distinct roles: (a) the expounder of the Qur'an, (b) the legislator, (c) one to be obeyed, and (d) the model for the Muslim behavior. Sunnah (means models for others) gives Muslims the examples of the prophet's actions, conduct, and practical application of Qur'anic law in day to day life. The Qur'an regards obedience to the prophet as obedience to and love for Allah. There is hardly any principle of the Qur'an which is left untranslated in the Sunnah. It is the perfect record of the implementation of the Qur'anic teaching. Hadith (means tradition) are the statements made by the Prophet in the light of Qur'anic law and recorded by his companions about a variety of issues confronting the Muslim Umma at that time. The Qur'an seeks to inculcate a healthy, middle-of-the-road attitude on morality. While its warnings of punishment are very strong, so is its hope in God's compassion and forgiveness.

THE FIVE PILLARS OF ISLAM

Every act performed by a Muslim aiming at fulfilling the Will of God is tanta-mount to an act of worship in Islam. The specific acts of worship are termed the "Pillars of Islam" and provide the framework of Muslim spiritual life. These are as follows:

1. Al-shahadah (the declaration of faith): "To bear witness that there is no one worthy of worship except God (Allah), and that Muhammad is His final servant and messenger." The Qur'an persistently condemns worshiping others than God or assigning partners to him.

2. Al-salah (prayers): Prayers are prescribed five times a day as a duty toward God. Prayer strengthens and enlivens belief in God and inspires man to higher morality. It purifies the heart and controls temptation, wrong-doing, and evil. The prerequisites for prayer include *Wudu* (ablution), purity of intention, body, dress, and environment, and facing Mecca where Ka'bah is situated.

3. Al-Sawm (fasting during the month of Ramadan): This means abstention from dawn to sunset from food, beverages, and sex and curbing evil intentions and desires. It teaches love, sincerity, and devotion. It develops patience, unselfishness, social conscience, and willpower to bear hardships.

4. Al-Zakah (alms tax): A proportionately fixed contribution collected from the wealth and earnings of well-to-do and the rich. It is spent on the poor and needy, in particular, and the welfare of the society in general. The payment of Zakah pu-rifies one's income and wealth and helps to establish economic balance and social justice in the society.

5. Al-Hajj (pilgrimage to the Ka'bah in Mecca): Pilgrimage taken once in a lifetime, provided one has the means to undertake the journey.

CONCEPT OF RIGHTEOUSNESS

All humans are accountable for their deeds. The task of the Islamic communi-ty is defined as "commanding good and forbidding evil with faith in God" (Qur'an 2: 142;110). Faith in God and performance of righteous deeds are the springboard of the Qur'an. The Qur'an proclaims humans as "the noblest of all creatures, they nevertheless come down to the lowest of the low" (Qur'an 95:488) unless they re-deem themselves through faith and good deeds.

Islamic values are aimed at establishing a very moral and practical attitude to-ward life and the central objective of the Qur'an is to influence and provide guid-ance for human conduct. God stands at the very basis of the Qur'an's entire doc-trinal teaching. God constitutes the integrity of every existence, particularly of humankind both individually and socially. God alone is infinite and original be-ing; all else is created by Him and suffers finitude.

The four most fundamental relational qualities of God vis-à-vis humans are cre-ation, sustenance, guidance, and judgment, and they are logically interconnected.

Creation of the universe constitutes the primordial mercy of God. Nature is therefore the handiwork of God created for humankind: "God has made subservient the heaven and the earth and whatever is in them to human kind" (Qur'an 31:20;cf. 2: 29;45:12). Human beings were alone created to serve God.

Three key terms in the Qur'an relate to human conduct, all of which means "to be safe" and "to be integral and sound": *Iman, Taqwa,* and *Islam.*

Iman means belief or faith but its root *aman* means "to be at peace" and "to be safe." A *momin* (one who has Iman) is one who believes in God, his angels, in the Qur'an as his book, his messengers with Mohammad being the last of them all, the day of judgment, and the absolute knowledge and wisdom of God. A momin always trusts God and enjoys unshakable confidence in him. A momin observes his daily prayers regularly and pays religious taxes (Zakah) to the rightful beneficiaries. A momin enjoys the right and good and combats the wrong and evil by all lawful means.

Taqwa means "piety" or "fear of God," but whose root *wqy* means "to protect from getting lost or wasted" or "guard against peril." One can protect oneself from peril by being righteous. God explains righteousness in the Qur'an (2:177) as follows:

> It is not righteousness that you turn your faces towards east or west, but it is righteousness to believe in God and the last day and angel and the book and the messenger, to spend of your wealth in spite of your love for it, do all you can for orphans, for the needy, for the wayfarer, of those who ask and for the ransom of slaves, to be steadfast in prayer and practice regular charity, to fulfill the contracts which you have made, and to be firm and patient in pain and adversity and throughout all years of panic such of the people should be God minded.

THE CONCEPT OF EQUALITY

The Qur'an asserts that all human beings are equal in the eyes of Allah. The Qur'an (49:13) states,

> O, mankind verily, we have created you from a single pair of the male and the female, and have made you into nations and tribes that you may know each other. Verily, the most honored of you in the sight of God is the most righteous.

There may be differences of abilities, potentials, ambitions, wealth, etc., but none of these can by itself establish a status of superiority or one man raised against another. The cast, color, creed, and status have no bearing on the character and the personality of the individual in Allah's eyes. Allah recognizes piety, righteousness, and spiritual excellence as the criteria for superiority in mankind. Equality is not just a matter of constitutional right, it is an article of faith that the Muslim takes seriously and to which he or she must adhere sincerely. The foundations of the Islamic value of equality are deeply rooted in the structure of Islam. It stems from the basic principles such as (a) all men are created by One and the same eternal God, the Supreme Lord of all; (b) all mankind belong to the human race and share equally in the common parentage of Adam and Eve; (c) God is just and kind to all His creatures; He is not partial to any race, age, sex, or religion; the whole universe is His dominion, and all people are His creatures; (d) all people are born equal in the sense that none brings any possession at birth and none takes back any of worldly belongings at death; (e) God judges every person on the basis of his or her own merit and deeds; and (f) God has conferred on man a title of honor and dignity. Islam describes itself as a theme, an all-encompassing description that goes way, way beyond the boundaries of religion. Thus, Islam is not just a religion; it is a political system and a method of social organization. It is a methodology of solving mankind's spiritual, practical, and intellectual problems. Islam therefore is a culture and civilization and a worldview—a living, dynamic total system.

This system maintains a unified structure through a matrix of internal values and concepts which gives Islam its unique character. Because Islam is a total system, these values and concepts permeate every aspect of human life and endeavor. Nothing is left untouched by these values, whether political structures or social organizations, economic concerns or educational curricula, environmental outlook, technological pursuit of needs, or requirements in management of physical or mental health needs.

The Qur'an proclaims "one God and one humanity." Islamic civilization was therefore the first international civilization on an almost global scale involving people of different faiths, races, and nationalities. This is best demonstrated during Hajj (pilgrimage to Mecca), when millions of people belonging to all races, color, and creed clad in a piece of cloth march around Ka-bah proclaiming the greatness of their creator. As such, Islam is the genuine precursor of modern Western civilization. It is not surprising to find striking similarities between Qur'anic laws and the Constitution of the United States of America.

CONCEPT OF WELLNESS AND ILLNESS

The Islamic strategy for the promotion of mental health and well-being is based on the recognition of the inherent human defects and calls for systematic and constructive enactment to overcome them. Essentially, in the five-time daily prayer, the Muslim recites the opening of the Holy Qur'an and appeals to the Lord of the world to "show us the straight path, and the path of those whom thou hast favored, not of those who earn thine anger nor those who go astray." The Qur'an has also dealt with some specific mental processes and behaviors. For example, problems such as suicide have been ordained with clear, precise, and firm directives. The Qur'anic verse emphatically states, "Do not kill yourself for God is merciful to you." This verse plays a great role in the prevention of self-injury and self-destruction of Muslim communities. Within the Islamic content the clearing up of guilt feelings is an exercise of faith and a practical process of learning by doing. It is a systematic, step-by-step enactment. First, the person has to recognize his or her sin. Second, the person has to face and apprehend his or her mistakes. Third, he or she should solemnly promise to give up and not repeat his or her wrongful behavior. Fourth, the person invokes the help of God in forgiveness and guidance. Fifth, this act of repentance has to be complemented by useful work.

The following values and practices are mandated by Qur'an for Muslims to enable them to cope with the trial and tribulation of life:

Al-Dhikr (remembrance of Allah): The Qur'an (13.28) says, "Verily in the remembrance of Allah do hearts find tranquility." Al-Dhikr is the very life of a Muslim; "Such as remember Allah, standing, sitting and reclining" (Qur'an 3:191). The believers find humility, tranquility, peace, and divine love in this noble exercise.

Al-Tawbah (repentance): Human beings are created innocent. They are accountable in the life hereafter for their deeds. Allah not only accepts repentance which is accompanied by faith, sincerity, and determination, but also loves such persons (Qur'an 39:53; 2:222).

Al-Du'a (supplication): It is a spiritual connection with Allah. Allah listens to the supplication done in humility and bestows His blessing on souls out of His benevolence. Al-Du'a always opens the door for divine mercy and forgiveness. Whatever exists in the universe exists because of divine mercy. His mercy encompasses everything. A Muslim therefore should always seek His mercy and forgiveness (Qur'an 40:60; 2:186).

Rida' Allah (pleasure of Allah): The attainment of Allah's pleasure is the ultimate goal of a believer's life. All other desires are trivial and should be sacrificed for the fulfillment of this cardinal desire (Qur'an 22:59; 2:207).

Al-Tazkiyah (purification): It is an inner purity which enables a person to act righteously. It can be attained by first doing all that Islam enjoins and abstaining from what Islam forbids; second, by doing more of what Islam encourages such as seeking Allah's pleasure and reward; and third, giving up much of the permissible desires (Qur'an 91:9; 3:164).

Al-Jihad (exertion): The human nature is prone to be subdued by temptations leading to a satanic path. Through Jihad (exertion) these temptations can be warded off, allowing mankind to follow the path of Allah's pleasure. Through spiritual Jihad the human soul is made submissive to the divine will, thus achieving the highest level of tranquility (Qur'an 89:27).

Al-Tawakkul (trust in Allah): Trust in Allah and total submission to His divine will at all times, in sickness or in health and in prosperity or in adversity, provides strength, courage, and determination and prevents disappointment, hopelessness, and guilt.

Al-Sabr (patience/perseverance): Muslims are encouraged to observe patience and endurance in the face of calamities. The Qur'an tells the story of Jobe to describe the importance of patience and submission and acceptance of Allah's will and trust in His divine mercy.

Al-Ihsan (goodliness/kindness): To act with kindness with the fellow human being and to give and share one's resources with the needy, all to please Allah, is highly demanded. "Allah commands justice, the doing of good and to giving to Kith and Kin and he forbids all indecent deeds and evil and rebellion" (Qur'an 16:90).

Al-Afu (forgiveness): Overlooking the faults of a fellow human being and forgiving his or her mistakes is a divine quality which each Muslim seeks to emulate. This practice makes a person kind, sympathetic, considerate, polite, and far-sighted (Qur'an 3:15, 4:48).

Al-Ukhuwwah (brotherhood): The bond of Islam can unite strangers into a brotherhood stronger than a blood relation. The spirit of Islamic brotherhood creates mutual love, cooperation, sharing, sacrifice, understanding, and tolerance (Qur'an 49:10).

PROPHETIC MEDICINE

A large mass of medical traditions are contained in Hadith and are called prophetic medicine. This medical knowledge is divinely revealed. In prophetic medicine, the natural causes of illness and natural effects of medication are recognized. The Qur'an and the Hadith recognize several divine purposes of illness and other misfortunes. God's trial of people and the cathartic effect of illness if it's bourne with patience are most frequently mentioned. According to several Hadith, a person who dies of a disease or a mother who dies in child birth attain a rank of a martyr.

There are spiritual therapies which utilize the faith in God and trust in Him, charity and prayer, repentance and seeking God's forgiveness, doing good to mankind, helping the helpless, and relief of the afflicted. It is believed that when the heart of a person becomes attuned to the Lord of the World, the creator of ailments and remedies who governs the nature according to His will, other medicines become available that cannot be experienced by an unbelieving person and indifferent heart. When a person's spirit becomes strong, and soul and bodily nature are strengthened, they cooperate in repelling disease and overcoming it. The prophetic medicine employs a preventive and holistic approach to illness.

THE ROLE OF PRAYER IN HEALING

The role of Islamic ritual prayers which involve changing physical postures are fourfold—spiritual, psychological, physical, and moral. According to the principles of prophetic medicine, prayer can cause recovery from pain of the heart, stomach, and intestine. The concentration of mind during prayer distracts the mind from perceiving pain. The physical aspect of prayer with changing postures has a very relaxing effect on the body. It is interesting to note that certain exercises prescribed by modern physicians for chronic lower back pain are similar to the posture acquired during part of the Islamic ritual prayer.

THE CONCEPT OF MENTAL ILLNESS

Islamic doctrine rejected the supernatural or demonic causation of mental illness and asserted that it is the product of imbalance of humors of the body. The psychic causation of illness is recognized and various forms of psychotherapy were practiced. The use of shock and shame therapies were Islamic inventions.

SPIRITUAL THERAPIES

The Islamic doctrine asserts that the constitution of the universe is basically spiritual and moral and the material existence is palpably under the impact of the spiritual reality. The Qur'an repeatedly points out that the rise and fall of civilizations are moral in nature. In prophetic medicine, volumes of spiritual prescription for cure are available. Recitation of Qur'anic verses and prayer have healing effects on a variety of illnesses.

MEDICAL ETHICS

Medical ethics (*adab*) constitute an important component of prophetic medicine. General piety and sincerity in the character of a physician are essential attributes and allow the physician to help both body and soul. The mental–moral–spiritual aspects of a physician's work are highly valued.

Al-Razi (Rhazes), the famous Muslim physician, identifies a number of moral ailments, the first being "love" (*ishq*). Falling in love played an important causative role in mental–moral malady among predominantly females. According to Al-Razi, people with high goals and ambitions in life seldom fall in love, and if they do they get out of it quickly. The love with a human is artificial love (*ishq-e-mijazi*) and should be a prelude to the eternal love (*ishq-e-haqiqi*) which is the love with God. The fear of death is another moral ailment which is caused by the desires for this life and disbelief in hereafter life.

THE FAMILY

The Qur'an emphasizes family as a social unit and declares that sex pairing is a universal law operative in all things. The Qur'an speaks of husband and wife relationship as that of "Mutual love and Mercy" (Qur'an 30: 21). The rights of parents are strongly emphasized to children and Hadith declares that "Heaven lies under the feet of one's Mother." Sexual intimacy is universal and is a gift of God, but chastity (sexual immunity) is introduced as a Qur'anic legislation whereby sexual intercourse is permitted between spouses by marriage only.

PROFILE OF A MUSLIM PATIENT

A Muslim:

Possesses faith and believes in the absolute power and mercy of Allah and submits to His divine will.

Believes that nothing happens without the will of Allah, including health and illness.

Allah and Allah alone has the power to heal. One of Allah's 99 names is "Al-Shaafi," The Healer.

Through illness and adversity, Allah sometimes tests His slaves. Response to illness with *sabr* (patience) and acceptance of His will and asking for His mercy in this world and hereafter are the expected reactions to illness.

Life and death are predetermined by the divine will. In life a Muslim is thankful for the time in this world. The Muslim views death as the beginning of life hereafter. The surviving family accepts the death of a loved one as the will of God. This is why in Islamic countries, the health care professionals are not held responsible for the death of a loved one. Suing a physician for causing the death of a patient is unheard of.

POINTS TO CONSIDER WHEN EVALUATING A MUSLIM PATIENT

A Muslim patient will seldom initiate contact with mental health professionals. The concerned relatives, however, will make that contact.

A Muslim patient will try religious approaches to achieve mental health concurrently with the modern methods. This should not be resisted or discouraged. If a faith healer is involved, work with that faith healer.

Muslims believe in the existence of the supernatural beings called the Jins who are made of fire and have powers of metamorphoses into different shape and form. Possession by a Jin is a legitimate possibility in the Muslim belief system. Such belief should not be considered a manifestation of psychosis.

CONCLUSION

Islam, in addition to being a religion, is also a sociopolitical system which offers a comprehensive methodology of solving mankind's spiritual, intellectual, and day to day problems. Allah is the absolute transcendent creator and the master of all things. Nothing happens without his permission. A total submission to His will and a trust in His mercy provide eternal peace. His laws are aimed at achieving peace, safety, and tranquility and to inculcate a healthy, moral, safe, and peaceful society. Illness and misfortunes may occur as Allah's tests for his slaves and enduring these tests with patience and piety elevate one's status in His eyes. Islamic traditions contain a very elaborate system of health care which promotes mental health and prevents mental illness. A health care provider to a Muslim must consider these factors in diagnosis and treatment.

REFERENCES

Al-Razi. (1978). *Introduction to Al-Tibb.* Cairo, Egypt: Abd al-Latif Al-td.
Horrie, C. and Chippendale, P. (1997). *What Is Islam? A Comprehensive Introduction.* Great Britain:
    Virgin Book.
Rahman, F. (1979). *Islam.* Chicago: University of Chicago Press.
Rahman, F. (1987). *Health and medicine in Islamic tradition.* New York: Crossroad.
Sayyid-Marsot, A. L. (1979). *Society and the sexes in medieval Islam.* Malibu, CA: Undena.

21

RELIGION AND CULTURE
IN PSYCHIATRY: CHRISTIAN
AND SECULAR PSYCHIATRIC
THEORY AND PRACTICE
IN THE UNITED STATES

ATWOOD D. GAINES

Case Western Reserve University and School of Medicine
Cleveland, Ohio 44106

This chapter analyzes religious and cultural aspects of professional (ethno)psychiatric theory and practice in the United States by focusing on two categories of professional "ethnopsychiatrists" (Gaines, 1992a); "Christian" and "secular" psychiatrists. Both may be termed ethnopsychiatrists indicating the cultural basis of theory and practice in each domain. The term ethnopsychiatry in the medical and psychiatric anthropological literature previously referred to folk or popular psychiatry when it was presumed, without any basis in research, that "their psychiatry" was based in and expressed a particular local culture, whereas "our" (professional) psychiatry was acultural, scientific, and, therefore, culturally neutral (Gaines, 1992a, 1992b). These are, of course, the same assertions made with reference to Western medicine when contrasted with the ethnomedicines of other cultures (Gaines & Hahn, 1982; Hahn & Gaines, 1985; Kleinman, 1988a; Mishler et al., 1981).

Contrary to these assertions and as is shown here and now widely elsewhere with the advent of the anthropology of biomedicine (see Gaines, 1979; Gaines & Hahn, 1982; Hahn & Gaines, 1985), cultural beliefs are regnant in professional, as well as popular or folk, medicine and psychiatry. The impress of culture is readily discernible in both the theory and the practice of the professional medicines and their psychiatries around the world (e.g., Gaines, 1992a; Gaines & Hahn, 1982; Hahn & Gaines, 1985; Lindenbaum & Lock, 1993; Lock & Gordon, 1988; Weisberg & Long, 1984; Wright & Treacher, 1982).

This chapter focuses on several elements of what Kleinman (1980b) calls "core clinical functions" of psychiatry, such as help-seeking, the cultural construction of illness and clinical realities, the hermeneutic nature of clinical encounters, and the logic of therapeutic modalities. Other issues receiving emphasis here are the culturally specific psychological constructs underlying practice, that is, the concept of person in psychiatric practice, and the symbolic construction of the corporateness of professional and, by implication, secular psychiatry. Lastly, this chapter considers some of the ethical implications of divergent beliefs for patient care in modern psychiatry. Because of the subject matter, this essay is theological (i.e., exegetical), ethnopsychiatric, and bioethical.

LA DIFFÉRENCE: DISTINGUISHING THE ONCE- AND THE TWICE-BORN

In the past decade, Christian psychiatrists were introduced into the growing anthropological literature on Western biomedical specialists (Gaines, 1982a, 1982c, 1985a). (In this chapter, I draw on my previous publications on Christian psychiatry; Gaines, 1982a, 1982c, 1985a.) Here I present Christian psychiatry in light of contemporary issues of boundaries, multiplicities, and constructions, all of which were foreshadowed in earlier work (Gaines, 1982a, 1982c, 1985a). The research I conducted on Christian psychiatry, as well as some secular psychiatry, took place in Mason Medical Center, located in the southern United States. Certain characteristics of the "group" of Christian psychiatrists practicing at Mason Medical Center appear key in its (self)definition. These central elements distinguish Christian psychiatrists from "secular" psychiatrists (e.g., Gaines, 1979, 1982a, 1992a, 1992b, 1992c, 1995a, 1995b).

CHRISTIAN PSYCHIATRISTS

My first task is to explain what my informants and I intend by the use of the term "Christian psychiatrist." I begin with a focus on the commonalities of belief and practice in this group in order to approach the bases for an ascribed common identity, i.e., Christian psychiatry. I then challenge the notion of corporateness by discussing the many points of similarity and contrast within the group and the lack of any attempt to develop a consensus concerning belief and action as Christian psychiatrists. As a consequence, the term Christian psychiatry is not employed. I shall further explain this terminological specificity below.

Because informants in the ethnographic research conducted at Mason Medical Center (a *nom de centre*) are practicing professional psychiatrists and practicing Christians, I have an additional database in their published writings. While I make references to positions taken or ideas held in the published works of my informants, I shall not provide citations for such works in order to preserve the authors' anonymity.

SELF IDENTITY: "ALIVE IN CHRIST"

A Christian psychiatrist represents the coincidence of at least two distinguishable identities, as is implied by the appellation, so the identity of a Christian psychiatrist is at least a dual one. For the sake of brevity, I leave aside the several other components of the total identity of these individuals. Other elemental identities central to an individual's configuration of unique identities include birth order, age, gender, marital status, ethnicity, regional and national identities, and religious identity. Psychoanalyst–classicist–anthropologist George Devereux's (1982) notion of human self-identity as constituted by a complex and unique combination of a number of identities is appropriately invoked here.

EXPERIENCE

The "Christian" identity assumes that the individual has developed an ongoing, personal relationship with "the Savior." The Savior is that divine entity capable of granting salvation and is the avenue to that salvation. The relationship is generally believed to develop as a result of a specific episode in which the individual is enlightened so that he or she "realizes the power of God," that "Jesus truly loves" him or her, or that "it is time to let Jesus into his or her life." However this event occurs, an individual has a personal experience of the Savior.

This personal experience of an aspect of divinity constitutes a second birth because the individual is said to be (re)born in Christ. Thus, an individual with this experience is said to have been "born again" and/or to be "alive in Christ." This is the key or core symbol (Ortner, 1973; Turner, 1974) for one-half of the focal identity of the Christian psychiatrist. The phrase "alive in Christ" among believers carries the connotation that Christ (and/or the Holy Spirit and/or God) is alive within the individual and that the individual is "enlivened" and "alive" (especially as relates to the vividness of the second birth) by virtue of that indwelling presence(s). As the foregoing qualifications indicate, the various spiritual entities are not always clearly differentiated in thought and action in the tradition.

In some ways, there is but one spiritual entity, "God." Jesus, the "Son of God," is conceptually distinct and a refraction of God. The Holy Ghost is likewise both individual and a refraction of a high god. Christian psychiatrists further believe that Jesus, God, and the Holy Spirit are, like the Nuer's notion of their high god, *kwoth,* refractions of a single divinity (Evans-Pritchard, 1940). This is referred to as the Trinitarian belief. They also believe that there is a connection between the world of their God and that of humans. (In some traditions, a high God created the world of humans but has receded and is no longer engaged in human affairs.) For Christian psychiatrists (and nonpsychiatrists), the connection to or with divinity is at least twofold: God may act in the lives of people and, indeed, dwell within them, or a refraction of its (or "His") spirit, i.e., Jesus Christ, may be indwelling. People may communicate with God (or Jesus) through the action of prayer; though, interestingly, people do not pray as often to the Holy Ghost, which is ostensibly an equal constituent of the Trinity. It may be that in the tradition, while God and Jesus have been anthropomorphized, the Holy Ghost has not. As a result, the Holy Ghost may not be conceived of in terms sufficiently human-like to motivate notions of communicative possibilities between humans and Holy Spirit as much as with God or Jesus.

The conversion experience, however cognitized, is of sufficient emotional significance to the individual that she or he feels motivated subsequently to frequently relate a narrative of the experience to others. This communicative act is called "testifying." In these events, one usually testifies to another believer. So it is that one frequently both will testify to others and bear witness to others' "testimony."

Some people, including one of my informants, prefer to describe the transformative experience as becoming alive in Christ. He believes that the phrase "born again" is "too commercialized." He refers to himself as alive in Christ, not born again. He avers that Christ is alive and, literally, dwelling within him. It is also his belief that a person is animated, enlivened by the indwelling, divine presence such as he experiences. In his view, and that of his cobelievers, a person has a dual nature; he or she is both physical and spiritual and sacred and profane.

These experiences and positions are but one-half of the identity. However, it requires the intersection of two sets of experiences to produce a Christian psychiatrist. One transforms the individual in terms of his relation to a perceived divinity and the other is a lengthy, secular educational experience in profane, accredited, secular institutions. Individuals known as Christian psychiatrists also may have had some rather lengthy educational experiences in seminary or Bible college, but such are not necessary to "receive" Christ in one's life. In fact, all my Christian psychiatrist informants had done missionary work for periods of a year or more, usually in other countries. Ironically, these cross-cultural experiences produced an interest in things anthropological in these psychiatrists that distinguished them from their secular peers.

KNOWLEDGE AND BELIEF

There is a tendency to invalidate "different" views of things by referring to them as "beliefs." Simultaneously, we refer to our beliefs in medicine and science as "knowledge" (Good, 1994). We implicitly assert that our beliefs as knowledge are certain, whereas others' beliefs are just that. The reader may be tempted to do the same with the Christian psychiatrists' ideology; I suggest that such a view is problematic and posits a false dichotomy.

Based on my interviews with six Christian psychiatrists at Mason Medical Center, I concluded that they hold many views in common. However, these views more apparently than actually distinguish them, individually and collectively, from oth-er, secular, psychiatrists. First, they all believe in "salvation" through being born again. By salvation, it is meant that the individual is "saved" and will ascend to heaven at death, including a death following some divinely inspired cataclysmic event. They believe that they, as individuals and collectivities, professional, fa-milial, and congregational, have an ongoing personal relationship with Jesus Christ, the Savior. It is through and by virtue of this relationship that they are saved and others are not.

Prayer may involve communication with divinity through thoughts or through speech. Prayer activity may be conducted in solitude or in groups, wherein indi-viduals may be praying for the same or different desires or goals. Related to the belief in communication with divinity is the notion that divinity may speak to the individual. This speech act often seems to be regarded as divine placement of words or thoughts into the mind of the individual. Communications thus may flow in two directions, each side "hearing" the other and potentially being affected by such communications.

Based on these beliefs, it is understandable that my informants believe that prayer is a potentially efficacious therapeutic tool. They do not, however, agree on the extent to which prayer should or could be used, nor do they agree on the appropriateness of specific contexts of prayer "with" or "for" their patients. How-ever, prayer with patients is a key symbol of difference for secular psychiatrists. Indeed, Post (1992), in an article sympathetic to new religious movements and religious ideas that do not receive a welcome in psychiatry, states that, "A secu-lar psychiatrist justifiably refuses to pray with patients who request prayer" (p. 81).

AUTHORITY IN THE PSYCHIATRIES

Christian psychiatrists believe that Scripture is the ultimate authority in med-ical as well as secular matters. Scripture serves as the final, unequivocal word. However, my informants are mostly Evangelical Christians and hence should be distinguished from Fundamentalist Christians. That is, while all of my Evangeli-cal informants (who in fact belong to several different denominations, including Baptist, Church of God, and Southern Presbyterian) share the view that Scripture is the final authority, none would accept literal interpretations of Scripture.

Their nonliteral interpretations distinguish them from Fundamentalists, though the two groups do in fact share many theological beliefs. Evangelicals do not seem to establish unitary doctrines or to exact conformity to particular theological con-ceptions. Hence, there are differences of opinion within the "group" and there seems little effort to exact unanimity on particular issues.

A final commonality of Christian psychiatrists is the belief that such individu-als should manifest "Christian love" toward all other people, whether they are be-lievers or not, whether patients, friends, or acquaintances. This notion of "love" suggests an element of tolerance for difference that may not always play itself out in behavior, however. It appears akin to the notion that one is to love others because the spirit of Jesus Christ dwells within them; hence, to love another, even the unacquainted, is to love Jesus.

The authority of secular psychiatry is a bit more complicated. It rests on several things. First, it stands on the authority of medicine. Second, it is based in the authority of science from which medicine in large part draws its own particular form of authority. Third, it draws authority from institutions with which and in which it works. Fourth, it rests on its historical professional genealogy which, in the popular mind, "goes back to the Greeks." Finally, it has legal authority to enforce some of its treatment decisions. All sources are this-worldly, in contrast with the Christian psychiatrists' source(s) of authority.

The first portion of the dual identity of the Christian psychiatrist involves a religious transformation. This experience and the associated beliefs ostensibly are not found associated with individuals to whom only the second half of the identity is applied and which I consider later, i.e., psychiatrists.

(SECULAR) PSYCHIATRISTS

Psychiatry is a specialty of Western biomedicine that deals with a number of problems considered in the West to comprise a single domain called "mental disorders" (or "illness"). To a lesser extent, this medical specialty is also concerned with questions of what is called "mental health." The field of action of this specialty is wide and includes diagnosis, management, research, and treatment of a host of often ill-defined "diseases" of the "brain," conceived as a physical entity, and the immaterial "mind," seen as the seat of emotion, perception, and cognition. The field also treats behavioral disorders of the young and of adults and the elderly [e.g., American Psychiatric Association (APA), 1980, 1994].

Psychiatric disorders may be present in the absence of abnormalities of the brain. However, abnormalities of the brain are not necessarily manifested as abnormalities of the mind. The specialty thus treats disorders said to be psychogenic (purely problems of mind), organic (problems of brain structure or processes), developmental (either problems of mind or brain seen developmentally), characterological (usually problems of mind but referring to distortions, disorders, malformations, etc. of the personality, i.e., the total psychological organization or being of a person), toxicological (acute or chronic problems of mind or of brain resulting from ingestion of noxious substances), and apparent social problems ("conduct disorders") that cannot be easily attributed to problems in either brain or mind (Gaines, 1992c).

Within this medical specialty, there exist a number of subspecialties, including child, consultation–liaison, geriatric, forensic, social, community, and anthropological or "cultural" psychiatry (Kleinman, 1980a). The latter has been redefined as the "new ethnopsychiatry" and incorporates sociocultural elements not usually construed as part of psychiatry (e.g., gender, violence, aging, disability, and self-concepts) (Gaines, 1992b). A practitioner in one or more of these subspecialties is a psychiatrist, though the approach to problems which a given psychiatrist will take may vary widely from that of his or her colleagues within any given subspecialty in a given country (e.g., Castel, Castel, & Lovel, 1982; Gaines, 1979, 1992a; Hershel, 1992; Johnson, 1985, 1987).

This part of the dual identity is, like the first, anchored in a set of experiences. However, here they are "medical education" and subsequently "psychiatric residency." In addition there must be externally manifest, disembodied certification (diplomas, board certification, etc.) of such educational experiences and knowledge acquisition. This portion of the identity takes some time to achieve. Its course is predetermined by forces outside of the individual and the attainment of the status is granted by individuals other than the self through processes that are institutionalized.

Social science research suggests that medical education and residency refine but do not produce psychiatrists' etiologic conceptions (e.g., Gaines, 1979; Light, 1976), though such experiences are powerful influences in terms of role behavior and the acquisition of pharmacological, therapeutic, management, diagnostic, and other knowledge and skills. Professional psychiatric training provides a context in which preexisting etiologic notions of mental illness are clarified and refined. Therefore, cross-cultural research demonstrates rather sharp differences among psychiatries but similarities between a culture's professional and its popular conceptions of mental health and illness (Gaines, 1992a; Gaines & Farmer, 1986; Kleinman, 1980b, 1986; Kleinman & Good, 1985; Reynolds, 1980; Townsend, 1978). We also see that the organization of psychiatric care is modeled on local social forms such as the family (e.g., Dwyer, 1987; Gaines, 1992a; Nomura, 1992).

Previous cultural experience establishes cultural conceptions of mental disorders. These conceptions remain relatively stable throughout residency training and have been noted to manifest themselves in clinical as well as didactic contexts (Gaines, 1979; Wen Shing Tseng, personal communication).

Christian psychiatrists appear to contrast with other psychiatrists in several ways. Christian psychiatrists often use this term for themselves which, taken literally, does not distinguish them from a host of others. That is, there are many psychiatrists with few, if any, of the beliefs noted previously, who nonetheless would describe themselves as Christians.

RELIGION AND IDENTITY

Several people I interviewed, some of whom were not psychiatrists and some of whom were, stated that they "resented" what they see as a "restricted" use of the term Christian. Some laypersons felt that the designation Christian is inappropriate for people such as my informants. For example, Catholics regard themselves as Christians and dislike the cooption of the term Christian by Protestant Fundamentalists and Evangelicals.

My informants are not the only Evangelicals or Fundamentalists who are psychiatrists. That is, not all individuals with "a personal relationship with God" (or the Savior) who are psychiatrists refer to themselves or are known as Christian psychiatrists, though they may be known as Christians. Many Christians, in fact, do not even regard my Evangelical informants as "proper" Christians but as rather strange birds who give a bad name to the larger flock, a flock which includes Catholics, Lutherans, Reformed (Calvinist), and other Christians.

The label implies for some that Christian psychiatrists are the only psychiatric professionals who have a regard for or interest in general religious or specifically Christian values in their practice. Other, ostensibly secular, informants stated that while they are not the same sort of Christians as my informants, they too are concerned with and take account of spiritual values and beliefs in their clinical practice. They may also do so in their private lives.

Several self-described atheists stated that they feel the appellation makes it appear that they, as labeled secular psychiatrists, are by apparent definition unconcerned with spiritual issues in their clinical work. In fact, these individuals say they often concern themselves with these issues in their clinical work. Because they are not Evangelicals or Fundamentalists does not mean that they are unaware or unappreciative of the role of religion in the lives of their patients. Also, they do not regard that role as entirely negative, though that negative view of things religious is rather well represented in the *Diagnostic and Statistical Manuals* of the APA (e.g., 1980, 1987, and 1994) (Gaines, 1992c, 1995a; Post, 1992).

Christian psychiatrists and secular psychiatrists upon closer inspection (re)appear less dissimilar than is initially apparent. In a survey conducted by the APA (1975), a subsample of 900 randomly selected psychiatrists were asked to state theological viewpoints in terms of three choices: "theistic," "agnostic," and "atheistic" (the total sample out of which the 900 were drawn was 14,843).

Fully 86% of the respondents answered the question: 70.3% classified themselves as theistic (APA, 1975, p. 19). Eleven percent stated that they had at least some theological training. Of this figure, half had received sufficient training, at least 3 years, to complete seminary education (APA, 1975, p. 18). A very substantial majority of respondents (75.3%) attended church or temple at least occasionally. A small minority (9.2%) "never" attended a place of worship (APA, 1975, p. 21). Christian psychiatrists are thus not alone in their belief(s) in divinity among psychiatric professionals in the United States.

DIFFERENCE AND ACTION: HELP-SEEKING AND CLINICAL REALITY

In this section I consider the means of help-seeking that lead individuals to psychiatrists in general and to Christian psychiatrists in particular. Examining some commonalities and dissimilarities may be enlightening as concerns several core clinical functions of the local health care system. It should be mentioned at the outset that Christian psychiatrists are by no means the only Christian (in the born again sense) medical professionals practicing in the South.

In addition to these professional ethnopsychiatrists, there are numbers of folk healers, including "power doctors," "root doctors," spiritual healers and readers, herbalists, and clergypersons of various denominations who provide help with various problems that might otherwise be presented to health care professionals. I have also encountered an elderly woman who is paid by others, usually in goods rather than cash, to pray for good results for health problems they themselves have or for those of their relatives. She is believed to have a "gift" (divinely given ability) for producing efficacious prayers. Finally, the popular, family based level of health care is alive and well in this area despite the presence in the area of Mason Medical Center, a tertiary care center.

HELP-SEEKING

In an earlier study, I examined how psychiatric patients found their way into the psychiatric emergency room and, hence, into the psychiatric system (Gaines, 1979). This work confirmed that of earlier researchers in showing that the diagnostic process that leads to the psychiatric system is, in its initial stages, a lay, not a professional, process. Friends, relatives, workmates, neighbors, or even the future patient him- or herself make the initial judgment that the problem at hand is psychological or mental and not "physical" (Mechanic, 1962). This determination is in accordance with the bifurcate division of disorders in the indigenous professional ethnomedical system which differentiates between mental and physical disorders. It is only after lay diagnosis and after (usually) nonpsychiatric medical diagnoses, as in the emergency room or clinic, that a psychiatrist is consulted. This may then lead to a diagnosis of a specific kind or type of psychiatric diagnosis, thus providing specification for what nonpsychiatric others have previously determined (Gaines, 1979).

In much the same way, individuals find their way to Christian and secular psychiatrists alike at Mason Medical Center. Both sorts of psychiatrists obtain their patients through referrals from laypersons and other physicians, including those in the emergency rooms and wards. In my work with them, Christian psychiatrists were receiving referrals increasingly from other Christian physicians and Christian laypersons.

In a number of cases, for example, Christian surgeons made referrals to Christian psychiatrists when some postoperative problem, usually depression, evidenced itself. There seemed to be developing an "in-house" or, rather, an "in-faith" referral and consult network. There are also cases of secular psychiatrists referring patients to Christian psychiatrists. Such referrals seem to occur when a patient's clinical presentation includes a considerable amount of religious ideation.

CLINICAL REALITY

I note here that religious orientation, or lack thereof, may be added to the list of factors affecting help-seeking, at least in the Bible Belt of the United States. However, one should also be aware that the definition of problems, the illness, will likewise be cultural, i.e., "meaningful" in local cultural terms (Good, 1977). Christians may seek aid for illnesses that appear to be nosologically distinct from those found in the dominant professional ethnopsychiatric culture. I will consider two such problems, the first of which is divorce.

Divorce as Clinical Reality

Divorce is seen as a problem on several levels and as such it is a problem that requires both spiritual and Christian psychiatric assistance. In the Christian tradition we are focusing on, divorce is both an illness and a disease, the latter in the sense that it is a problem seen as a clinical entity as conceived of by the professional Christian ethnopsychiatric healers.

Because of the strong male bias of the tradition, which is consistent with the Mediterranean culture area from which it comes, the desires of a woman seeking divorce may lead her to be treated by a Christian psychiatrist, though many Christian psychiatrists would not accept such an occurrence as a "case." It should be understood that divorce is both illness (popularly recognized malaise) and disease (professionally recognized malaise). (In using this distinction, I assume these two realities are independent of one another, not mirror images.) We must recognize the sacred nature of this institution among some Christian psychiatrists.

Marriage is an institution that is a key to the social order. Marriage creates families (as informants define that institution; Finkler, 1991; Gaines, 1985b; Gaines & Farmer, 1986). Families, not individuals, are the constituent elements or building blocks of society. The maintenance of the marital union is, therefore, of utmost importance to society as it maintains the principal social unit.

Cross-culturally, familism is quite common but involves much larger social units than a nuclear family. Therefore, while those of the tradition assume their family centeredness is unique to them, it is not and, indeed, appears rather anemic in its narrowness when considered in light of familism in other traditions, even some in the West such as France and Italy (Gaines, 1985b, n.d.; Gilmore, 1982).

In one case involving divorce as a clinically significant disorder, a woman of about 35 years of age was admitted to Mason Medical Center for emotional and behavioral problems with which her family and friends could not cope. She had decided to leave her husband of 15 years. One might think she had good reason to leave him; he had a drinking problem, had affairs with other women, and he physically abused the patient. However, it was reported to me secondhand by a psychiatric nurse that the case was referred to a very well-known Christian psychiatrist on the staff of Mason Medical. This psychiatrist's "therapeutic recommendation" was that the woman return to her husband and that such was her

"Christian duty." She "should ask God" for the ability to understand her husband and to allow her to have "Christian patience and endurance."

In a sense, the Christian psychiatrist suggested that the patient would be a better Christian and a better person if she returned to her husband and endured the hardship. Here there is an element of the notion of the saint who endures the slings and arrows of outrageous fortune with equanimity. The specific role of the saint is not, however, nearly as developed as in the Mediterranean tradition in which long-suffering individuals may receive lay canonization (Gaines & Farmer, 1986). Such recommendations did not appear to be uncommon. There is suggested the view that in marriage, whatever problem arises is to be corrected or borne by the woman; the male prerogative is to be preserved.

A psychoanalytically trained psychiatrist on the staff of Mason made his feelings about such cases quite clear. He felt strongly that such recommendations were wrong; they served only to "confirm and validate the sadistic tendencies of the husband in question. He argued that such dealings were unethical as well. His argument, apparently a principalist one, suggests that harm was being done to the patient by having her continue in an abusive relationship. Also, there is a conflict with a second principle, the autonomy of the patient in the (re)identification of the locus of the problem as afflicting her (lack of patience, Christian love, endurance, etc.) rather than her husband.[1]

Homosexuality as Disease

There is another sort of case that may be placed in the care of a Christian psychiatrist. These are "cases" of homosexuality. Interestingly, these cases, and those of divorce, are referred not only by other professionals but also often by members of the congregations or fellowship groups of the Christian psychiatrists. This is a source of referrals which other psychiatrists would be less likely to have.

Homosexuality is considered a sin, an "abomination," to Evangelicals and Fundamentalists alike. One of my informants has had great success "treating homosexuality." His major tools are prayer and conversion, the leading of the patient to God. If a person undergoes the born again experience, he or she often may cease the practice of homosexuality (Gaines, 1982c). Homosexuality, whether ego-syntonic or dystonic, is thus seen as both a moral illness and a disease that a Christian psychiatrist might be very effective in treating.[2]

The following section explores notions of person that distinguish the two categories of psychiatrists and which seem to be responsible for discernible differential interpretations and subsequent action in the clinical sphere. Later I examine aspects of psychiatric practice among both the Christian and secular psychiatrists. In that regard, the focus will be on the logic of praxis in psychiatry for these two categories of psychiatrists and also their respective notions of therapeutic efficacy. Several cases will illustrate the belief of Christian psychiatrists that a Christian perspective made a difference in the clinical outcome. We shall see the essentially hermeneutic nature of clinical interactions grounded in cultural assumptions and conceptions which preexist but which may be refined in, and brought to bear on, particular interactional encounters. A key cultural conception appearing in clinical contexts is that of the person.

BOUNDARIES AND TRANSGRESSIONS: RELIGION, PERSON AND PSYCHIATRY'S SELF, PERSON AND OTHER

Early in the 1950s, and again recently, anthropological researchers focused their attention on cultural conceptions of the person and self (Conner, 1982; Gaines, 1982a; Geertz, 1973; Hallowell, 1955; Lee, 1959; Schweder & Bourne, 1982). It now seems beyond doubt that different cultures hold differing conceptions of the person. These conceptions vary radically across cultures in ways unrelated to economic, developmental, or educational differences (Shweder & Bourne, 1982).

SELVES AND PERSONS IN THE WEST

It was Clifford Geertz (1977), the dean of interpretive anthropology in the United States, who may be said to have rekindled, among many other topics, our interest in cross-cultural constructions of self and person. He gives us some insights into our own "Western" conception of self in the course of his examination of Balinese, Moroccan, and Javanese concepts of self. Geertz describes the Western self as

> A bounded, unique, more or less integrated motivational and cognitive universe; a dynamic center of awareness, emotion, judgment, and action organized into a distinctive whole and set contrastively both against other such wholes and against a social and natural background. (p. 9)

Geertz assumes a unitary notion in the West though his own work on the pervasiveness of religious orientations (Geertz, 1973) would suggest a division in the West into at least several traditions. Some of the author's research in France focused on this and shows the presence of at least two major cultural traditions in the West, the Northern European Protestant and the Mediterranean tradition, each with distinctive conceptions of person and self (Gaines, 1982a, 1985a, 1992c).

Geertz's description of a concept of person clearly refers to the European Protestant psychocultural construction. In my own work I have labeled this traditions' notion the "referential self" (Gaines, 1985a). This concept of the person is part of the dominant cultural ideology in the United States, including that of medicine and psychiatry (Gaines, 1982a, 1985a, 1992c). I emphasize some of the features of this conception.

The first distinction to make is that this sort of Protestant ethnopsychology is not isomorphic with U.S. Protestantism. The Protestant traditions of the six Christian psychiatrists that I interviewed are not forms of European Protestantism, i.e., they are not spiritual kin to Calvinism, Lutheranism, Methodism, or Presbyterianism. Their sort of Protestantism is a U.S. creation based not on the ideas of Luther or Calvin but on literal interpretations of the Bible. That is, their form of Protestantism is largely sculpted out of the Mediterranean Latin ideology which is the very tradition that, nominally, they "protest."

The person in the Protestant (European) tradition is a bounded, psychophysical entity; personhood is coterminous with the extent of a physical body. That body is the domain of the core of medicine, internal medicine (Hahn, 1982), and parts of it receive the attention of the gaze of medicine's other branches. The person, furthermore, is seen as unique, though a combination of "typical" features. The person is a center of awareness, judgment, and action whose organizational integrity stems from inner affective and cognitive, i.e., psychological, resources and strengths. The self is whole, complete unto itself, and it is thought to exist in an environment consisting of other such unique, distinct, separate "individuals"—a word that well conveys the notion of boundedness, uniqueness, and autonomy/independence (Gaines, 1979, 1982a; Geertz, 1977; Shweder & Bourne, 1982).

Disorder conceived of in a worldview containing such a notion of person logically must locate the problem within an "individual," that is, within the physical confines of a person so conceived. Therapy logically must be directed toward the individual and healing activities focused on the body and mind (as constituents) of the individual person. A concrete, constant person exists that is referred to in discourse; hence, I have termed this person conception the referential self (Gaines, 1982a).

In contrast, the conception of person which can be elucidated from expressed thought and action of our Christian psychiatrist informants provides a rather different view of personhood. The Christian person is in fact that psychocultural notion outlined for the Mediterranean tradition, the "indexical" person construct (Gaines, 1982a). This should not be surprising because people of the Mediterranean are, as Arensberg (1963) once called them, "people of the Book" (Davis, 1975). Also, of course, the same book is the guide for and of this and the next life. The Bible is the literal Word for Fundamentalists and the figurative Word for Evangelicals.

Let us contrast the two notions. First, the Christian self and the reflection of the self seen in others, the person, is fundamentally a spiritual, partly otherworldly, self. That is, the self is not solely, or even primarily, a physical entity—a unique, corporeal object. The boundary, if indeed there is a boundary in the same sense as that found in the contrastive notion of self considered later, is drawn around other persons, relatives, both living and dead. The very notion of a boundary demarcating and setting off each individual self appears to be a product of a particular cultural psychology's construction of the person. In the Northern European Protestant tradition, the boundary is drawn around, but can be permeated by, extracorporeal, invasive elements of a natural, though pathological sort (e.g., viruses, bacteria, and pathophysiological processes). That is, the presence of other than self within self is pathological.

Among the Christian psychiatrists I interviewed, the notion of self incorporates a spirit or spirits. The incorporation of spiritual elements is found commonly in other cultures such as Native American (Hallowell, 1955), Balinese (Conner, 1982) and Indian (Karkar, 1982; Nuckolls, 1992). In Christian psychiatrists' cosmology, one sees incorporated into the self construct several elements of and/or the totality of the Trinity.

The in- and extradwelling spirits observe and involve themselves in peoples' lives. They may listen to them, hold expectations, and direct and even tempt the person. For the latter, it should be noted that there are "evil" as well as good spirits. Not the least of these evil spirits or "demons" is the devil. It is believed that the devil can move people to act and is thought to be capable of residing within an individual. Malevolent spirits can direct the actions of the person. These beliefs are also found in the Catholic Charismatic Renewal Movement (Csordas, 1992; Favazza, 1982).

Likewise, good spirits are believed to be indwelling as well as external. As Saint Paul said, "I live, yet not I, but Christ liveth in me." The spirit dwells within the believer from the moment of his or her second birth. The indwelling spirit is seen as animating the person and "leading" the person in his or her life.[3]

The presence of a unified, indwelling overseer and sovereign implies several things of importance for an understanding of the contrastive nature of the Christian psychiatrist's notion of self. First, the uniqueness of a person is in some sense diminished because all believers share an indwelling and animating spirit. Second, the sharing of a spiritual dimension makes an individual a part of a total Christian community and family. Also, it is the family that is considered a sacred social unit, not the individual (or his or her rights, wants, or needs).

According to this view, what animates an individual and what is good and positive about a person are things not unique to a given person; they are elements shared by all believers. The focus of thought is not on that which is unique about a person but that which is held in common. The individual is a refraction of the Christian community and family and, as such, the self is not the center of awareness, as in the case of the referential conception of person. Nor is the person or self seen as complete. On the contrary, a person without the spirit is, by definition, incomplete. Furthermore, this person would not be the source of personal action, whether good or bad, since the person is animated by spiritual entities. Rather, the self is a sort of shell filled and even animated by benevolent superior spiritual forces and entities. Clearly, the person is conceived of as neither independent nor autonomous.[4]

All this makes for a person who is "sociocentric" rather than "egocentric" (Shweder & Bourne, 1982) or "indexical" rather than "referential" (Gaines, 1982a). The person is both self and other in this tradition, just as Lacan has claimed in his formulations in his French version of psychoanalysis (Turkle, 1978). Importantly, White and Marsella (1982) have pointed out that when behavior is seen to emanate from an individual conceived of as bounded (a corporeal self), agency and responsibility are attributed to either the self or to another or other, bounded selves. That is, agency or responsibility are not attributed to social relations or to spirits.

In cultures in which persons are considered as more than mere physical entities, agents are located in one or more of several places outside of the physical limits of the person: for example, in family networks or ancestors, as in China (Kleinman, 1980b) and Japan (Lebra, 1976), or in disrupted community relations, as is
found among the Ndembu of Africa (Turner, 1969). These examples highlight the
interrelation of self and other, the latter in the form of family and community. The
individual, then, is more an expression of a larger family/community than an autonomous "individual."

This is not to say that these other cultures have a single relational concept of
self while the West holds a unitary individualistic notion of self. As is noted here
and elsewhere, the West is not a single cultural area. Also, the concepts of self in
all those cultures noted here may have a few things in common, such as extraper-
sonal elements incorporated, but they are not at all otherwise similar; the Japanese self, while social, is not all like that of India, China, Bali,, specific African cultures, nor are these like individual other self constructs (Gaines, 1982a, 1985a,
1992b, 1992c).

The individual in the Christian tradition, which is a Mediterranean psychocultural construct and not a general western one, is not the primary social unit. Primacy is accorded those aspects of the tradition seen as (symbolically) representing its sacred units, the family, and hence marriage and the (Christian) community.
This point lays bare the logic underlying treatment recommendations for the two
clinical entities discussed earlier—divorce and homosexuality.

There are other important features to consider with regard to the Christian concept of person. Most notably these are aspects of the personality or dimensions of
inner psychological resources, such as "strength, "will," "patience," and "endurance." What is important here is that these qualities and resources are seen as
the property of an indwelling spirit, not as personal qualities of an individual *qua*
individual. Success or luck (good or bad) are seen as ultimately stemming from a
spiritual source, i.e., outside the domain of personal responsibility.[5] These ideas
have some import for clinical praxis among Christian psychiatrists, including diagnosis and therapeutic activities.

CLINICAL PRAXIS OF CHRISTIAN
PSYCHIATRISTS: PERSON, PRACTICE,
AND INTERACTION

It is of central importance to recognize the hermeneutic, interpretive nature of
clinical practice. Just as all illness episodes must be seen as essentially semantic
or meaningful episodes (Good, 1977), so too must clinical interactions be seen as
essentially hermeneutic or interpretive encounters (Good & DelVecchio Good,
1981, p. 4). Diagnosis should be seen as a process of interpretation of symbolic elements and not as a reading of signs of distress which have clinical import *sui
generis*. One result of clinical interactions is a definition of the nature of the cur-

rent situation or condition of the patient, that is, the EM of the physician. The condition which is thought to exist is "clinical reality." It is thought to exist as a feature of the patient, as an individual, at the time of presentation in the clinical context (Kleinbaum, 1980b) and as such manifests a referential view of persons.

If the construction, through interaction in clinical contexts, of clinical reality were a mere decoding of signs and not a semantic, hermeneutic encounter, the bringing to bear of different perspectives on clinical reality, especially nonbiomedical perspectives, should not alter that constructed clinical reality. However, research indicates that clinical reality can be changed by the introduction in clinical settings of aspects of anthropological science, including knowledge, methodology, and theory (Gaines, 1982b; Good & DelVecchio Good, 1981). New information, or a different perspective, can change the clinical reality because it can alter the meaning of the signs of sickness, signs which are actually symbols— things which stand for, but do not resemble, their referents.

As Schutz (1967) pointed out, people interpret current interactional encounters through a process of negotiations in interactions. These negotiations are based on their understandings of the meaningful elements (symbolic) brought to and exchanged in those encounters (words, acts, and gestures). Individuals' meanings brought to encounters are grounded in their respective "stock(s)-of-knowledge at hand" (Schutz, 1967). Those stocks of knowledge, in Schulz's phenomenology, are built up or "precipitated" from previous social experiences. Here I raise the issue of the meanings of presenting complaints as symbolic constructions of and for both patient and healer (Kleinman, 1980b). Phrased another way, this is the issue of transference in clinical practice (Good, DelVecchio Good, & Moradi, 1985). Just as (secular) psychiatrists view their patients in terms of unconscious assumptions such as the "racial" categories (Gaines, 1995c), the biology of disease, and the corporeal nature of persons, so too do Christian psychiatrists. As the psychiatrist seeks to treat a disorder believed to be located within the physical boundary of the person, the Christian psychiatrist sees not just a physical person but also a spiritual being. Whether the patient himself or herself is aware of one's own spiritual nature is not important; the Christian understands that this side or dimension or social reality is a copresent, vital aspect of being.

Among Christian psychiatrists, patients, and people in general, are seen and perceived in meaningful terms according to a remembered past and an assumed (conception of) self (and, hence, of the other). The distinct construction of self is reflected in Christian psychiatric practice.

(RE)THINKING DIVORCE AND HOMOSEXUALITY

The emphasis on this dependent relationship is reflected in the phrase, "believe on God" (or Jesus) rather than "in" God or Jesus. Therapeutic or diagnostic action in the Christian tradition appears based on a notion of the incompleteness of the person, necessitating action to maintain dependence, including "enduring" a bad relationship.

The primacy of community (including family) fosters a therapeutic approach that maintains community rather than splinters it. In their therapeutic relationships, Christian psychiatrists believe that God is ever-present and is an active agent in the therapeutic process, though His role varies somewhat according to my informants. It is seen to vary from that of an assistant of the psychiatrist to that of the sole, prime mover in the therapeutic process (Gaines, 1982c). Since divinity is part of the therapeutic process (and part of the therapist as well), it should not be surprising that elements of the religious sociocentrism would often prevail over the usual egocentric approach which posits that improvement depends on individual actions and efforts, both of which are an individual's responsibility (Gaines, 1985a, 1992c, 1995a, 1995b; Nunnerly, 1961; Townsend, 1978).

The ideal situation for the Christian is in fact a state of dependency, that is, "dependence on" Jesus. Autonomy, as in the case of a woman seeking divorce, is thus not viewed favorably in this tradition as it is in the dominant (European Protestant) tradition in the United States and in its professional ethnopsychiatry (Gaines, 1992c). The exercise of autonomy is doubly problematic when it threatens the sacred bond, marriage, that unites the "Holy Family."

It is important to note that the view of female autonomy now seen in the dominant culture is rather new in that context despite the fact that its appearance is a rather obvious and logical outcome of Northern European Protestant theology from the time of the Reformation. That theology stressed an ungendered individuality in its relation to divinity, hence leaving no theological basis for gender inequality (Gaines, 1982a, 1992c, 1995b, n.d.). Given the previous understandings, one can also understand the abortion and autonomy debates in the United States as a conflict of Western traditions, the Northern European and the Mediterranean, about autonomy and gender roles. The belief in the autonomy of the individual is to be found not only in secular psychiatry theory and practice but also in bioethics of the principalist type. There, it is seen as one of the four principals of principalist bioethics (Beauchamp & Childress, 1994).

CLINICAL ACTION IN THE NAME
OF THE SPIRIT

Several other diagnostic, therapeutic, and management activities are undertaken by Christian psychiatrists which may not be seen among "secular" psychiatrists. The first activity I discuss here concerns an aspect of the diagnostic assessment which some Christian psychiatrists may employ, the "Spiritual History."

SPIRITUAL HISTORY

A development among some Christian psychiatrists in the mid-1980s was the "Spiritual History." Rather than a personal history, the Christian psychiatrist would take a spiritual history (SH). The SH is clearly predicated on the belief that people are spiritual creatures. The SH is distinct from the initial interview (Rittenberg & Simons, 1985), the mental status examination, or the usual medical history.[6] Those who take SHs feel that they are relevant for an understanding of the resources which an individual may draw on, or may have drawn on in the past, when confronted with a crisis.

The SH includes information on the general background of the individual, especially his or her education, church affiliations and attendance, and the like. The history focuses on crisis situations in an effort to explore the family, community, and whatever specifically religious resources the patient has drawn on in times past. The Christian psychiatrist taking a SH would want to know how particular crises were handled—how they were "endured." It should be noted here that enduring and suffering are very much a part of this tradition. Here, as in the Mediterranean, its parent tradition, suffering is seen as enobling and is thus positively viewed (Gaines & Farmer, 1986; Good et al., 1985). This is another element of counseling against divorce in Christian psychiatry.

In addition to the general background information, data on crises, and sources of support, the SH serves to highlight the role and value of religion in the patient's life. However, the Christian psychiatrist also wishes to explore whether or not the patent has been religious in the past and/or to sensitize the patient to the positive potential of religion (the psychiatrist's specific notion thereof) in his or her life. In fact, it appears that a major reason of the taking of the SH is the sensitization of non- or "under"-religious people and the confirmation of the importance of the dependent relationship with respect to divinity. This sensitization may be useful in dealing with the patient's current clinical issue(s).

In a presentation by a Christian psychiatrist to a group of Christian mental health workers, a speaker explained the use of the SH and gave an illuminating example. The speaker, a Christian psychiatrist from California, stated that the Spiritual History was not only for "the religious," but also for the "atheistic." The SH can point out, for the patient and the healer, a certain (spiritual) lacuna in the patient's life, the satisfaction of which might be helpful in overcoming the current problem.

The speaker related an episode from his clinical experience. The case concerned a friend of the speaker who, it was pointed out, was an atheist. The friend had experienced a life-threatening illness requiring hospitalization for surgical intervention to deal with his problem. Postoperatively, the patient evidenced marked depressive affect, the recognition of which led to a psychiatric consultation. The patient's interpretation of his illness, his EM, was that his life, as he had lived it up to that point, was over. His formerly active lifestyle would no longer be possible given his cardiac condition, even after surgery.

Prior to surgery, a consultation had been called for and a SH taken. Postoperatively, the consulting Christian psychiatrist continued to work with the patient. The outcome was that the patient survived the ordeal and could look forward to a new, though altered, lifestyle as a born again Christian. In this case, the Spiritual History was shown to have converted an atheist in crisis, thus demonstrating the proselytic utility of a spiritual history. However, it also demonstrated "empirically" the positive benefits for the patient, i.e., his discovery of new meaning and value in his new, previously devalued, inactive lifestyle. This example points up another therapeutic modality which Christian psychiatrists employ—religious conversion.

CONVERSION

The use of conversion is neither universally accepted nor employed by all Christian psychiatrists. As mentioned earlier, one practitioner has found conversion quite useful as a therapeutic tool for "curing" homosexuality. The use of conversion as a therapeutic goal, which does indeed alter people's lifestyle as long as they do not "backslide," again points to the conception of the person as spiritual—potentially a vessel filled by an animating divinity.

PRAYER WITH AND PRAYER FOR

The use of prayer has been discussed elsewhere (Gaines, 1982c) and the distinction has been drawn between "prayer with" and "prayer for." The former describes prayer involving patient and healer in the clinical context. Such activity dramatically symbolizes the presence and interest of divinity in the healing process, His power to influence that process, and the fact that the healing context is not dyadic but triadic. Both patient and healer submit themselves to the ultimate power, thus effacing the individual basis of the relationship as understood in traditional psychiatry. Prayer for a patient is that which is done by the physician in the absence of the patient, usually in nonclinical contexts. Christian psychiatrists will pray for all their patients, regardless of the faith, or lack of it, of those patients. The patient is usually not made aware of these prayers, whereas in the case of the use of prayer with a patient, the patient is aware, and must be a party to, the communication with God, the Holy Spirit, or Jesus. However, my informants indicated a newer and distinct conceptualization of prayer as a therapeutic tool.

PRAYER OBSERVED

Another innovation among my informants in the mid-1980s was the use of prayer by Christian psychiatrists. The particular usage has its analog in the early use of hypnosis in psychoanalysis. In what I term "prayer observed," the patient is asked if he or she feels like praying to God about his or her problems and concerns. Unlike prayer with a patient, the psychiatrist in this instance observes the prayer but does not participate. The purpose of the observation is to gain insight into the genuine, conscious and unconscious concerns of the patient. The underlying idea was summed up by Dr. Davis (a pseudonym). He explained that having the patient pray about his or her problems and feelings allowed the therapist to get to the heart of the matter much more quickly than would otherwise be the case. The reason for this more efficient means for problem identification was, as he said, "They may lie to me, but they won't lie to God."

Dr. Davis demonstrated a recognition that his patients, whether Christian or not, may not be candid and honest with him. The observation of patients in prayer thus allows him access to feelings, thoughts, and beliefs that might otherwise remain concealed from him for some time. The therapeutic process may move more rapidly, he said. In the case of one patient, Dr. Davis and his supervisor (Dr. Davis had recently finished his residency at the time of the research) believed that the therapeutic process was completed successfully at least a year earlier than would have been possible without the use of prayer observed.

In considering prayer here, I have raised another issue of importance for the practice of Christian psychiatrists: the issue of the meaning of the religious orientation of the patients of these professional healers. Dr. Davis is an example of a Christian psychiatrist who does not expect his patients, even if Born Again, to be truthful with him. How deep does cynicism run among Christian psychiatrists, and how widespread is it among them?

PRACTICE AND CYNICISM

An outside observer, especially an atheistic one, might suggest, as have many secular psychiatrist informants, that the religious presentations of the patient may be a mask—a form of resistance to the therapeutic process. Surprisingly, many Christian psychiatrists wholeheartedly agreed. I posed the question to two of my informants because of its relevance to their clinical practice. Both informants, Dr. Lane from my earlier study (1982c) and Dr. Davis, stated categorically that in fact they assumed, "unless otherwise proven," that any patient seeking their aid *because* they were Christian psychiatrists was more than likely using his or her religion to conceal other problems. That is, at least initially, the presentation of the patient as Christian to a Christian therapist who was sought out because of his or her religious orientation was assumed by them to indicate psychological problems that were cloaked by a religious guise.

My informants went on to say that, contrary to others' ideas about them, they do not expect every clinical problem that they encountered to be a religious one. Informants stated that when they began their residency, they assumed that "all problems were religious." With experience, they had to "learn to be cautious about employing prayer with patients" and other Christian psychiatric practices. In their initial work as Christian psychiatrists, they had a tendency to "jump right in" with their religious orientation. Experience, however, tempered their enthusiasm and made them wary of the veracity of the religious dimension of the problems with which some of their patients presented.

Moreover, none of my informants has any interest in working in a purely Christian environment. Several have turned down very lucrative positions in Christian clinics and universities for lower paying positions at other universities that did not have a Christian orientation. The practice of psychiatry, including training, appeared to make Christian psychiatrists less religious in their approach to patients rather than the reverse. However, the diminution of clinical religious enthusiasm does not affect their notion of the nature of persons or their relationship with the divine. What is affected are their ideas regarding the general utility of religiously influenced diagnostic, therapeutic, and management strategies.

SUMMARY AND CONCLUSIONS

The foregoing account has provided some data and interpretations about the nature of psychiatry as a profession, about bioethical issues, and about anthropological theory's (especially interpretive types of theories) attempts to comprehend such collectivities in terms of their defining features of belief and action. I have considered psychiatrists and Christian psychiatrists in terms of their defining features of belief and action, including their respective conceptions of persons. In looking at the defining characteristics, which would seem to delimit the boundaries of two distinct groups, the distinctiveness of the groups actually begins to blur; the groups seem to lose their individuality, their initially apparent distinctiveness.

For example, not all Christians who are psychiatrists are Christian psychiatrists. Not all secular psychiatrists are uninterested in religion in their practice and, as noted previously, Christian psychiatrists through experience come to define many, if not most, of their patients' presenting complaints in nonreligious terms. There are individuals with religious training, such as Bible college, who do not practice a personal version of Christian psychiatry. Many secular psychiatrists were shown to be believers (APA, 1975) rather than atheistic. There is even the reference to the Lord and His power in the core of biomedicine, internal medicine, by a practitioner who most likely does not regard religion as central or even relevant in his medical work (Hahn, 1985).

The Christian ideology of my informants is held by others, both nonprofessionals and professionals; the latter includes members of such organizations as the Christian Lawyers' Association or that of Christian Realtors. Christian psychiatrists' beliefs do not in fact distinguish them from all other psychiatrists or nonpsychiatrists; the boundaries of the group are quite indistinct. A specific religious orientation employed in their practice is likewise without uniqueness because I am aware of practicing priest psychiatrists and rabbi psychiatrists in the northeastern United States.

In terms of training, in the mid-1980s there were at least two American psychiatric residency programs that offered, within the context of secular state-supported medical education, Christian psychiatric residency training much as any other subspecialty training would be offered. These advertise in Christian journals and magazines as well as use informal channels. At least one program provided a rotation in a Christian hospital for both Christian and secular residents. The patient population of the hospital is largely Christian (e.g., Evangelical and Fundamentalist Protestant).

Examining help-seeking, some differences emerge in the ways in which Christian psychiatrists obtain their patients. However, the means by which patients find their way to Christian psychiatrists are not wholly dissimilar to those of other psychiatrists. As I have pointed out, secular psychiatrists and other specialists do receive and make referrals to Christian psychiatrists despite the tendency for intrafaith referrals. In fact, many of the patients received by Christian psychiatrists doubtless come from secular sources.

Two forms of sickness in the Christian tradition, divorce and homosexuality, seem at first to distinguish this group of healers. Divorce, however, is considered by secular psychiatry to be a stressful event because it causes major life disruptions, some positive and some negative, as well as engendering very strong emotions such as loss, frustration, guilt, anger, and abandonment. While secular psychiatry may locate a disease, e.g., depression, in a person that is a result of divorce, there is clearly considerable overlap in the secular and Christian viewpoints, especially if one notes feelings of guilt or failure (of culturally defined roles.) For both, there is a close relationship between divorce and disease.

Homosexuality, while considered a sin and, as such, both an illness and a disease in the Christian tradition, has only recently been perceived very differently by secular psychiatry. *DSM-III* (APA, 1980) makes a new distinction between egosyntonic and egodystonic homosexuality, with the latter only being a psychiatric disease; and most laypeople still believe either form indicates serious problems. It was certainly not long ago that homosexuals were handed over to the mental health industry for "cures." Again, the difference between those called Born Again and the secular psychiatrists turns out to be more apparent than real.

I have argued here for the centrality of the concept of person for an understanding of EMs of patient and healer and for an understanding of clinical praxis. I hasten to point out, as is implied in the foregoing, that while we can contrast the conception of person among Christian psychiatrists with that of secular psychiatrists, neither is unique. The Christian view is actually that of the people of the Mediterranean, or the Book; it is shared with the vast majority of the patients attending Mason Medical Center located in the Bible Belt. Also recall that 30–40% of Americans say they have experienced something equivalent to being born again as reported in the popular media. A key belief in terms of Christian psychiatric clinical practice thus does not distinguish them from some other professionals and nonprofessionals in the larger society.

Among those called Christian psychiatrists, then, we find, as we do among secular psychiatrists, a wide range of beliefs and practices. For example, the use of conversion as a therapeutic tool is found among Christian psychiatrists, but as far as I am able to determine, its use is quite rare. Of my six informants, only one uses conversion as a tool; the other informants all strongly disavow its use in their practice. Some of them view conversion as proselytizing, which should not be a point or part of psychiatry practice which seeks to "heal the emotions." I also pointed out the variety of beliefs about the role of divinity in the therapeutic process and the differing views of prayer with and prayer for (Gaines, 1982c) as well as the innovation of prayer observed.

In the use of conversion and prayer as therapeutic modalities, Christian psychiatrists represent the beliefs and values of their cultural tradition, just as do practitioners of other branches of Western biomedicine (Gaines & Hahn, 1982; Hahn & Gaines, 1985; Lock & Gordon, 1988), thus falsifying the political economic (and evolutionist) assertions that "only in tribal societies are values unseparated from medical facts" (e.g., Taussig, 1980). I also note that psychiatric ideology, whether secular or Christian, is widely shared vertically in the social body. Ideas in medicine may be more refined, but they are nonetheless fundamentally cultural ideas that are widely shared with culture-mates of various social categories (Gaines, 1985a, 1992a; Reynolds, 1976; Townsend, 1978).

More important, just as some in medicine (and others outside of it) adhere to an "empiricist theory of language" (Good & DelVecchio Good, 1981), others seem to adhere to an empiricist theory of medicine and medical practice (e.g., Illich, 1975; Taussig, 1980). Research presented here and elsewhere in recent years reveals the cultural basis of medical practice; medicines are everywhere cultural systems and, hence, all are equally ethnomedicines and ethnopsychiatries (Gaines, 1992b). The great heterogeneity of belief and praxis within specialties of medicine and the overlap in belief and practice with folk and popular sectors of local health care systems are evident (Gaines, 1979, 1982a, 1982b, 1982c; 1992a, 1992b, 1992c; Gaines & Hahn, 1982; Hahn & Gaines, 1985; Kleinman, 1980b; Lock & Gordon, 1988; Townsend, 1978; Wright & Treacher, 1982).

Diversity of opinion and practice characterizes the ideology and praxis of any medical specialty. The same ideas and practice may be found among other specialties in whole or in part, often in different guises. For example, psychiatrists treat mental sickness, but so do general practitioners, psychologists, and the clergy. Psychotropic drugs may be, and currently are, given by other medical specialists, and psychotherapy is provided by any number of professional and quasiprofessional mental health workers.

What distinctive qualities are there for psychiatrists? Are the qualities of a good psychiatrist unique and can they serve to differentiate him or her from other medical specialists? Sir Denis Hill (1978) considered all the aspects of psychiatric practice, i.e., teaching, administration, leadership, treatment, research, etc. He concluded that the qualities of good psychiatrists are empathy, responsibility to patients, and open-mindedness. However, such characteristics hardly distinguish psychiatrists, even good ones, from other physicians. Such qualities also fail to differentiate psychiatrists from folk healers and/or laypersons concerned with the ill (e.g., family members).

The apparent reality, the existence "out there" of Christian psychiatrists or secular psychiatrists or any other such group, is a function of empiricist theories of groups as coherent, distinctly labeled social entities that can be contrasted with other such entities. The natural distinctiveness of entities is similar to conceptions

of the notion of person in the Northern European Protestant tradition and the notion of distinct "races" as seen in both science and society (Duster, 1990; Gaines,
1982b, 1992d, 1995c, 1997, n.d.; Gould, 1981). The reality of psychiatry is a matter of abstract conceptualization as are the "realities" of such entities as human
"races" and social classes; these exist in researchers' minds, not in the external environment. Such conceptions are cultural products. We must therefore apprehend
social and cultural complexity in our research rather than abstracting neat social
categories, labeling them, and thereby giving them the cloak of reality such that
we can then go about "explaining" them or comparing and contrasting them with
other realities.

In recognizing the cultural construction of both groups, we also address the
problem of the ethics of care among Christian and secular psychiatrists. Both define and construct reality in terms of their beliefs; one is not more culturally constructed than the other. We cannot therefore argue for the moral primacy of one
over the other. We must accept a relativist stance, seeing clinical reality and therapy from each vantage point. I note here that the relativist position as represented
in bioethics is generally mischaracterized. In anthropology, the articulation that
there are distinct, local moral worlds is not an argument or a theoretical position.
It is a statement of empirical cross-cultural reality.

In addition, the anthropological relativist account does not accept heinous individual actions as unobjectionable because it recognizes that all humans are members of local cultures and as such are members of local moral worlds. Therefore,
such random behavior is not to be condoned. Bioethicists opposed to relativism
fail to recognize that between the individual and the universal lies the cultural (e.g.,
Post, 1993; Ridley, 1998; Wong, 1993). With the recognition of the level of culture, we find that antirelativist arguments about the moral chaos of individualism,
if we do not accept universal ethics, are misplaced and miscast. They fail to understand the concept of culture. In the examples here, it is clear that there are two
distinct moral worlds. Hence, we confirm the reality of local cultural constructions
of reality and of morality and cannot give primacy to one or the other on rational,
or moral, grounds.

I have tried to move back and forth between demonstrating the distinctiveness
and, therefore, corporate character of Christian psychiatry and effacing the view
of a group reality so constructed. The complexity of social and cultural realities of
biomedicine suggests that we would do best not to resort to stereotypic, and generally distorted, macro critiques of a putatively monolithic and ideologically and
behaviorally distinct social group, whether such critiques come from the political
left (e.g., Navarro, 1976a; Taussig, 1980) or right (e.g., Illich, 1975; Szasz, 1961).

A second point is more straightforward. The concept of person used by professionals and laypersons is critical for an understanding of health-related actions,
though the conception is neither conscious nor limited in its relevance only to sickness episodes.

Much thought relevant to clinical contexts or sickness episodes is unconscious
and involves understandings, conceptions, and assumptions not easily articulated

because they form the foundation on which other thoughts, such as the conscious EMs, are built. The interpretation of illness realities for patient and healer occurs within broad cultural semantic domains, in what Good (1977) has discerned as Semantic Illness Networks. We may say that broad cultural conceptions, such as that of person, anchor understandings and knowledge about function and dysfunction and significance and insignificance of specific symptoms and illness (and define them as such) and also provide nodes of attachment for webs of significance such as Semantic Illness Networks. From these understandings and cultural knowledge are drawn models (EMs) about specific illness episodes.

Sickness befalls persons certainly, but persons are not construed homogeneously across cultures. The statement that "a person is sick" is an explanation rather than a description precisely because the meaning and the references of each of the terms vary with the cultural context. What a person is or is not greatly shapes what are thought to be the possibilities of sickness and its cause, outcome, and processes. These notions in turn shape the conception of sickness, the experience of it, and what is deemed appropriate and sufficient therapeutic action in lay, folk, and professional circles as individuals manipulate elements of their particular symbolic domains to deal with malaise.

In approaching the meaningful elements of sickness cross-culturally, it is important to address the symbolic nature of distress and the symbolic construction of relevant social sectors concerned with the alleviation thereof. Without such a perspective, we overlook the meaning of sickness, healing, patients, healers, and their symbolic relationship(s) to one another and to the wider domains of human culture to which they are intimately related. It is in these terms that we should understand culture and religion in psychiatry

EDITOR'S COMMENT

Based upon over 15 years of research and clinical practice, I would like to respond to Dr. Gaines' thoughtful and articulate essay. My comments represent a different view that the reader should consider. Each comment is referenced to that section of Dr. Gaines' essay to which it is relevant.

[1]A "Christian psychiatrist," as described in this chapter, might make a wide range of recommendations in response to an abusive family situation. Many Christian psychiatrists who practice today (1998) would support a woman's decision to separate from her abusive, alcoholic husband. The Christian psychiatrist, however, would encourage the woman to make this decision for a reason other than anger, rage, and desire for revenge. The reason for leaving would be based on the over-riding principle of "love thy neighbor as thyself." In other words, leaving her husband and not returning until his behavior changed could be viewed as an act of *love.* The alcoholic, abusive husband is on a self-destructive and other-destructive path. If the wife does not leave her husband or "set limits" in some other way, then this would support and enable evil to continue. Leaving him and withdrawing her support may help him to see the error of his ways and bring about change and healing in both the husband and family.

[2]Not all "Christian psychiatrists," even the Fundamentalist-Evangelical types, would make as their primary goal the transformation of a homosexual to a heterosexual. Many—perhaps the majority—

would first help the homosexual obtain healing in their relationship with Christ. They would focus on Christ's love, complete acceptance of the person, and understanding of the suffering the patient was experiencing. The Christian psychiatrist would then help the patient clarify what the patient's goals were, and then help him or her to achieve those goals. For some patients, transformation to heterosexuality would not be desirable or even possible; achievement and maintenance of celibacy is one of a number of alternative goals that might be pursued. If the psychiatrist felt the patient's goals were not those that he or she could ethically support, then the patient would be referred to someone whose theology was more in line with the patient's.

[3]There is an implication that the person did not have an "in-dwelling spirit" prior to being "born again." Many Evangelical-Fundamentalist Christians would take issue with this implication, emphasizing that all persons have a spirit and a spiritual nature, but on being "born again" that spirit becomes transformed or regenerated.

[4]Most members of the Evangelical-Fundamentalist Christian community would not agree with the notion that the individual is not important and his or her needs are less important than the needs of the social group (see Matthew 18:12–14, where the story is told of the shepherd who leaves his entire flock of sheep to possible danger in order to find the one sheep that has strayed). Most members of the Evangelical-Fundamentalist Christian community would also not agree with the concept that the "self" or "person" is simply a "sort of shell filled and even animated by benevolent superior spiritual forces and entities . . . . [and that] . . . the person is conceived of as neither independent nor autonomous." Rather, they would argue that personal responsibility and accountability are the foundations upon which the concept of "sin" (and judgement) is based.

[5]While success may often be attributed to Christ's working within a person's life, this attitude of gratefulness and humble recognition of Christ's role in their success does not eliminate the "personal" role or responsibility. The New Testament clearly emphasizes that "strength, will, patience, and endurance" are qualities that the individual must earn through diligent effort (James 1:12), although they may be difficult to obtain alone without Christ's help. To attribute success to the person or self only, however, may result in spiritual pride (which all major religious traditions condemn).

[6]Today, Spiritual Histories are usually not separate, but performed as part of the routine psychiatric evaluation and are included as part of the developmental history, where information is collected on spiritual issues along with social and sexual issues (see Larson DB, Lu F, Swyers JW (1996). *Model Curriculum for Psychiatric Residency Training Programs.* Rockville, MD: National Institute for Healthcare Research). The SH's purpose is not intended as a tool for coercing religious conversion, but rather to inform the psychiatrist about religious or spiritual factors that may influence the patient's illness.

Final Thought: While they may inquire about the religious background of patients and perhaps even suggest its utility in addressing certain problems, most professional psychiatrists who would call themselves "Christian psychiatrists" do not attempt to force their views upon or proselytize their non-religious or non-Christian patients. Rather, these clinicians try to be sensitive to the religious background and beliefs of their patients, and allow *the patient* to determine whether or not these factors should be included in therapy. If religious or spiritual factors are important to the patient (often the reason for their consulting a Christian psychiatrist), then these factors will be considered by the psychiatrist as a resource (rather than a liability) which he or she will help the patient draw on for healing.

REFERENCES

American Psychiatric Association. (1975). *Psychiatrists' viewpoints on religion.* Washington, DC: Author.
American Psychiatric Association. (1980). *Diagnostic and statistical manual,* 3rd ed. Washington, DC: Author.

American Psychiatric Association. (1994). *Diagnostic and statistical manual.* 4th ed. Washington, DC: Author.

Arensberg, C. (1963). The old world peoples. *Anthropological Quarterly, 36*(3).

Beauchamp, T. L., & Childress, J. F. (1994). *Principles of biomedical ethics,* 4th ed. Oxford, UK: Oxford University Press.

Boissevain, J. (1979). Toward an anthropology of the Mediterranean. *Current Anthropology, 20,* 81–93.

Castel, R., Castel, F., & Lovell, A. (1982). *The psychiatric society.* New York: Columbia University Press.

Conner, L. (1982). The unbounded self. In A. J. Marsella and G. M. White (Eds.), *Cultural conceptions of mental health and therapy.* Dordrecht: Reidel.

Csordas, T. (1992). The affliction of Martin: Religious, clinical and phenomenological meaning in a case of demonic oppression. In A. D. Gaines (Ed.), *Ethnopsychiatry: The cultural construction of professional and folk psychiatries.* Albany: State University of New York Press.

Csordas, T. (1994). *The sacred self. A cultural phenomenology of charismatic healing.* Berkeley: University of California Press.

Davis, J. (1975). *People of the Mediterranean.* London: Routledge & Kegan Paul.

Devereux, G. (1982). Ethnic identity. In G. DeVos & L. Romanucci-Ross (Eds.), *Ethnic identity: Cultural continuities and change.* Chicago: University of Chicago Press.

Duster, T. (1990). *Backdoor to eugenics.* New York: Routledge.

Dwyer, E. (1987). *Homes for the mad.* New Brunswick, NJ: Rutgers University Press.

Evans-Pritchard, E. E. (1940). *Nuer religion.* Oxford, UK: Oxford University Press.

Favazza, A. (1982). Modern Christian healing. *American Journal of Psychiatry, 139,* 728.

Finkler, K. (1991). *Physicians at work, patients in pain: Biomedical practice and patient response in Mexico.* Boulder, CO: Westview Press.

Gaines, A. D. (1979). Definitions and diagnoses. *Culture, Medicine, and Psychiatry, 3*(4), 381–418.

Gaines, A. D. (1982a). Cultural definitions, behavior and the person in American psychiatry. In A. J. Marsella & G. M. White (Eds.), *Cultural conceptions of mental health and therapy.* Dordrecht: Reidel.

Gaines, A. D. (1982b). Knowledge and practice. In N. Chrisman & T. Maretzki (Eds.), *Clinically applied anthropology.* Dordrecht: Reidel.

Gaines, A. D. (1982c). The twice-born: "Christian psychiatry" and Christian psychiatrists. *Culture, Medicine, and Psychiatry, 6*(3), 305–324.

Gaines, A. D. (1985a). The once- and the twice born: Self and practice among psychiatrists and Christian psychiatrists. In R. A. Hahn & A. D. Gaines (Eds.), *Physicians of Western medicine: Anthropological approaches to theory and practice.* Dordrecht: Reidel.

Gaines, A. D. (1985b). Faith, fashion and family: Religion, aesthetics, identity and social organization in Strasbourg. *Anthropological Quarterly, 58*(2), 47–62.

Gaines, A. D. (Ed.). (1992a). *Ethnopsychiatry: The cultural construction of professional and folk psychiatries.* Albany: State University of New York Press.

Gaines, A. D. (1992b). Ethnopsychiatry: The cultural construction of psychiatries. In A. D. Gaines (Ed.), *Ethnopsychiatry: The cultural construction of professional and folk psychiatries.* Albany: State University of New York Press.

Gaines, A. D. (1992c). From DSM I to Ill-R: Voices of self, mastery and the other: a cultural constructivist reading of U.S. psychiatric classification. *Social Science and Medicine, 35*(1), 3–24.

Gaines, A. D. (1992d). Medical/psychiatric knowledge in France and the United States: Culture and sickness in history and biology. In A. D. Gaines, (Ed.), *Ethnopsychiatry: The cultural construction of professional and folk psychiatries.* Albany: State University of New York Press.

Gaines, A. D. (1995a). Culture specific delusions: Sense and nonsense in cultural context. In M. J. Sedler (Ed.), *Delusional disorders.* Philadelphia: Saunders.

Gaines, A. D. (1995b). Mental illness II: Cross-cultural perspectives. In W. T. Reich (Ed.), *Encyclopedia of bioethics* (Vol. 3). New York: Macmillan.

Gaines, A. D. (1995c). Race and racism. In W. T. Reich (Ed.), *Encyclopedia of bioethics* (Vol. 4). New York: Macmillan.

Gaines, A. D. (1997). Culture and values at the intersection of science and suffering: Encountering ethics, genetics and Alzheimer disease. In S. G. Post & P. J. Whitehouse (Eds.), *Genetic testing for Alzheimer disease: Clinical and ethical issues.* Baltimore: Johns Hopkins University Press.

Gaines, A. D. (n.d.). *The word and the cross: The cultural construction of Alsatian ethnic and religious identity in France.* Unpublished manuscript.

Gaines, A. D., & Farmer, P. A. (1986). Visible saints: Social cynosures and dysphoria in the Mediterranean tradition. *Culture, Medicine and Psychiatry, 10*(3), 295–330.

Gaines, A. D., & Hahn, R. (Eds.). (1982). Physicians of Western medicine: Five cultural studies. *Culture, Medicine, and Psychiatry, 6*(3), 10. (Special issue)

Geertz, C. (1973). *The interpretation of cultures.* New York: Basic Books.

Geertz, C. (1977). On the nature of anthropological understanding. In *Annual editions in anthropology.* Guilford, CT: Dushkin.

Gilmore, D. (1982). Anthropology of the Mediterranean area. In *Annual reviews in anthropology.* Palo Alto, CA: Annual Reviews.

Good, B. (1977). The heart of what's the matter. *Culture, Medicine, and Psychiatry, 1*(1), 25–58.

Good, B. (1994). *Medicine, rationality and experience.* Cambridge, UK: Cambridge University Press.

Good, B. & DelVecchio Good, M.-J. (1981). The meaning of symptoms. In L. Eisenberg & A. Kleinman (Eds.), *The relevance of social science for medicine.* Dordrecht: Reidel.

Good, B., DelVecchio Good, M.-J., & Moradi, R. (1985). The interpretation of Iranian depressive illness and dysphoric affect. In A. Kleinman & B. Good (Eds.), *Culture and depression: Cross-cultural studies in the anthropology and cross-cultural psychiatry of affect and disorder.* Berkeley: University of California Press.

Gould, S. J. (1981). *The mismeasure of man.* New York: Norton.

Hahn, R. A. (1982)."Treat the patient, not the lab": Internal medicine and the concept of "person." *Culture, Medicine, and Psychiatry, 6*(3), 219–236. (Special issue)

Hahn, R. A. (1985). A world of internal medicine: Portrait of an internist. In R. A. Hahn & A. D. Gaines (Eds.), *Physicians of Western medicine: Anthropological approaches to theory and practice.* Dordrecht: Reidel.

Hahn, R. A., & Gaines, A. D. (Eds.). (1985). *Physicians of Western medicine: Anthropological approaches to theory and practice.* Dordrecht: Reidel.

Hallowell, A. I. (1955). The self and its behavioral environment. In A. I. Hallowell (Ed.), *Culture and experience.* Philadelphia: University of Pennsylvania Press.

Hershel, H. J. (1992). Psychiatric institutions: Rules and the accommodation of structure and autonomy in France and the United States. In A. D. Gaines (Ed.), *Ethnopsychiatry: The cultural construction of professional and folk psychiatries.* Albany: State University of New York Press.

Hill, D. (1978). The qualities of a good psychiatrist. *British Journal of Psychiatry, 133,* 97–105.

Illich, I. (1975). *Medical nemesis.* New York: Pantheon.

Johnson, T. (1985). Consultation–liaison psychiatry: Medicine as patient, marginality as practice. In R. A. Hahn & A. D. Gaines, (Eds.), *Physicians of Western medicine: Anthropological approaches to theory and practice.* Dordrecht: Reidel.

Johnson, T. (1987). Premenstrual syndrome as a Western culture-specific disorder. *Culture, Medicine, and Psychiatry, 11*(3), 337–356.

Karkar, S. (1982). *Shamans, mystics and doctors: A psychological inquiry into India and its healing traditions.* Chicago: University of Chicago Press.

Kleinman, A. (1980a). Major conceptual and research issues for cultural (anthropological) psychiatry. *Culture, Medicine, and Psychiatry, 4*(3), 3–13.

Kleinman, A. (1980b). *Patients and healers in the context of culture.* Berkeley: University of California Press.

Kleinman, A. (1986). *Social origins of distress and disease: Depression, neurasthenia, and pain in modern China.* New Haven, CT: Yale University Press.

Kleinman, A. (1988a). *The illness narratives: Suffering, healing and the human condition.* New York: Basic Books.

Kleinman, A. (1988b). *Rethinking psychiatry: From cultural category to personal experience.* New York: Free Press.

Kleinman, A., Eisenberg, L., Good, B. (1978). Culture, illness, and care. *Annals of Internal Medicine, 88,* 251–258.

Kleinman, A., & Good, B. (Eds.). (1985). *Culture and depression: Studies in the anthropology and cross-cultural psychiatry of affect and disorder.* Berkeley: University of California Press.

Lebra, T. (1976). *Japanese patterns of behavior.* Honolulu: University Press of Hawaii.

Lee, D. (1959). *Freedom and culture.* Englewood Cliffs, NJ: Prentice Hall.

Light, D. (1976). Work styles among American psychiatric residents. In J. Westermeyer (Ed.), *Anthropology and mental health.* The Hague: Mouton.

Lindenbaum, S., & Lock, M. (Eds.). (1993). *Knowledge, power and practice.* Berkeley: University of California Press.

Lock, M., & Gordon, D. (Eds.). (1988). *Biomedicine examined.* Dordrecht: Kluwer.

Mechanic, D. (1962). Some factors in identifying and defining mental illness. *Mental Hygiene, 46,* 66–74.

Mishler, E., AmaraSingham, L. R., Hauser, S., Liem, R., Osherson, S., & Waxler, N. (1981). *Social contexts of health, illness and patient care.* Cambridge, UK: Cambridge University Press.

Nanji, A. (1993). Islamic ethics. In P. Singer (Ed.), *A companion to ethics.* Oxford, UK: Blackwell.

Navarro, V. (1976). *Medicine under capitalism.* New York: Prodist.

Nomura, N. (1992). Psychiatrist and patient in Japan: An analysis of interactions in an outpatient clinic. In A. D. Gaines (Ed.), *Ethnopsychiatry: The cultural construction of professional and folk psychiatries.* Albany: State University of New York Press.

Nuckolls, C. (1992). Notes on a defrocked priest: Comparing South Indian shamanic and American psychiatric diagnosis. In A. D. Gaines (Ed.), *Ethnopsychiatry: The cultural construction of professional and folk psychiatries.* Albany: State University of New York Press.

Nunnerly, J. C. (1961). *Popular conceptions of mental health.* New York: Holt, Rinehart & Winston.

Ortner, S. (1973). On key symbols. *American Anthropologist, 75*(3), 1338–1346.

Post, S. G. (1992). DSM-III-R and religion. *Social Science and Medicine, 35*(1), 81–90.

Post, S. G. (1993). *Inquiries in bioethics.* Washington, DC: Georgetown University Press.

Reynolds, D. K. (1976). *Morita psychotherapy.* Berkeley: University of California Press.

Reynolds, D. K. (1980). *The quiet therapies: Japanese pathways to personal growth.* Honolulu: University Press of Hawaii.

Ridley, A. (1998). *Beginning bioethics.* New York: St. Martins.

Rittenberg, W., & Simons, R. C. (1985). Gentle interrogation: Inquiry and interaction in brief initial psychiatric evaluations. In R. A. Hahn & A. D. Gaines (Eds.), *Physicians of Western medicine: Anthropological approaches to theory and practice.* Dordrecht: Reidel.

Schutz, A. (1967). *Collected papers I: The problem of social reality* (M. Natanson Ed.). The Hague: Nijhoff.

Shweder, R., & Bourne, E. (1982). Does the concept of person vary cross-culturally? In A. J. Marsella & G. M. White (Eds.), *Cultural conceptions of mental health and therapy.* Dordrecht: Reidel.

Szasz, T. (1961). *The myth of mental illness.* New York: Hoeber & Harper.

Taussig, M. T. (1980). Reification and the consciousness of the patient. *Social Science and Medicine, 14B,* 3–13.

Townsend, J. M. (1978). *Cultural conceptions and mental illness.* Chicago: University of Chicago Press.

Turkle, S. (1978). *Psychoanalytic politics.* New York: Basic Books.

Turner, V. W. (1969). *The ritual process.* Chicago: Aldine.

Turner, V. W. (1974). *Dramas, fields and metaphors: Symbolic action in human society.* Ithaca, NY: Cornell University Press.

Weisberg, D., & Long, S. O. (Eds.). (1984). Biomedicine in Asia: Transformations and variations. *Culture, Medicine and Psychiatry, 8*(2). (Special issue)

White, G., & Marsella, A. (1982). Introduction: Cultural conceptions in mental health research and

2

practice. In A. J. Marsella & G. M. White (Eds.), *Cultural conceptions of mental health and therapy.* Dordrecht: Reidel.

Wong, D. (1993). Relativism. In P. Singer (Ed.), *A companion to ethics.* Oxford, UK: Blackwell.

Wright, P., & Treacher, A. (Eds.). (1982). *The problem of medical knowledge: Examining the social construction of medicine.* Edinburgh, UK: University of Edinburgh Press.

CLINICAL APPLICATIONS

22

RELIGION AND
PSYCHOTHERAPY

HAROLD G. KOENIG

Department of Psychiatry
Duke University Medical Center
Durham, North Carolina 27710

JOHN PRITCHETT

Private Practice of Psychiatry
Charleston, South Carolina 29412

In this chapter, we examine the religious and spiritual needs of psychiatric patients and how therapists might utilize the patient's religious beliefs to complement and facilitate the process of psychotherapy. Parts of this topic have been addressed elsewhere (Miller & Martin, 1988; Pattison, 1966; Propst, 1987). Here, we provide some practical information and guidelines that will help the therapist address religious issues in psychotherapy and, where appropriate, utilize the patient's spiritual resources to enhance mental and emotional healing. While this can be admittedly treacherous ground for psychiatrists and other mental health specialists, addressing spiritual issues with patients is becoming an increasingly accepted part of whole person care. While clinicians will differ in the extent to which they decide to utilize and delve into religious issues with their patients, a new minimal standard is beginning to emerge. This new standard has arisen from several sources.

First, the American Psychiatric Association (APA) published *Practice Guidelines for the Psychiatric Evaluation of Adults* (APA, 1995a), which states that (a) "important cultural and religious influences on the patient's life" (p. 71) be collected as part of the initial evaluation of the psychiatric patient; (b) "evaluation ought to be performed in a manner that is sensitive to the patient's individuality, identifying issues of development, culture, ethnicity, gender, sexual orientation, familial/genetic patterns, *religious/spiritual beliefs,* social class, and physical and social environment influencing the patient's symptoms and behavior" (p. 74); and (c) assessment must include "information specific to the individual patient that goes beyond what is conveyed by the diagnosis . . . [including] issues related to culture, ethnicity, gender, sexual orientation, and *religious/spiritual beliefs*" (p. 76).

Second, the diagnostic nomenclature has changed from *DSM-III-R* to *DSM-IV.* It now includes religious or spiritual problems as an "additional condition that may be a focus of clinical attention" (Lukoff, Lu, & Turner, 1992); thus, clinicians now have a diagnostic code for such problems that is akin to major psychiatric disorders and thus deserving of attention by mental health specialists.

Third, in March 1994, the American College for Graduate Medical Education included in its Special Requirements for Residency Training (Accreditation Council on Graduate Medical Education, 1994) in psychiatry that all training programs comply with the following: (a) didactic training in the "presentation of the biological, psychological, sociocultural, economic, ethnic, gender, *religious/spiritual,* sexual orientation and family factors that significantly influence physical and psychological development in infancy, childhood, adolescence, and adulthood" (pp. 11–12), and (b) "the residency program should provide its residents with instruction about American culture and subcultures, particularly those found in the patient community associated with the training program. This instruction should include such issues as sex, race, ethnicity, *religion/spirituality,* and sexual orientation" (p. 18). Likewise, psychology training programs are required to "include exposure to theoretical and empirical knowledge bases relevant to the role of cultural and individual diversity," (p. Iw-27) which includes religion (American Psychological Association, 1995b).

Thus, prior to any form of psychotherapeutic intervention, initial psychiatric evaluation at the very minimum must explore the patients' religious beliefs and background (taking a "religious history"; see Chapter 25) and assess how these might either contribute to the development of psychopathology or, in contrast, facilitate its resolution. This, of course, does not demand or encourage the use of religious beliefs and practices as part of psychiatric intervention. It may be useful at times, however, particularly with religious patients or patients whose disordered religious beliefs stand in the way of successful psychotherapy, for the therapist to directly address religious issues and perhaps even utilize the patient's religious beliefs, if healthy and affirming, to help effect emotional healing. How a prudent therapist may sensitively and delicately do so is the subject of this chapter.

SPIRITUAL NEEDS OF PSYCHIATRIC PATIENTS

Recent studies indicate that psychiatric patients have spiritual needs that, if addressed, might aide the process of psychological healing. In Fitchett, Burton, and

Sivan's (1997) survey of psychiatric and medical inpatients (ages 20–89 years), 80% of psychiatric patients considered themselves a religious or spiritual person (vs 86% for medical patients), and 88% reported they had three or more religious or spiritual needs (vs 76% of medical patients). These needs were divided into religious belief needs, religious practice needs, and religious social support needs. Religious belief needs included "to know God's presence" (84%), "purpose and meaning in life" (75%), and "relief from fear of death" (51%). Religious practice needs included prayer (80%), receiving sacraments or communion (39%), and attending religious services (84%). Religious social support needs included "care and support from another" (90%), "chaplain visit and pray" (65%), and "visit from a clergyperson" (59%). Table 22.1 provides an expanded list of psychological and spiritual needs of patients that therapists should consider addressing (Koenig & Weaver, 1997).

Furthermore, 68% of psychiatric patients and 72% of medical patients in Fitchett et al.'s (1997) study responded "a great deal" to a statement indicating that re-

TABLE 22.1   Psychological and Spiritual Needs of Psychiatric Patients[a]

Needs related to self
 A need for meaning and purpose
 A need for a sense of usefulness
 A need for vision
 A need for hope
 A need for support in coping with loss and change
 A need to adapt to increasing dependency (older adults)
 A need to transcend difficult circumstances
 A need for personal dignity
 A need to express feelings
 A need to be thankful
 A need for continuity with the past
 A need to accept and prepare for death and dying (older adults)

Needs related to God
 A need to be certain that God exists
 A need to believe that God is on their side
 A need to experience God's presence
 A need to experience God's unconditional love
 A need to pray alone, with others, or for others
 A need to read and be inspired by scripture
 A need to worship God, individually and corporately
 A need to love and serve God

Needs related to others
 A need for fellowship with others
 A need to love and serve others
 A need to confess and be forgiven
 A need to forgive others
 A need to cope with the death of or separation from loved ones

[a]Some of these needs may apply only to patients from a Judeo-Christian background.

ligion was a source of strength and comfort to them. Interestingly, only 24% of psychiatric patients had talked to a clergyperson about their hospitalization compared with 81% of medical patients. These findings suggest that many psychiatric patients have spiritual needs which they may not be able to meet through traditional routes (due to embarrassment, inaccessibility, etc.).

Kroll and Sheehan (1989) also reported in their study of 52 psychiatric inpatients a high prevalence of belief in God (95%), the devil (69%), and an afterlife (80%), and that they had recently sinned (43%). Religious activities were likewise prevalent, with 65% indicating membership in a church or synagogue, 53% attending religious services at least weekly, and 53% consulting the Bible or praying about decisions. Again, this relatively high prevalence of religious beliefs and practices among psychiatric inpatients suggests that spiritual needs related to these beliefs and practices are prevalent.

There is some preliminary evidence that meeting those spiritual needs by addressing religious issues and concerns may have a positive impact on mental health outcomes. Chu and Klein (1985) studied factors related to discharge from the hospital, community adjustment, and rehospitalization in a sample of 128 black schizophrenic inpatients in Missouri. They reported that patients were less likely to be rehospitalized if their families encouraged them to continue religious worship while they were in the hospital, and patients were more likely to be readmitted if their families had no religious affiliation. Chu and Klein concluded that there was a positive correlation between religious worship and favorable community outcomes.

Likewise, Koenig, George, and Peterson (1998) found that among 87 depressed medical inpatients, almost two-thirds of patients indicated they used religion at least to "a large extent" to help them cope with their medical problems and other life stressors; in that study, patients with higher intrinsic religiosity remitted from depression significantly faster than those with lower scores (70% faster for every 10-point increase on an intrinsic religiosity scale administered at baseline). Finally, two clinical trials that have used religious-oriented psychotherapy for treating religious patients with either anxiety or depressive disorder report that patients receiving religious-oriented therapy experienced significantly better short-term outcomes (Azhart, Varma & Dharap, 1994; Propst, Ostrom, Watkins, Dean, & Mashburn, 1992). These data suggest that addressing religious or spiritual needs during the course of psychotherapy might facilitate the healing process.

CONDUCTING A RELIGIOUS/SPIRITUAL ASSESSMENT

Many patients because of guilt or shame over their psychiatric problems will be reluctant to approach their ministers over spiritual issues that relate to those problems. This often leaves the therapist as one of the few persons with whom the patient can safely talk about their spiritual struggles. How does the therapist conduct religious or spiritual assessment that will both obtain relevant information and communicate to the patient that the therapist is open to addressing such issues?

The following four questions (Dale Mathews, personal communication) are nonoffensive and easily remembered:

F. Is religious faith an important part of your life?
I. How has your faith influenced your life (past and present)?
C. Are you a part of a religious or spiritual community?
A. Are there any spiritual needs that you would like me to address?

Briefly exploring the answers to each of these questions (if yes, why; if no, why not) will provide a wealth of information that will help the therapist develop a therapeutic plan.

WHY ADDRESS RELIGION IN PSYCHOTHERAPY?

Why address religious or spiritual factors during therapy with emotionally disturbed patients? Addressing religious issues with patients will help the therapist (a) better understand the patient's psychological conflict, (b) design interventions that are more acceptable to the patient and congruent with their worldview (and thus more likely to be complied with), (c) identify healthy religious resources that may bring comfort and support, (d) recognize psychological roadblocks that prevent the patient from utilizing potentially powerful spiritual resources, and (e) strengthen the therapeutic relationship (because this demonstrates sensitivity to an area that may be very meaningful to the patient).

First, knowing about the religious background and experiences of patients may help the therapist to better understand the conflicts that patients struggle with. For example, a patient is struggling with extreme guilt that seems to be resistant to traditional psychotherapy. On exploration of the patient's religious background, the therapist learns that the patient was raised in a strict fundamentalist religious family in which eternal damnation was taught as a consequence of unrepented sin. On further exploration, the patient admits that after his or her spouse left 6 months ago, the patient became angry at God and committed the unpardonable sin of blaspheming the Holy Spirit. Since that time, the patient had developed a very deep depression which at the core was the guilt over having cursed God over his or her distressing circumstances. Including the patient's minister in the psychotherapy sessions helped to clarify the theological question involved here and allowed the patient to confess and accept forgiveness in the tradition of his or her faith. Before understanding the central religious conflict involved, the therapist was unable to make much progress. In other cases, however, guilt related to committing unpardonable sins is delusional in origin and must be treated with antipsychotic medication rather than spiritual clarification. Other patients may believe that some other sin is directly responsible for their present psychiatric difficulties and may even feel the need to continue suffering as penance or the need to "work through" their actions by repentence. Sheehan and Kroll (1990) found that 23% of 52 psychiatric inpatients believed that sin-related factors (such as sinful thoughts or acts) had affected the development of their illness.

Second, knowing the patient's religious background and the role that it currently plays in a person's life can help the therapist to intervene cognitively and behaviorally in a manner that is acceptable to the patient's belief system and is thus more likely to be complied with. For example, the religious female patient involved in a codependent, destructive relationship with an abusive husband may be reluctant to set limits or follow through with consequences because of the religious belief that a wife should honor and submit to her husband. Without understanding the patient's motivation for such behavior, the therapist may be unsuccessful in altering her behaviors that enable the destructive behaviors on her husband's part. Addressing this religious concern directly and challenging this belief in a gentle though persistent manner, with support from the patient's clergyperson, may help the patient to break out of this destructive relationship pattern. For other patients who have strong beliefs based on religious scriptures (such as the Bible), the therapist can utilize those beliefs for confronting cognitive distortions and for limit setting with regard to unacceptable behaviors.

Third, knowledge of the religious beliefs, behaviors, and commitments of the patients will help to identify healthy religious resources that can be relied on to complement traditional therapy. We now know that many patients, both psychiatric and medical, report they derive great comfort from their religious faith, and the presence of a strong religious faith predicts faster resolution of psychiatric symptoms (Koenig et al., 1992; 1998). Helping the patient tap into these religious resources while at the same time addressing the patients psychological conflicts using traditional forms of psychotherapy can bring about a more rapid healing.

Fourth, previous negative religious experiences may block the patient's utilization of faith resources in coping with their present problems. Learning about and helping the patient work through such negative experiences with religion can help free him or her to once again utilize these religious resources. Prior negative experiences with religion in their family (overly strict or punitive) or in prior experiences with church, a pastor, or a disappointment with God or unanswered prayer can place a roadblock for the patient in accessing spiritual resources.

Finally, addressing religious issues will communicate to the patient that the therapist is not only being very thorough and inclusive in his or her diagnostic assessment but also that he or she is sensitive to an area of the patient's life that is very meaningful to that person (and will address issues in this area the person may be struggling over but is unable to talk freely about with others). When done in a sensitive and patient-centered way, this invariably strengthens the therapeutic relationship.

WHO SHOULD HANDLE RELIGIOUS ISSUES IN PSYCHOTHERAPY?

Because of difficulty with definitions and language, and perhaps because of overlap of the concepts themselves, the separation of psychological and spiritual needs has not always been clear (Table 22.1). Even the definition given for the word "psychology" itself, according to Webster's original 1928 (1983) dictionary, is "A discourse or treatise on the human soul; or the doctrine of the nature and properties of the soul." For that reason, there has been some controversy over who is responsible for meeting what needs. This controversy has raged over the past 35 years, as there has been increasing interaction between mental health and religious professionals (Klausner, 1964).

Klausner (1964) discusses four different ideological positions on who should address religious issues. The secular "reductionist" claims that mental health is entirely in the realm of scientific psychology, whereas the religious reductionist claims that mental health is entirely within the province of religious belief and practice. The "dualist" argues that there are both psychological and spiritual problems and that a single qualified therapist can deal with both. "Alternavists" claim that there is only one problem which is primarily psychological, and that either a minister or a psychotherapist can deal with it. Finally, the "specialist" maintains that there are spiritual problems and psychological problems, and each area should be dealt with by a specialist in that domain.

From our perspective, it is likely that no one ideological position is applicable to all patients in all clinical situations. In certain disorders, such as schizophrenia, the secular reductionist's claims may be more true because of the overwhelming biological component to the disease. In other conditions, such as existential depression or issues related to death or dying, religious or spiritual factors may predominate and require the expertise of the clergy. In most conditions, however, both spiritual and psychological issues are present that overlap and are difficult to separate, requiring the expertise of either a mental health professional with background and interest in spiritual needs or a religious professional with considerable training in psychology. Often, one professional will need to consult with the other and together treat the patient as a team. Sometimes, however, situations will demand that the mental health professional address religious or spiritual issues because the patient will not see a religious professional or a religious professional must address psychological issues because the patient refuses to see a mental health professional. In any case, it is our belief that most psychiatric and spiritual conditions involve a mixture of psychological and spiritual issues, both of which need addressing to allow for the total healing of the person.

RELIGIOUS INTERVENTIONS IN PSYCHOTHERAPY

We will address six specific religious interventions that therapists may utilize when treating religious patients and, in some cases, when treating nonreligious patients who give explicit permission to the therapist to use such methods. These interventions are primarily based in the Judeo-Christian religious tradition, which we are most familiar with; thus, they may not be applicable to patients from other religious backgrounds. The interventions include (a) listening to and validating healthy forms of religious coping; (b) pointing out religious scriptures that provide hope, a positive self-esteem, and a sense that they are loved and cared for; (c) challenging maladaptive religious cognitions or behaviors; (d) use of the patient's religious worldview to alter maladaptive, dysfunctional cognitions and encourage healthy behaviors; (e) referral of the patient to a minister, chaplain, or pastoral counselor; and, (f) most controversial, praying with patients. Each of these interventions will be discussed below.

First, listening to and validating the patient's use of religion to facilitate adaptation and coping is consistent with the underlying principle of supportive psychotherapy. According to Dewald (1971), the function and technique of supportive therapy involves the following:

> One of the therapist's tasks in supportive treatment is to survey the various defenses available to the patient and determine which of these can most effectively be introduced, strengthened, encouraged or reinforced. . . . He tries to help the patient more effectively use preexisting defenses which for him are familiar, rather than introduce new ones the patient is not able to use himself. (p. 105)

This principle is particularly applicable in situations in which the patient is experiencing an acute psychosocial or situational stressor. Even if the therapist is of a different religious background than the patient or is of the same religious background but disagrees with the patient's particular view, the therapist can still listen to the patient and be supportive. The therapist may also explore with the patient how his or her religious faith helped him or her deal with and overcome some past stressor. This will serve as a reminder of the usefulness of their faith in coping with present difficulties.

Second, the therapist may point out religious scriptures to the patient in a nonthreatening, nonjudgmental manner that foster hope, encourage, and portray a sense of being cared for. These scriptures may bring comfort to the patient during times between sessions when he or she must deal with painful feelings without the therapist. Repeating a particular scripture at certain times of the day or during stressful circumstances may bring comfort to some patients. For example, a patient was having difficulty crossing streets alone because of an unreasonable fear that he would be hit by an automobile. By repeating a particular passage of scripture suggested by his therapist he was able to reduce his anxiety sufficiently to allow him to cross the street unaided. Scriptures also contain role models of people overcoming depression, anxiety, hopelessness, and difficult life problems that can inspire patients to do the same. Finally, promises contained in scripture address issues such as meaning, isolation, guilt, and mortality; pointing out these promises may provide comfort and support, assist with cognitive restructuring, build self-esteem, and promote hope.

Third, once the acute stressor has passed, and the patient has achieved some type of emotional equilibrium, then reeducative therapies that focus on changing dysfunctional attitudes, altering maladaptive behaviors, or uncovering and processing deep-seeded psychological conflict become the primary mode of treatment. Paul Pruyser (1977) points out that not all uses of religion are healthy, particularly when they involve a sacrifice of the intellect; rationalization for hatred, aggression, and prejudice; promotion of excessive dependency; surrender of agency, dissociation, and disavowal (the devil made me do it); justification for being judgmental and insensitive to situations; displacement to the body (excessive asceticism); or obsessional thinking (excessive focus on sin and guilt). These negative uses of religion must at some time be addressed in therapy without alienating the patient or too quickly removing a needed psychological defense. The therapist may need to gently and sensitively challenge religious beliefs that are clearly maladaptive or are being used as a defense to avoid dealing with other issues. The assistance of the patient's minister may be helpful in this regard to ensure that doctrinal issues are being interpreted correctly by both therapist and patient.

Fourth, the therapist may use the religious belief system of the patient to further the goals of psychotherapy. For example, Propst (1987) has developed a religious form of cognitive–behavioral psychotherapy (CBT) that uses Christian rationales for restructuring thought processes, religious arguments for countering irrational thoughts, and religious imagery as part of the behavioral component. This method has been shown to be equally effective as secular psychotherapy and more rapidly effective in treating mild to moderate forms of depression in religious patients (Propst et al., 1992). The remarkable finding from this study was that religious CBT when administered by nonreligious therapists was as effective, if not more effective, than when delivered by religious therapists. Thus, either religious or nonreligious therapists can use the patient's religious belief system as a tool to effectively alter distorted cognitions.

Finally, in circumstances in which the therapist feels incompetent to deal with religious issues, the patient expresses discomfort over addressing religious issues with the therapist, or the therapist feels that addressing religious issues would interfere with the therapeutic relationship, then referral to a minister, chaplain, or pastoral counselor is indicated. Before referring the patient, however, the therapist must first conduct a thorough evaluation to learn about the patient's religious background and prior negative and positive experiences with religion and perform a preliminary evaluation of the patient's current spiritual needs. This will allow the therapist to make an informed referral to the appropriate religious professional. Follow-up with patients on the results of the referral is also important (was the appointment kept, how was the patient treated, and was there any perceived benefit?).

GUIDELINES FOR PRAYING WITH PATIENTS

Praying with patients remains a controversial intervention, particularly with psychiatric patients who have deep, complex, emotional issues. Introducing religion into the therapeutic relationship through prayer may have unpredictable consequences on that relationship. Traditional therapists may gasp even at our mention of the topic and view it as a clear violation of patient–therapist boundaries. We do not have a final answer to this difficult question, and most of the information provided here is primarily anecdotal. Prayer is more delicate of an issue with psychiatric patients than it is with medical patients because of boundary issues involved. Praying with patients can produce an intimacy that is threatening to both patient and therapist. There have been no studies on how frequently mental health professionals pray with patients let alone studies on how to pray with patients or the consequences of doing so. In a random sample of 160 family physicians in Illinois, we found that about one-third of physicians prayed with their elderly patients; the vast majority of physicians indicated prayer was helpful "somewhat" (33.9%) or "a great deal" (55.4%) (Koenig, Bearon, & Dayringer, 1989). Frequency of prayer, for the reason mentioned previously, between therapists and patients is probably not as high as that among physicians and patients in general medical practice. The absence of any guidelines in this area for mental health professionals is problematic, even if the practice is relatively rare, given its potential impact on the therapeutic relationship between therapist and patient. With some trepidation, we make an attempt to provide reasonable recommendations on how to proceed.

A therapist may choose to pray with some patients in certain circumstances. On the one hand, prayer can bring deep comfort and hope that lasts beyond the therapeutic session, convey a sense of caring and commitment by the therapist, combat the patient's isolation and loneliness, and build trust in the therapist–patient relationship. On the other hand, praying with psychiatric patients during a therapeutic session can in some circumstances be dangerous, threaten the therapeutic alliance, and adversely affect the psychological stability of the patient. This is particularly worrisome in fragile patients with poor ego boundaries who may have difficulty coping with the intimacy that prayer can involve. Furthermore, in certain types of psychotherapy, prayer may disturb the therapist's neutrality and objectivity. Thus, routinely praying with all patients (whether religious or not) is unwise, and if the therapist feels at all uncomfortable, then the best procedure is to find a religious professional to pray with the patient.

Some indications that prayer might be useful are (a) the patient makes clear to the therapist that religion is an important way he or she copes with problems; (b) the patient and therapist are from the same religious background (although this is not always necessary); (c) the patient either asks for prayer himself or herself or shows no hesitation when the therapist asks for permission to pray; (d) the patient has sufficient ego strength and general psychological stability that disturbance of boundaries is not an issue; and, most important, (e) the situation indicates that prayer would help advance the therapeutic goals. Prayer is often appropriate when the patient is going through some type of acute situational stressor—the death or serious injury of a spouse, child, or loved one; deep personal disappointment (fired from a job or marital separation); severe, life-threatening medical illness that is out of the patient's control (diagnosis of cancer or need for major operation); or some other type of discrete stressor. Prayer can also be helpful to patients struggling with chronic behavioral problems that seem impossible to overcome (such as a chronic alcoholic or compulsive gambler); in those instances, prayer may counteract the sense of hopelessness that would otherwise paralyze further efforts to overcome the problem.

From our limited experience, there is a method of approaching patients about this topic that is nonoffensive, nonintrusive, and reduces the risk of adverse consequences. The therapist should first assess if prayer is congruent with the patient's worldview. If so, than he or she might say the following: "Some of my patients find comfort in prayer, others do not. Would my praying with you over this situation be helpful to you, or do you feel that it would not be particularly helpful?" In whatever manner this subject is broached, the patient must be given clear and explicit permission to reject the offer for prayer without feeling uneasy or feeling like they have disappointed the therapist. Even if the therapist has prayed with the patient previously, the same cautious approach should be taken every time a new occasion for prayer arises.

If the patient agrees and shows sincere interest in proceeding, then we suggest that prayer be conducted in the following manner. First, we suggest that the prayer be brief (typically less than 1 minute, particularly if the therapist does the praying). Long prayers are more distracting then they are helpful. Second, we suggest that the patient do the praying, not the therapist. The therapist should simply listen attentively and offer support at the end of the prayer with an "Amen." The patient, not the therapist, is the best person to determine the content and form of the prayer (although personal and spontaneous, rather than memorized prayers, should be encouraged). Also, by carefully listening to the patient's prayer, the therapist may learn things about the patient's motivation and priorities that may otherwise not be revealed. Third, if the patient asks the therapist to pray, then the prayer should be general, supportive, affirming, and hopeful (e.g., prayer for strength and support; prayer for a sense of being loved and cared for; and prayer for successful resolution of a specific problem that the patient wishes to be resolved). Fourth, during the next session, explore with the patient how he or she felt about the prayer, allowing the patient to report both negative and positive experiences.

TRANSFERENCE AND COUNTERTRANSFERENCE ISSUES

A number of transference and countertransference issues arise when introducing religion into the therapeutic relationship between patient and therapist. Moshe Spero (1981) addressed this topic, focusing on the problems that might arise when religious therapists treated religious patients. When the patient and therapist share the same religious beliefs, there may often be "idiosyncratic" and "conflicting" differences based on differing needs (neurotic and healthy) for religion in the patient and therapist. For example, the religious patient may have expectations and fantasies of magical cure by the therapist or, alternatively, may see the therapist as punitive, demanding, and judgmental as a religious figure or parent in their past. The religious therapist, on the other hand, may experience countertransference reactions to the patient that range from fantasies of rescuing the patient to neurotic projections resulting in feelings of disdain for the patient. The therapist's own religious beliefs may cause him or her to reject or harshly judge the patient who, for example, continues in an adulterous affair, persists in abusing alcohol, or refuses to alter a lifestyle that conflicts with religious principles.

Spero (1981) provides therapists with seven ways of managing countertransference issues that arise in these situations. First, the therapist needs to develop an understanding of the patient's neurotic and nonneurotic needs for religion. Second, the therapist must identify neurotic forms of religious belief (e.g., how religion is used as a defense mechanism for aggressive drives or as a front for excessive dependency needs) that reflect underlying psychological conflict and must separate these immature forms of belief from mature forms that are adaptive. Third, the therapist must perform a self-examination in order to identify his or her own neurotic needs for religion and immature beliefs that arise from those needs; recognizing how these are similar to or different from the patient's needs and beliefs will help the therapist to avoid or at least be conscious of countertransference reactions during therapy.

Fourth, when the therapist experiences negative feelings toward the patient, he or she should try to recognize if overconcern or overidentification with the patient is the cause for such feelings. Fifth, similar religious backgrounds of therapist and patient should not be grounds for either more or less appreciation of the patient. Avoiding "special treatment" will help the therapist maintain the therapeutic neutrality and objectivity necessary for therapy to be successful. Sixth, the therapist must recognize the limits placed on therapeutic goals when religious commitments are similar between patient and therapist, because this may restrict the therapist's ability to see how such commitments are used as unhealthy defenses by the patient. Finally, the therapist should try to avoid providing the patient with his or her own religious insights into the patient's problems since this may distract from a major goal of therapy, which is to identify how the patient's religious beliefs are involved in his or her neurotic conflict. This does not mean, however, that the therapist should avoid pointing out and reinforcing adaptive forms of religious coping that may facilitate emotional healing.

CONCLUSIONS

Religious and spiritual needs are common among psychiatric patients and may influence the course of mental disorder. Addressing spiritual issues in the context of the therapist–patient relationship requires great sensitivity on the part of the therapist, who must approach this subject delicately and proceed at all times following cues given by the patient. We have provided reasons why spiritual needs should be addressed during psychotherapy and have suggested a nonoffensive way of spiritual assessment. We have also listed 25 psychological and spiritual needs that therapists might consider addressing (Table 22.1) and have proposed a number of spiritual interventions that might be used to help meet those needs. Some interventions, such as praying with patients, are more controversial than others, such as inquiring about and supporting the patient's healthy beliefs. Therapists must seek a level of comfort in addressing both psychological and spiritual needs of patients and develop a referral system for meeting the needs of patients which they feel less competent to address. Finally, therapists who choose to address religious issues with patients must be conscious of transference and countertransference issues likely to arise when religious beliefs of patient and therapist are similar.

REFERENCES

Accreditation Council on Graduate Medical Education. (1994, March). *Special requirements for residency training in psychiatry.* Author.

American Psychiatric Association. (1995a). American Psychiatric Association practice guidelines for psychiatric evaluation of adults. *American Journal of Psychiatry Supplement 152*(11), 64–80.

American Psychological Association. (1995b). Guidelines and principles for accreditation of programs in professional psychology. In *American Psychological Association Committee on Accreditation Site Visitor handbook* (pp. 5, Iw-27). Washington, DC: Author.

Azhart, M. A., Varma, S. L., & Dharap, A. S. (1994). Religious psychotherapy in anxiety disorder patients. *Acta Psychiatric Scandinavica, 90,* 1–3.

Chu, C. C., & Klein, H. E. (1985). Psychosocial and environmental variables in outcome of black schizophrenics. *Journal of the National Medical Association, 77,* 793–796.

Dewald, P. A. (1971). *Psychotherapy: A dynamic approach.* New York: Basic Books.

Fitchett, G., Burton, L. A., & Sivan, A. B. (1997). The religious needs and resources of psychiatric patients. *Journal of Nervous and Mental Disease, 185,* 320–326.

Klausner, S. Z. (1964). *Psychiatry and religion: A sociological study of the New Alliance of Ministers and Psychiatrists.* Glencoe, NY: Free Press.

Koenig, H. G., Bearon, L., & Dayringer, R. (1989): Physician perspectives on the role of religion in the physician–older patient relationship. *Journal of Family Practice, 28,* 441–448.

Koenig, H. G. Cohen, H. J., Blazer, D. G., Pieper, C., Meador, K. G., Shelp, F., Goli, V., & DiPasquale, R. (1992). Religious coping and depression in elderly hospitalized medically ill men. *American Journal of Psychiatry, 149,* 1693–1700.

Koenig, H. G., George, L. K., & Peterson, B. L. (1998). Religiosity and remission from depression in medically ill older patients. *American Journal of Psychiatry, 155,* 536–542.

Koenig, H. G., & Weaver, A. J. (1997). *Counseling troubled older adults: A handbook for pastors and religious caregivers.* Decator, GA: Abingdon Press.

Kroll, J., & Sheehan, W. (1989). Religious beliefs and practices among 52 psychiatric inpatients in Minnesota. *American Journal of Psychiatry, 146,* 67–72.

Luckoff, D., Lu, F., & Turner, R. (1992). Toward a more culturally sensitive DSM-IV: Psychoreligious and psychospiritual problems. *Journal of Nervous and Mental Disorders, 180,* 673–682.

Miller, W. R., & Martin, J. E. (1988). *Behavior therapy and religion: Integrating spiritual and behavioral approaches to change.* Newbury Park, CA: Sage.

Pattison, E. M. (1966). Social and psychological aspects of religion in psychotherapy. *Journal of Nervous and Mental Disease, 141,* 586–597.

Propst, L. R. (1987). *Psychotherapy within a religious framework: Spirituality in the emotional healing process.* New York: Human Sciences Press.

Propst, L. R., Ostrom, R., Watkins, P., Dean, T., & Mashburn D. (1992). Comparative efficacy of religious and nonreligious cognitive–behavioral therapy for the treatment of clinical depression in religious individuals. *Journal of Consulting and Clinical Psychology, 60,* 94–103.

Pruyser, P. (1977). The seamy side of current religious beliefs. *Bulletin of the Menninger Clinic, 41,* 329–348.

Sheehan, W., & Kroll, J. (1990). Psychiatric patients' belief in general health factors and sin as causes of illness. *American Journal of Psychiatry, 147,* 112–113.

Spero, M. (1981). Countertransference in religious therapists of religious patients. *American Journal of Psychotherapy, 35,* 565–575.

Webster, N. (1983). *American dictionary of the English language* (3rd ed.). San Francisco: Foundation for American Christian Education. (Original work published 1828).

23

THE ROLE OF NONPARISH

CLERGY IN THE MENTAL

HEALTH SYSTEM

LARRY VANDECREEK   DAVID CARL

Department of Pastoral Care   *Department of Pastoral Care*
The Ohio State University Medical Center   *Carolinas Medical Center*
Columbus, Ohio 43210   *Charlotte, North Carolina 28232*

DUANE PARKER

Interfaith Health Care Ministries
Rhode Island Hospital
Providence, Rhode Island 02903

In the mental health system not much attention is given to the services produced by clergy. At least one reason for this is clear: Religion is regarded as a negative influence on mental health (Ellis, 1980; Freud, 1927). Given this attitude, the clergy do not merit attention. This attitude toward religion is changing, however. Its positive contributions are increasingly described (Pargament, Maton, & Hess, 1992; for annotated bibliography of journal articles see Matthews, Larson, & Barry, 1993; for review see Worthington, Kurusu, McCullough, & Sandage, 1996). A recent review concluded, "The overwhelming mass of research evidence suggests far more beneficial associations between religion and mental well-being than adverse effects of religion on mental health" (Hood, Spilka, Hunsberger, & Gorsuch, 1996, p. 408).

Given this discovery of religion, can further exploration of how clergy support and mobilize these benefits be far behind? We hope not! A remaining problem before the ministry of clergy can be appreciated, however, is the research results that describe them as possessing a wide variety of intrapsychic, interpersonal, and identity problems (Hood et al., 1996, p. 429). Thus, mental health professionals often think of clergy in negative terms. Most of these studies date back to the antireligious era in psychology and many clinicians seem unaware of recent results (Hunt, Hinkle, & Malony, 1990).

In this chapter we describe three contexts outside the traditional parish setting in which clergy provide mental health services (for an empirical study of counseling activities by parish clergy, see Mollica, Streets, Boscarino, & Redlich, 1986). These settings include ministry as chaplains in psychiatric inpatient facilities, as pastoral counselors in church-based or community centers, and as mental health care brokers who mobilize communication between parish clergy, mental professionals, and consumers. We comment on relevant research literature and describe future concerns.

We make at least three assumptions. First, we construe "religion" in the broadest terms. The word connotes not only formal, traditional beliefs and practices or new styles of spirituality but also each individual's response to the ultimate questions of life, e.g., "What is my purpose in life?" "Why is my life worth living?" and "What happens at death?" These questions require at least implicit responses in how life is construed as meaningful and worthwhile; this ultimate character makes such questions and answers religious.

Second, we assume that religious concerns are relevant to the diagnosis and treatment of mental illness. If they are wholly separate from illness or irrelevant to its treatment, there is no need for chaplains.

Third, the contributions described here are created by clergy who are theologically educated, are endorsed for this ministry by a recognized faith group, have received supervised training in ministry to the mentally ill in nationally accredited programs, and are certified for this ministry by a national body of peers. There is no room in this ministry for theologically uneducated, untrained, self-declared clergy who wish to operate independent from a relationship to a recognized faith group.

CLERGY AS CHAPLAINS IN PSYCHIATRIC INPATIENT FACILITIES

Here we describe four contributions which chaplains make as part of psychiatric inpatient treatment teams: (a) spiritual assessments, (b) responses to and uses of religious psychological material, (c) interactions with clinical staff members, and (d) liaisons with communities of faith.

SPIRITUAL ASSESSMENTS

Psychiatric patients take their religious needs, beliefs, and practices into the hospital and these can contribute to or complicate recovery (Kroll & Sheehan, 1989; Pruyser, 1984). Religious assessments upon admission and throughout hospitalization are relevant. In an obvious example, one study found that 10% of psychiatric patients believes they were in the hospital because they had sinned and 19% believed penances were necessary before they could get better (Sheehan & Kroll, 1990).

The literature contains multiple spiritual assessment models, ranging from lengthy interviews to self-administrated paper-and-pencil instruments (Berg, 1994; Eimer, 1989; Hall & Edwards, 1996; Pruyser, 1971; VandeCreek, Ayres, & Bassham, 1995; see Fitchett, 1993, for review of selected approaches and instruments). Many of these models have not been tested with psychiatric populations, however.

Assessments can also be less formal and deliberate. For example, a young woman in a closed unit began a public worship service to Satan in the middle of the dayroom. This was upsetting to other patients, but the staff—not wishing to violate her religious rights—allowed her to dominate that area while they waited for the chaplain to arrive. The chaplain interrupted the patient, verifying that she had no historical roots with that faith group and thus no foundation upon which to call for such special treatment. This was an important incident for this patient because her worship activity was a pathological religious coping effect that merited therapeutic attention.

RESPONSES TO AND USES OF RELIGIOUS PSYCHOLOGICAL MATERIAL

Patients, whether or not they are involved in a church or synagogue, frequently report religious concerns and want to talk about them (Fitchett, Burton, & Sivan, 1997; Kroll & Sheehan, 1989). If religion is unhealthy, attention to and support of these concerns should be discouraged. As noted previously, however, religion often promotes mental health. Religious teachings seek to make clear the stance and intention of an Ultimate toward the creation and beliefs about this can be helpful in the face of illness and other perplexing problems. In one study (Berg, Reed, Fonss, & VandeCreek, 1995) which examined patients with a major affective disorder, the presence of an active religious faith and practice were associated with a reduced length of time in the hospital. Results suggested three important spiritual concerns positively related to a longer stay: a sense that life was unfair, that life's meaning was unclear, and a history of infrequent worship attendance.

What contributions do chaplains make in treatment? We describe three ways in which they function. First, given the role and power of religion, chaplains mobilize a patient's faith perspective so that it can assist them in their treatment and recovery. Consider the following example:

A 27-year-old unmarried male entered a psychiatric facility after a schizophrenic episode. His history suggested that he had separated himself from his family of origin, thus compromising a major source of social support. He worked as a manager of a recreation facility and his schizophrenic episode was precipitated by the death of a child who had fallen from playground equipment. In the priestly atmosphere of the conversation with the chaplain, the patient was able to share how he could not reach out to his family because of the way he had left home. When the chaplain tenderly reminded him of the prodigal son story (which was within his Christian heritage), the patient gained sufficient courage to contact his family. In large part, his family's loving response contributed to his recovery and shortened stay.

A second way in which chaplains function within the team is as leader of pastoral care groups which weave mental health principles into discussion groups and worship experiences. For example, in one weekly group, patients examined two biblical stories about St. Peter. At one time he seemed able to walk on water, but later he quickly denied Jesus three times. Wrestling with these two stories about a revered saint encouraged patients to be less rigid in splitting good from bad, perfect from imperfect. This discussion taught tolerance, both for themselves and for others, when personal standards were not met.

Leadership of worship experiences constitutes a variation of these pastoral care groups. Participation in worship and private devotions among community populations are significantly related to life satisfaction and happiness (Ellison, 1991; Williams, Larson, Buckler, Heckmann & Pyle, 1991) and clinical experiences suggest that they are also important for some psychiatric patients. The contributions of such worship experiences merit additional research.

Chaplains also lead less formal worship experiences. An example includes the opportunity to sing favorite hymns. Some patients find that this music for the soul expresses their inner feelings, longings, and religious commitments. This, in turn, enhances their well-being (St. George & McNamara, 1984). Such activities are not simply entertainment or ways to pass the time; they can mobilize religious coping and take on treatment implications. When patients suggest favorite hymns, they disclose something about their momentary moods but also open themselves to the music and lyrics. For example, one patient loved the hymn "What a Friend We Have in Jesus" and repeatedly suggested that the group sing it. At the same time, she compromised her recovery from depression by refusing to talk about her feelings and experiences. At the end of one of these worship experiences, the chaplain invited her reflection on the lyrics of this song:

Oh, what peace we often forfeit,
Oh, what needless pain we bear.
All because we do not carry,
Everything to God in prayer.

The chaplain further suggested the potential benefits of such a prayerful conversation, both with God and with others. This was a uniquely persuasive pastoral intervention and the patient was able to share her feelings more openly in the context of prayer and conversation with the chaplain.

A third way in which chaplains participate in the team is as interpreter of religious thoughts and actions that are unfamiliar in our secular culture. This becomes increasingly important as society and mental health providers become more sensitive to multicultural issues, including religious diversity (Lukoff, Lu, & Turner, 1992). As the following example shows, some behaviors which seem bizarre in secular society are religious coping efforts:

The 28-year-old patient became violent in an inpatient acute unit and was placed in seclusion. The staff dutifully checked on him every 15 min and noticed that after awhile he was laying quite still in the middle of the room. After several more observations at 15-min intervals, they noticed he had not moved and they entered the room, concerned that something was wrong. The patient greeted them warmly and was soon released from seclusion. He immediately picked up a broom and went around the adjacent dayroom and slightly tapped other patients on the head, ever so gently. The staff was ready to place him back in seclusion when the chaplain suspected that he was responding to a religious experience. In response to that question from the chaplain, this Jewish man quickly offered a religious interpretation. During the seclusion he had remembered the story of Moses and the thirsty Israelites in the desert; Moses had tapped the rock and water that lowed out for the people to drink. In seclusion, he had first felt like that lifeless rock. However, then he began to feel a flowing sense of warmth and peace; it was like living water. He now wished the same for the other patients and that light touch on the head was intended to bring it about.

Other staff members did not understand this patient's reference to the biblical story and the chaplain provided the context and continued conversation with the patient. While this episode suggests the patient's many continuing problems, a religious understanding avoided another period of seclusion and opened the door for further religious coping efforts.

Another example suggests the same theme. A patient treated for clinical depression began to raise issues concerning her inability to experience forgiveness. The therapist invited the chaplain to a session in which the patient more fully expressed her concerns about her "unforgivable sin." The chaplain then helped her clarify this scriptural reference and, with the help of the therapist, engaged the patient in a confession and absolution rituals. This patient's effort to manage her guilt required a clergy whom the faith community had set apart as an expert on sin, guilt, and forgiveness.

INTERACTIONS WITH CLINICAL STAFF MEMBERS

In the previous discussion, it was suggested at several points that chaplains as members of psychiatric teams contribute not only to patients but also to other staff members. Given the ubiquitous nature of religious concerns, this interprofessional contribution appears to be a more evident role for chaplains than most other mental health professions. Such conversations with staff members can include not only discussions about patient religiosity but also open dialogue with those who are religiously rooted and those who are skeptical about the place of religion and spirituality. This aspect of the chaplain's ministry requires additional research.

LIAISONS WITH THE COMMUNITIES OF FAITH

More than any other health care profession, chaplains represent (and are part of) the faith communities within which many patients themselves live. Chaplains, like all professionals, live in the community, but far more important, they officially extend the religious community into the mental health facility. Thus, they link psychiatric facilities to faith communities and their leaders. At a superficial level, this offers public relations opportunities. At a more profound level, chaplains can draw faith communities into the after-hospital care of patients. This is described later.

This liaison with the community also promotes public education concerning the complexities of mental illness and its treatment. Such contacts can encourage helpful, early interventions and address stereotypes and stigmas too long tolerated by religious communities. This at once reinforces the perception that mental health facilities can be helpful. It seems likely that the religious community will increasingly be discovered as an important resource in the era of managed psychiatric care. The chaplain will be a key staff member in that relationship.

CLERGY AS PASTORAL COUNSELORS

Formal pastoral counseling constitutes a second way in which clergy provide mental health services. The character of this ministry varies widely. On the one hand, some use a prescriptive approach drawing on scripture passages to instruct clients on how to resolve problems. At the opposite extreme, others use a more psychodynamic approach. Clergy who give priority to their counseling tend to cluster in two national organizations.

The American Association of Christian Counselors consists of approximately 16,000 members, although it is unclear how many are clergy. It sponsors active promotional and educational endeavors particularly among evangelical Christians. Its purposes are informational, educational, and affiliative; membership does not imply certification of the individual. They sponsor two journals: *Christian Counseling Today* is a glossy discussion-oriented quarterly, and *Marriage and Family: A Christian Journal* is intended for those who focus on marriage and family issues.

The American Association of Pastoral Counselors [AAPC] (North, 1988) was formed in 1963 to promote this ministry and the professional counseling competence of clergy. The ministry of many of its members consists entirely of in-office counseling. With a membership of approximately 3200 clergy and more than 100 free-standing or church-related pastoral counseling centers, it reports over 3 million treatment hours annually in individual, group, marital, and family therapy (American Association of Pastoral Counselors [AAPC] n.d.). It accredits training centers which conduct supervised training programs, certifying members, fellows, and diplomates. It participates in a consortium of pastoral organizations that sponsor the *Journal of Pastoral Care*. Posavac and Hartung (1977) describe reasons why clients choose a pastoral counselor instead of another type of therapist.

Two features of the services provided by these certified AAPC counselors merit note. First, educational and clinical requirements are as high, or higher, than those for peer professionals in other disciplines (AAPC, n.d.). Requirements include a bachelor's degree, a 3-year professional degree from a seminary, a specialized masters or doctoral degree in the field, and extensive counseling with clients under interdisciplinary supervision. This training appears to be unique because it requires in-depth supervision from mental health professionals outside the field of pastoral counseling. Membership in the organization is obtained only after sustaining a face-to-face interview with a committee who listens to tape recordings of client counseling and questions the applicant about his or her therapeutic decision making.

Second, the nationwide average fee collected per 50-min hours is approximately $50 (AAPC, n.d.). Thus, pastoral counselors offer more cost-effective services.

Worthington et al. (1996) have reviewed the empirical literature concerning religion, psychotherapeutic processes, and outcomes. They note that evaluations of the outcomes of clergy counseling—and religious counselors generally—is "notably missing." They add, "At present, we can conclude only that much religious counseling may be occurring, but we do not know how effective it is" (p. 466).

CLERGY AS MENTAL HEALTH BROKERS

In this section we describe chaplains who assume the role of "pastoral care broker," functioning as "an intermediary and interpreter within and amongst organizations, be they congregation, parish, hospital, or agency" (Anderson, 1985). These brokers facilitate interdisciplinary contact and build alliances between them. Their expertise is not that of creating a product but of linking persons and organizations so that new and better relationships can produce improved, more comprehensive mental health care.

This broker activity is important as mental health systems implement models of recovery and integrate consumers into the community. The recovery model usually gives attention to spirituality as one of the cornerstones for movement from illness to health, but as others (Larson et al., 1988, p. 1065) have observed, "An alliance between mental health professionals and clergy . . . appear(s) to be . . . distant." Clergy are experts in spiritual matters and can lead the way in incorporating spirituality into recovery programs.

The stumbling block, however, is usually the lack of meaningful working relationships between mental health professionals, clergy, and consumers. Mental health professionals often view themselves as experts; clergy and consumers are recipients of their expertise. Some clergy view mental health professionals with skepticism, undercutting effective working relationships with consumers in their congregations. Consumers, aware that they are the dependent partner in this triangle, begin to believe that they have no voice in what would be helpful.

Here we describe an organization which is a third example of how clergy function within the mental health system. In this model the participants work from equal footing in establishing partnerships with each viewed as a potential resource for the other. This model, the East Bay Interfaith Mental Health Alliance of Providence, Rhode Island, creates an expectation of interdependence, not dependency.

The mission of the alliance is "to build a collaboration of interfaith and mental health communities and to enhance the integration of spiritual and mental health resources to improve the lives of children, adults, and families affected by mental illness" (Interfaith Health Care Ministries, 1997). It assumes that each of these partners values the mental health of the community and consequently all meetings and program planning include significant input from each of the partners. Events are not planned by one partner for the other.

One highlight of the partnership formation process came when members of the alliance decided to put programming and reporting aside to share individual spiritual journeys. In these meetings, consumers, family members, clergy, and mental health professionals shared their spiritual journeys focusing on how faith or struggles with faith influenced their lives.

The alliance sponsored a public forum on mental health services, an interfaith religious service, advocacy with the legislature, support for the development of the consumer drop-in centers, and a workshop for consumers, clergy, and professionals. One aspect of the alliance is the Interfaith Health Care Ministries, which was funded to carry out three projects: (a) a national literature search concerning religion and mental health relationships: (b) interviews with area clergy, mental health professionals, and consumers concerning program development: and (c) the development of consumer drop-in centers using the resources of the faith communities.

THE LITERATURE SEARCH

The search identified significant literature resources that support the following conclusions concerning working partnerships in mental health:

1. Faith communities can have an important role in the deinstitutionalization process and attempts to move mental health services to the community.
2. Faith resources are important in recovering from mental illness.
3. Consumers can play an important role in providing services and education.
4. Clergy and mental health professionals can work effectively together in a community mental health setting.

A copy of the annotated bibliography produced by the search is available (Interfaith Health Care Ministries, 1997).

THE INTERVIEW COMPONENT: CLERGY

After developing an instrument, interviews with clergy and mental health professionals were conducted; those with consumers are under way. Interview results from 39 clergy (75% of the 49 available in the alliance area) suggested the following:

1. Faith communities offer a wide variety of programs with mental health implications, including youth activities, prayer groups, soup kitchens, emergency services (funds for food and/or shelter), and pastoral visitation and counseling.

2. Faith community facilities host many self-help groups.

3. Clergy have significantly more education related to serving the mentally ill and their families than anticipated. A majority (70%) had completed a pastoral care and counseling course in seminary and 57% reported completing a supervised clinical pastoral education program. Many (40%) were multidisciplinary in their training, possessing a graduate degree or clinical experience in a related profession such as nursing or marriage and family counseling.

4. Clergy were considerably more positive about the services of mental health professionals than anticipated. Most were supportive of mental health endeavors and open to exploring new cooperative pathways.

5. Five congregations expressed interest in hosting consumer-run drop-in centers.

THE INTERVIEW COMPONENT: MENTAL HEALTH PROFESSIONALS

Thirty-two mental health center staff members were interviewed. Selection was based on their center's administrative and clinical responsibilities, availability, and potential interest in the project. Results suggest the following:

1. Intake interviews ask clients about their religious affiliation as part of identifying community resources for them and their family.

2. Staff members ($n = 13$) had referred clients to faith communities for diverse reasons, including social contact, discussion with clergy about spiritual issues, and utilizing services such as soup kitchens.

3. Most staff had not worked with clergy directly as part of a treatment program. Confidentiality was cited most frequently as the reason for lack of clergy contact.

4. Some staff members (40%) reported at least some educational experience concerning faith as a resource to the mentally ill and their families. Two staff members had theological degrees, whereas others had taken courses in undergraduate or graduate degree programs. Others were active participants in faith communities.

5. Most staff members were supportive of working more closely with clergy and 28 of the 32 reported interest in participating in educational events with clergy.

Subsequent to the interviews, mental health center statistics reflected more requests for consultation from area clergy as well as referrals. Three congregations created consumer drop-in centers. The mental health center placed a chaplain on their staff 1 day per week. One seminar for clergy, mental health professionals, and consumers took place and others are planned.

This project also generated disappointments. The number of clergy participants in the monthly alliance meetings has declined. Several reported that other duties made their continuing attendance impossible. Others said they had little direct contact with seriously mentally ill persons and hence were putting their efforts into other projects. Some were impatient with the slow progress in moving from discussion to action. The optimism about consumers taking responsibility for the drop-in centers has been challenged by the reality that most consumers are dependent on staff-run programs and have difficulty planning meetings and special events without staff involvement. Mental health staff find the confidentiality issue to be a major concern in considering new ways of working with clergy around specific cases.

FUTURE DIRECTIONS AND PRIORITIES

At the beginning of the chapter, we indicated that we would comment on relevant research results. A number of references are scattered throughout the text, but the lack of research is a serious problem; publications tend to describe the role of religion rather than that of clergy. References to mental health benefits produced by clergy are almost uniformly anecdotal.

Additionally, the literature does not address the impact of managed care on pastoral services provided by these clergy. Both inpatient and outpatient mental health treatment are changing rapidly and dramatically. We know of no empirical literature that addresses the effects of the changes on these services.

Most important, research needs to demonstrate not only that clergy provide competent and helpful services but also that these services are clinically so efficacious that the broader system cannot afford to ignore them. It is one thing to demonstrate, even empirically, that psychiatric chaplains, pastoral counselors, or pastoral care brokers are helpful. It is something else to demonstrate that they are so helpful that the system can ill afford to ignore them. Until that is demonstrated, the broader mental health system will likely view the contributions of clergy as optional.

What directions can this ministry take in the future and how can research elucidate this effort? We suggest the following possibilities:

1. Increasingly, mental health professionals affirm that religion, generally, is good for people. The crucial question that follows from this affirmation, however, is whether clergy are good for mental health consumers. Answering this question will be complicated because the practice of ministry across faith groups possesses no "standard of practice." Ministry varies widely and some styles are likely more helpful than others. The mental health system will likely continue to marginalize the clergy until the influence of ministry styles is clarified.

2. There is evidence that highly religious individuals tend to avoid the mental health system. Some researchers believe that this is related to the devaluation of religion among mental health professionals (Larson et al., 1986, 1989) and is likely related to the rise of Christian psychiatry (Galanter, Larson, & Rubenstone, 1991). Can wider acceptance of the proposition that religion is good for mental

health and further development of the chaplain's role within the system ameliorate this difficulty?

3. Clergy are based in traditions that emphasize community. One manifestation of this is the role of home visits, a practice which is particularly welcomed during illness. In fact, parish pastors usually go to the parishioners/patients, whether in the home or hospital, rather than waiting for them to make an appointment at the office. This is a unique feature of the chaplain's professional tradition which points to a possible contribution in the current health care system with its increasing emphasis on early hospital discharge and outpatient treatment. It appears that mental health administrators have not sufficiently explored this unique possibility for the chaplain's ministry.

The responsibility for developing the future of this ministry is twofold: Clergy must demonstrate their effectiveness in empirical ways, and mental health professionals must be open to the possibility that clergy, including those in nonparish settings, can be significantly helpful in the mental health system.

REFERENCES

American Association of Pastoral Counselors. (n.d.). *Pastoral counseling: A national mental health resource*. Advisory Committee on Advocacy, American Association of Pastoral Counselors, 9504A Lee Highway, Fairfax, VA 22031-2303.

Anderson, R. (1985). The assessment of systems in promoting collaborative aftercare: Religious and mental health organizations in partnership. *Journal of Pastoral Care, 39*(3), 236–248.

Berg, G. (1994). The use of the computer as a tool for assessment and research in pastoral care. *Journal of Health Care Chaplaincy, 6*(1), 11–25.

Berg, G., Reed, A., Fonss, N., & VandeCreek, L. (1995). The impact of religious faith and practice on patients suffering from a major affective disorder: A cost analysis. *Journal of Pastoral Care, 49,*(4), 359–363.

Eimer, K. (1989). The assessment and treatment of the religiously concerned psychiatric patient. *Journal of Pastoral Care, 43*(3), 231–241.

Ellis, A. (1980). Psychotherapy and atheistic values: A response to A. E. Bergin's "Psychotherapy and religious values." *Journal of Consulting and Clinical Psychology, 48*(5), 635–639.

Ellison, C. (1991). Religious involvement and subjective well-being. *Journal of Health and Social Behavior, 32,* 80–99.

Fitchett, G. (1993). *Spiritual assessments in pastoral care: A guide to selected resources*. Decatur, GA: Journal of Pastoral Care Publications.

Fitchett, G., Burton, L., & Sivan, A. (1997). The religious needs and resources of psychiatric in-patients. *Journal of Nervous and Mental Disease, 185,* 320–326.

Freud, S. (1927). *The future of an illusion*. New York: Norton.

Galanter, M., Larson, D., & Rubenstone, E. (1991). Christian psychiatry: The impact of evangelical belief on clinical practice. *American Journal of Psychiatry, 148*(1), 90–95.

Hall, T., & Edwards, K. (1996). The initial development and factor analysis of the Spiritual Assessment Inventory. *Journal of Psychology and Theology, 24*(3), 233–246.

Hood, R., Spilka, B., Hunsberger, B., & Gorsuch, R. (1996). *The psychology of religion: An empirical approach* (2nd ed.). New York: Guilford.

Hunt, R., Hinkle, J., & Malony, H. (1990). *Clergy assessment and career development*. Nashville, TN: Abingdon.

348 VANDECREEK ET AL.

Interfaith Health Care Ministries. (1997). Rev. Duane Parker, Director, Rhode Island Hospital, Gerry House No. 36, 593 Eddy Street, Providence, RI 02903–4970.

Kroll, J., & Sheehan, W. (1989). Religious beliefs and practices among 52 psychiatric inpatients in Minnesota. *American Journal of Psychiatry, 146,* 67–72.

Larson, D., Donahue, M., Lyons, J., Benson, P., Pattison, M., Worthington, E., & Blazer, D. (1989). Religious affiliations in mental health research samples as compared with national samples. *Journal of Nervous and Mental Disease, 177,* 109—111.

Larson, D., Hohmann, A., Kessler, L., Meador, K., Boyd, J., & McSherry, E. (1988). The couch and the cloth: The need for linkage. *Hospital and Community Psychiatry, 39*(10), 1064–1069.

Larson, D., Pattison, M., Blazer, D., Omran, A., & Kaplan, D. (1986). Systematic analysis of research on religious variable in four major psychiatric journals, 1978–1982. *American Journal of Psychiatry, 143,* 329–334.

Lukoff, D., Lu, F., & Turner, R. (1992). Toward a more culturally sensitive DSM-IV: Psychoreligious and psychospiritual problems. *Journal of Nervous & Mental Disease, 180,* 673–682.

Matthews, D., Larson, D., & Barry, C. (1993). *The faith factor: An annotated bibliography of clinical research on spiritual subjects.* Rockville, MD: National Institute for Healthcare Research.

Mollica, R., Streets, R., Boscarino, J., & Redlich, F. (1986). A community study of formal pastoral counseling activities of the clergy. *American Journal of Psychiatry, 143*(3), 323–328.

North, W. (1988). The American Association of Pastoral Counselors. *Journal of Pastoral Care, 42*(3), 197–201.

Pargament, K., Maton, K., & Hess, R. (Eds.). (1992). *Religion and prevention in mental health: Research, vision, and action.* New York: Haworth.

Posavac, E., & Hartung, B. (1977). An exploration into the reasons people choose a pastoral counselor instead of another type of psychotherapist. *Journal of Pastoral Care, 31*(1), 23–31.

Pruyser, P. (1971). Assessment of the patient's religious attitudes in the psychiatric case study. *Bulletin of the Menninger Clinic, 35,* 272–291.

Pruyser, P. (1984). Religion in the psychiatric hospital: A reassessment. *Journal of Pastoral Care, 38*(1), 5–16.

Sheehan, W., & Kroll, J. (1990). Psychiatric patients; Belief in general health factors and sin as causes of illness. *American Journal of Psychiatry, 147*(1), 112–113.

St. George, A., & McNamara, P. (1984). Religion, race, and psychological well-being. *Journal for the Scientific Study of Religion, 23*(4), 351–363.

VandeCreek, L., Ayres, S., & Bassham, M. (1995). Using INSPIRIT to conduct spiritual assessments. *Journal of Pastoral Care, 49*(4), 83–89.

Williams, D., Larson, D., Buckler, R., Heckmann, R., & Pyle, C. (1991). Religion and psychological distress in a community sample. *Social Science & Medicine, 32,* 1257–1262.

Worthington, E., Kurusu, T., McCullough, M., & Sandage, S. (1996). Empirical research on religion and psychotherapeutic processes and outcomes: A 10-year review and research prospectus. *Psychological Bulletin, 119*(3), 448–487.

24

MENTAL HEALTH PROFESSIONALS WORKING WITH RELIGIOUS LEADERS

ANDREW J. WEAVER

Department of Psychology
University of Hawaii
and
Hawaii State Hospital
Kaneohe, Hawaii 96744

In this chapter, I call for greater collaboration and mutual learning between clergy and mental health professionals. I spell out the reasons for potential collaboration and suggest some specific ways mutual learning can occur. Mental health professionals and clergy need to regard each other as valuable resources to increase the effectiveness of their care. Multiple studies over three decades have demonstrated that tens of millions of Americans with mental health and family problems first seek the help of clergy. However, research indicates that linkage between mental health professionals and religious leaders is too often lacking. This chapter identifies barriers to clergy and mental health professionals working together and suggests several unique opportunities for collaboration.

THE IMPORTANCE OF FAITH

Religion and spirituality are important factors in the lives of most Americans, providing meaning, support, and affiliation. There are nearly 500,000 churches, temples, and mosques with a presence in virtually every community in the United States. Forty percent of Americans attend one of these places of worship weekly and 60% attend monthly (Gallup, 1993). The more than 400,000 clergy and religious workers in the United States (Weaver, 1995) are among the most trusted professionals in society (Gallup, 1990), and churches and organized religion rank near the top among institutions in which Americans have confidence (Hastings & Hastings, 1994). These opinions and rates of religious involvement have remained fairly constant in the United States over the past 60 years (Gallup, 1990).

CLERGY AS FRONT-LINE MENTAL
HEALTH WORKERS

Given the importance of religion in American life, it is not surprising that clergy act as counselors for millions of Americans. The National Institute of Mental Health Epidemiological Catchment Area surveys found that a person with a *DSM-III-R* mental health diagnosis is more likely to seek assistance from the clergy than from psychologists and psychiatrists combined (Hohmann & Larson, 1993). This frequent use of the clergy by the public should not be a surprise given their availability, accessibility, and the high trust that Americans have in the clergy (Gallup, 1990). Young adults rank clergy higher in interpersonal skills, including warmth, caring, stability, and professionalism, than either psychologists or psychiatrists (Schindler, Berren, Hannah, Beigel, & Santiago, 1987).

According to the United States Department of Labor (1992), there are approximately 321,000 Jewish and Christian clergy serving congregations in the United States (4000 rabbis, 53,000 Catholic priests, and 255,000 Protestant pastors). Clergy report in 10 separate studies that they devote between 10 and 20% of their working time to pastoral counseling (Weaver, 1995). Annually, this allocation of hours totals 148.2 million hr of mental health services, a volume of services that is equivalent in time to each of the 38,000 members of the American Psychiatric Association (1993) delivering services at the rate of 78 hr per week. This estimate does not take into account the nearly 100,000 nuns in full-time religious vocation in the Roman Catholic Church (Ebaugh, 1993) and chaplains or clergy from other religious traditions about whom we have no research.

In addition, clergy are often in long-term relationships with individuals and their families. This enables them to observe changes in behavior that may indicate early signs of distress. Furthermore, within communities, clergy are accessible helpers who offer a sense of continuity with centuries of human history and experience of being a part of something greater than oneself. Religious communities also have established patterns of responding to crises. Clergy can help mental health specialists gain access to individuals and their families in crisis who would otherwise not receive psychological care. Clergy are also in a unique position of trust to assist persons in connecting to support systems available through their faith communities and beyond (Koenig & Weaver, 1997).

WHAT ARE THE BARRIERS
TO COLLABORATION?

Given the high levels of involvement in the religious community and the primary role of clergy in American mental health, why has there not been more linkage between the mental health and religious communities? Part of the answer to this question is found in studies showing that practicing religious people are underrepresented in mental health professions when compared to the population as a whole (Bergin, 1991). For many mental health professionals, a religious worldview is outside their experience. Five of 10 psychologists in an academic setting report having no religious preference, a figure seven times greater than that found in the general population (50 vs 7%) (Shafranske, 1996). In a separate survey, when the general public was asked to respond to the statement, "My whole approach to life is based on my religion," 72% agreed. When mental health professionals were asked to respond to the same statement, 33% of psychologists, 39% of psychiatrists, 46% of social workers, and 62% of marriage and family therapists agreed (Bergin & Jensen, 1990). These lower levels of religious involvement, especially among psychologists, psychiatrists, and social workers, stand in marked contrast to the much higher pattern of religious beliefs and practice reported by the general public.

In addition, few mental health professionals receive training in any aspect of religion or spirituality while in graduate school and few seek postgraduate continuing education in the topic (Sheridan, Bullis, Adcock, Berlin, & Miller, 1992). A survey of 409 clinical psychologists who were members of the American Psychological Association (APA) revealed that for only 5% were religious or spiritual issues addressed in their professional training (Shafranske & Malony, 1990). In a national survey of counseling programs accredited by the APA, one in four indicated they had a course component that addressed religious or spiritual issues (Kelly, 1994). In a separate national survey, clinical training directors working in Association of Psychology Internship Centers indicated that none of their internship programs offered education or training in spiritual/religious issues, while at the same time almost three of four acknowledged that they addressed such issues in their own clinical practice (Lannert, 1991). Similarly, when members of the American Association of Directors of Psychiatric Residency Training were asked if their program had a course on any aspect of religion, 19% responded "occasionally" and 12% responded "frequently or always." These low rates remained the same even when the residency program was located in a religiously affiliated institution (Sansone, Khatain, & Rodenhauser, 1990). It is not surprising that psychiatrists refer patients to clergy less frequently than do other medical specialities (Koenig, Bearon, Hover, & Travis, 1991) or that all mental health specialities infrequently make referrals to clergy (Meylink & Gorsuch, 1987). This trend is largely due to a lack of education about the powerful role that nonpunitive religion can play in helping people as well as a lack of knowledge about what clergy can offer to those in distress.

CLERGY, RELIGION, AND MENTAL HEALTH RESEARCH

An additional obstacle to linking the clergy and the religious community to the mental health network is the small amount of research found in mental health literature on the role of clergy in mental health or on the psychological dynamics of religious coping. In a review of 2468 quantitative articles in eight major APA journals from 1991 to 1994, a mere 1 in 600 included and assessed the role of the clergy in mental health (Weaver et al., in press-b). Only one of these studies placed its primary focus on clergy activities in mental health (Pargament et al., 1991). Despite abundant evidence that clergy are extensively involved with counseling families and individuals, there is a virtual absence of published research on the role of clergy in primary mental health journals.

This lack of basic research into the role of clergy in mental health can be further highlighted by a major study of family violence assessment skills among a variety of family helpers. The study was published in the prestigious *American Journal of Public Health* (Tilden et al., 1994). In this article, University of Oregon researchers investigated the knowledge levels of nurses, physicians, psychologists, social workers, dentists, and even dental hygienists, while altogether ignoring clergy members who are mandated by law in Oregon to report child abuse under penalty of a $1000 fine (Gil & Edwards, 1988). Given the major responsibility clergy assume within the mental health network for families in turmoil (Weaver, 1992; Weaver, Koenig, & Larson, 1997), neglect of the subject of clergy in mental health research needs to be replaced with a more inclusive approach.

Similar results have been found when examining religion/spirituality in empirical research. In systematic reviews of quantitative research on religion in several health and mental health disciplines, including psychology (Weaver et al., in press-a), psychiatry (Larson, Pattison, Blazer, Omran, & Kaplan, 1986), clinical geriatrics (Sherrill, Larson, & Greenwold, 1993), and family medicine (Craigie, Liu, Larson, & Lyons, 1988), such reviews have consistently found that religious variables are infrequently considered, and when they are considered, most of these studies are of limited clinical or research value. One needs to ask, should more be required in the training of mental health professionals in religion/spirituality since we are so poorly informed about how patients' religious beliefs affect their health and illness?

CLERGY NEED TRAINING IN CLINICAL
EVALUATION AND REFERRAL SKILLS

Clergy are often unprepared to recognize the mental health problems of persons who seek their help. In a comprehensive national study of almost 2000 Protestant pastors in which 95% endorsed having some counseling training in seminary, about two of five rated the overall quality of pastoral counseling as poor (Orthner, 1986). Four additional studies indicate that diverse groups of Christian and Jewish clergy perceive themselves as inadequately trained to meet the mental health needs of the persons that come to them for help (Abramczyk, 1981; Ingram & Lowe, 1989; Lowe, 1986; Virkler, 1979). Interestingly, unlike growth in other areas of pastoral ministry (e.g., administration, preaching, and teaching), pastors indicate that no matter how long they serve in their parish, they believe their counseling skills do not increase without continuing education (Orthner, 1986). More promising, many surveyed clergy see the need for additional training in mental health issues (Nichols, 1995; Weaver, 1995).

Referral skills are closely related to evaluation skills since the clinical evaluation usually guides the course of action. In 1987, Meylink and Gorsuch published a review of all research involving the referral patterns of clergy over a 20-year period. Of persons coming to clergy with problems, clergy referred <10% to mental health specialists. This means that more than 90% of those who seek clergy help are counseled in isolation from mental health professionals. Research indicates that training clergy in clinical evaluative skills significantly enhances their counseling skills and increases the effectiveness of mental health referrals (Ingram & Lowe, 1989; Wasman, Corradi, & Clemens, 1979). Clergy who have attended a workshop or seminar in the area of mental health in the past year are much more likely to refer a person or family to a mental health specialist (Clark & Thomas, 1979; Rumberger & Rogers, 1982; Wright, 1984). Clergy referrals are currently being made with little training in the required skills (Virkler, 1979).

The following reasons have been cited to explain why clergy do not refer more people to mental health professionals: lack of feedback after the referral is made (Meylink & Gorsuch, 1987; Wright, 1984), inability to assess the type and quality of resources available, absence of referral skills, financial considerations (Virkler, 1979), lack of perceived or actual common values (Ruppert & Rogers, 1985), a lack of collegiality shown toward clergy by mental health practitioners (Mollica, Streets, Boscarino, & Redlich, 1986), fear of overmedication of parishioner (Mannon & Crawford, 1996), and, most important, inadequate diagnostic skills (Koenig & Weaver, 1997; Wasman et al., 1979). One expert in pastoral counseling estimates that improved referral and evaluative skills could increase clergy referrals by almost three times the current rate (Lee, 1976).

HOW CAN THESE HELPING PROFESSIONS INCREASE THEIR LINKAGE?

Studies indicate many areas in which linkage between mental health specialists and religious leaders needs to be expanded, including addiction treatment (Turner, 1995), child maltreatment (Weaver, 1992), genetics counseling (Steiner-Grossman & David, 1993), psychosocial rehabilitation (Walters & Neugeboren, 1995), and hospice care (Millison & Dudley, 1992). The following sections focus on four major mental health emergencies in which research has shown an immediate need for collaboration, training, and additional research—depression awareness and suicide prevention, spousal abuse, elder abuse, and psychological trauma.

CLERGY RESPONSE TO DEPRESSION AND SUICIDE

The significant involvement of clergy in mental health and the need for collaboration and training is illustrated when we examine research on the role of clergy in response to depression and suicide. Depression is the most common and treatable mental disorder. According to the noted psychologist Marty Seligman (1990), depression has increased 10-fold in the United States since World War II. Approximately 1 of 10 Americans experiences a major depression in their lifetime and 15% of those who go untreated attempt suicide. There is a completed suicide in the United States every 20 min and someone attempts suicide every 2 min (Stillion, McDowell, & May, 1989). Suicide is the second leading cause of death among teenagers. Teen suicide increased more than 400% between 1950 and 1990 and continues to climb (National Center for Health Statistics, 1993).

Given these epidemic levels of depression and suicide, it is not surprising to learn that in five separate studies clergy have indicated that affective disorders are either at the top or near the top among presenting problems brought to pastors (Abramczyk, 1981; Ingram & Lowe, 1989; Lowe, 1986; Virkler, 1979; Wood, 1996). Again, most of these same studies reveal that clergy perceive themselves as inadequately trained to meet the mental health needs of persons who come to them for counseling, and many are willing to pursue continuing education in mental health issues including suicide prevention and depression awareness.

These reports by clergy regarding their inability to adequately recognize someone in emotional distress are further supported by a study published in 1990 by George Domino. Using a geographically representative sample of 157 American clergy, the study found that Protestant, Catholic, and Jewish clergy had about the same level of knowledge of the symptoms of emotional distress (such as depression) as a group of undergraduates in an introductory psychology class. These findings are further confirmed by research showing that even experienced clergy are woefully unprepared to assess suicide potential in persons at risk. When compared to mental health specialists, clergy scored much lower in their ability to assess suicide lethality (Domino, 1985; Swain & Domino, 1986). Most clergy agree that there is a pressing need by them for training in the recognition of depression (Weaver, 1993a) and suicide risk factors (Ingram and Lowe, 1989; Weaver, 1993b; Wylie, 1984). This point is further illustrated in the following section.

PASTORAL CARE, DEPRESSION, AND SUICIDE AMONG THE ELDERLY

The religious community is central to the lives of most older Americans. Eighty percent of the elderly are members of a church or synagogue and over half (52%) worship at least once a week (Gallup, 1994). The mental health needs of older persons are increasingly becoming the central counseling concern of Christian and Jewish clergy. By the Year 2000, about 50% of the members of mainline Protestant churches and American Judaism will be 60 years of age or older (Custer, 1991; Gallup, 1990). A National Institute of Mental Health study found that a person with a mental health problem, including major depression, age 65 or older is more likely to seek clergy help than help from a mental health specialist (Hohmann & Larson, 1993). A Gallup survey found that seniors are more willing to turn to clergy than medical doctors or mental health specialists for help when a friend is contemplating suicide (Gallup, 1992).

Current research indicates that the suicide rate among Americans 65 years and older is 50% higher than that in the rest of the population, and this rate is rising rapidly among older males (Osgood, 1991). If the present trends continue, the rate of suicides among seniors will double by the Year 2030 (McIntosh, 1992). Senior suicide and depression is an issue that clearly warrants the attention of the mental health and religious communities, especially when one expert argues that 50% of suicides are preventable if helpers, such as clergy, are properly trained (McIntosh, 1988). Unfortunately, national programs designed to train helping professionals in depression awareness have omitted the clergy (Weaver, Samford, & Koenig, 1997). In a survey of 242 United Methodist pastors in West Virginia, over half (57%) said they felt their knowledge of aging issues was inadequate and two-thirds said they would like additional training regarding the elderly (Nichols, 1995).

FAMILY VIOLENCE AND PASTORAL COUNSELING

The clergy's contribution to front-line mental health care is illustrated further by the number of women seeking pastoral assistance as a result of domestic violence. It has been well documented that clergy are often the first professionals whom battered women seek for help (Horton, Wilkins, & Wright, 1988). In a survey of 1000 battered women, Bowker and Maurer discovered that one in three received help from clergy, as did 1 in 10 of their battering husbands. The researchers conclude that "clergy probably has contact with a much larger number of battered wives than was previously recognized and are perceived to be relatively ineffective in their efforts on behalf of the battered women" (Bowker, 1988; p. 233). Five additional studies between 1979 and 1988 reported similar findings, indicating that clergy tended to be among the least effective helpers for abused women and need more training in this area (Gordon, 1996).

A recent nationally representative survey of reform, conservative, and orthodoxy rabbis provides evidence that the knowledge and attitudes of clergy on the issue of spousal abuse may be improving (Cwik, 1997). In the study, 80% of rabbis felt that physical injury of a wife should be prosecuted as a felony and most agreed that feminist understandings of spousal abuse best explained the reason for abuse (i.e., the abuser's mental and emotional problems). The rabbis also stated a general willingness to intervene immediately on behalf of abused wives to put a stop to maltreatment and most advocated assertive action on the part of women. About half the rabbis had preached a sermon on wife abuse and had counseled at least one victim of abuse in the past year.

Again, most clergy express a need for additional training in spousal abuse (Cwik, 1997; Ingram & Lowe, 1989; Lowe, 1986; Martin, 1989; Virkler, 1979). Educational modules dealing with domestic violence and its aftermath, designed for clergy by mental health specialists, could be an effective training strategy that may foster collaboration and mutual learning. Working with clergy appears particularly important, given that almost 100% of American clergy provide premarital counseling prior to performing 75% of all weddings; only one-half of clergy, however, have any formal training in premarital counseling (Jones & Stahmann, 1994). Specifically, therapists need to help clergy members develop questions they can use in premarital counseling to screen for couples at risk for domestic violence, work with them on ways to help these couples understand the need for further counseling, and take clergy though the steps to make an effective referral. Clergy need help to develop a plan of action for women's safety if violence appears likely and to work with women in the aftermath of violence (Gross & Stith, 1996; Weaver, Koenig, & Ochberg, 1996).

Fortunately, several texts provide useful information on domestic violence in the context of religious values and concerns, any of which would be helpful to mental health professionals preparing workshops for clergy and other spiritual caregivers (Adams, 1994; Aldsdurf & Alsdurf, 1989; Clarke, 1986). Marie M. Fortune, a pastor and director of the Center for the Prevention of Sexual and Domestic Violence in Seattle, has developed a manual that offers a step-by-step approach for those designing a workshop for clergy on domestic violence prevention (Fortune, 1991).

Finally, there is research evidence showing that religious involvement can be a factor in reducing the risk of domestic violence. In an extensive 6-year study of 1084 New Zealand couples, higher levels of church attendance in the family were predictive of significantly lower levels of reported cases of wife assault (Fergusson, Horwood, Kershaw, & Shannon, 1986). This is an area needing additional research.

ELDER ABUSE

Elder abuse is a second form of domestic violence that urgently calls for collaboration between clergy and mental health professionals. Nearly as prevalent as child abuse, elder abuse is a form of domestic violence that involves the mistreatment or neglect of an older person usually by a relative or other caregiver. This may include physical violence, threats, verbal abuse, financial exploitation, neglect, or sexual abuse (All, 1994). Elder abuse is largely a hidden problem. Among the risk factors for elder abuse are being female, advanced age, dependency, past abuse, intergenerational conflict, lack of support system, cognitive impairment, and shared living arrangements with the abuser (Lachs & Pillemer, 1995). The National Center on Elder Abuse estimates that only 1 in 14 of the 1.5–2 million annual cases of elder abuse are actually reported (Tatara, 1995).

Pastors can play a critical role in the prevention of elder abuse and neglect by learning to identify and appropriately respond to the problem. Research indicates that clergy are one of the most likely groups of caregivers to encounter cases of elder abuse (Crouse, Cobb, Harris, Kopecky, & Poertner, 1981). Unfortunately, when a national study compared 14 groups of professionals working with seniors, clergy were rated as the least effective counselors when addressing elder abuse issues and were among the least likely to refer abuse or neglect cases to helping agencies (Blakely & Dolon, 1991). Training clergy to recognize and actively respond to elder abuse and neglect is imperative (Koenig & Weaver, 1997).

PSYCHOLOGICAL TRAUMA

People frequently look to clergy for counseling in crisis situations associated with severe grief, reactions to trauma, personal illness or injury, death of a spouse or close family member or friend, divorce or marital separation, and change in health of a family member or friend. Clergy respond to persons exposed to a wide range of acute stressors, including domestic violence (Bowker & Maurer, 1987), natural disasters (Chinnici, 1985), rape (Golding, Siegel, Sorenson, Burham, & Stein, 1989), child abuse (Weaver, 1992), elder abuse (Pratt, Koval, & Lloyd, 1983), war (Jacob, 1983), and torture (Lernoux, 1980). All these forms of violence can bring on psychological trauma or posttraumatic stress disorder (PTSD). People in "crisis" involving the "death of someone close" were almost five times more likely to see a clergyperson (54%) than all other mental health professionals combined (11%) (Veroff, Kulka, & Douvan, 1981). Despite research evidence that most PTSD survivors (Green, Lindy, & Grace, 1988; Weinrich, Hardin, & Johnson, 1990) and those who work with the traumatized (Backus, Backus, & Page, 1995) use religion as a primary coping strategy, there is almost no research on the role of clergy working with the traumatized (Weaver, et al., 1996).

Mental health professionals can play an important role in educating clergy about the first signs of PTSD, enabling them to more effectively screen members of their congregation for this disorder. Such education needs to be available to all clergy but especially to clergy located in the inner cities, where near-epidemic levels of violence and psychological trauma prevail (Breslau, Davis, Andreski, & Peterson, 1991).

FOUR GROUPS THAT NEED
SPECIAL ATTENTION

Briefly, I highlight four groups for which there is already a natural link between clergy and mental health specialists which can be developed further: ethnic minorities, rural Americans, adolescents, and women. These groups provide many creative opportunities for religious leaders and mental health professionals to work together.

ETHNIC MINORITIES

In 1986, Mollica and colleagues found that African American pastors were much more likely to go into the community and seek out people in crisis than their non-African American colleagues. These authors summarized their findings, published in the *American Journal of Psychiatry* (p. 328), as follows: "Parish-based clergy, especially the black clergy, function as a major mental health resource to communities with limited access to professional mental health service." Similarly, Mexican Americans are more than twice as likely to seek help with personal problems from clergy than from psychologists and psychiatrists combined (Chalfant et al., 1990). In fact, the study found that the degree of identification with Mexican ethnicity was strongly related to seeking pastoral help as a primary resource. Mental health specialists could provide an important service to the community by training clergy, particularly ethnic minority pastors, in crisis intervention and preventive mental health care (Weaver & Koenig, 1996; Weaver et al., 1996). The mental health benefits of religious practices and beliefs for both African American (Levin, Chatters, & Taylor, 1995; Maton et al., 1996) and Hispanic Americans (Levin, Markides, & Ray, 1996; Maldonado, 1994) have been well documented.

RURAL AMERICANS

Clergy are particularly important as counselors in rural or small community settings where mental health services are sparse and churches often function as one of few community counseling resources (Rowles, 1986). Protestant and Catholic churches are found in almost every county in America (Bradley, Green, Jones, Lynn, & McNeil, 1990). Because of fewer rural mental health services, rural clergy are more likely to be used as a counseling resource than are clergy in larger urban congregations in which more mental health services are available (Orthner, 1986; Wylie, 1984). One reason for the great demand for rural pastoral counseling services is that the poor, elderly, chronically ill, and others at high risk for emotional distress are disproportionately represented among the 62 million Americans who live in rural areas (Human & Wasem, 1991). Mental health specialists working in rural America are in a particularly advantageous position to find ways of connecting with congregations and clergy, especially those working with seniors (Weaver, Koenig, & Switzer, 1997).

Research on the role of clergy in rural mental health care, however, is rare (Weaver et al., in press-b). One exception is a recent study conducted by the University of West Virginia Gerontological Center. It shows the value of clergy working together with educators and social services workers to plan and implement large-scale collaborative programs for the rural elderly (Nichols, 1995).

ADOLESCENTS

Researchers have discovered that religious practices may have a greater influence on American youth than had been previously thought. A Gallup survey found that about half of adolescents in the United States (ages 13–17) report attending church or temple weekly and 27% of the polled teens report a higher interest in religion than their parents (Gallup & Bezilla, 1992). Studies consistently indicate adolescent religious involvement is positively associated with prosocial values (e.g., time spent helping others and volunteering) and negatively related to suicidal thinking and behavior, substance abuse, involvement in violence, and premature sexual behaviors (Donahue & Benson, 1995). A better understanding of the role of clergy working with families with teenagers as well as more collaboration between those clergy and mental health professionals who specialize in adolescent care are needed. A Gallup survey revealed that while the great majority of teens hold clergy in high regard, a mere 1% would seek counseling from clergy when they have serious problems (Gallup & Bezilla, 1992).

WOMEN

According to the National Institute of Mental Health Epidemiological Catchman Area surveys, women are more likely to seek help from clergy than help from mental health specialists (Hohmann & Larson, 1993). A large percentage (63%) of female clergy more frequently counsel women than men, and many of the presenting problems brought to clergy by women are gender related—eating disorders, unplanned or unwanted pregnancies, spouse abuse, and adult survivors of sexual abuse (Wood, 1996). Rapid increases in the number of women clergy and female mental health specialities offer growing opportunities for these two historically underrepresented groups to work together. Currently, one-third of the total 66,000 seminary students in Canada and the United States are women, which is up from a low of 10% in 1972 (Bedell, 1997). In addition 45% of the members of the APA are female (APA, 1995). Promotion and development of more collaboration and training between female mental health professionals and female religious leaders offer many creative opportunities for collegiality while at the same time addressing important issues affecting women.

CONCLUSIONS AND SUMMARY

In this review, it has been shown that clergy play a central role in the mental health care of persons in America. Clergy clearly need more training in mental health evaluative and referral skills, and mental health professionals often lack the knowledge and experience needed to sensitively address religious issues with their clients. Learning from each other would be of mutual benefit to mental health and religious professionals. Clergy could be invited to take part in the training of mental health specialists and vice versa. By mixing clergy and mental health students together in the same learning forum, clergy could learn more about mental health approaches to mental health care and mental health specialists could reexamine their preconceived beliefs about the role of clergy in mental health care. In addition, this learning experience would allow clergy and mental health professionals to formulate ways to develop more effective working relationships in order to better serve those who come to them for help.

REFERENCES

Abramczyk, L. W. (1981). The counseling function of pastors: A study in practice and preparation. *Journal of Psychology and Theology, 9,* 257–265.

Adams, C. J. (1994). *Woman-battering.* Minneapolis, MN: Fortress Press.

Aldsdurf, J., & Alsdurf, P. (1989). *Battered into submission: The tragedy of wife abuse in the Christian home.* Downers Grove, IL: Inter Varsity Press.

All, A. C. (1994). A literature review: Assessment and intervention in elder abuse. *Journal of Gerontological Nursing, 20*(7), 25–32.

American Psychiatric Association. (1993). *Directory of the American Psychiatric Association.* Washington, DC: Author.

American Psychological Association. (1995). *Women in the American Psychological Association.* Washington, DC: Author.

Backus, C. J., Backus, W., & Page, D. I. (1995). Spirituality of EMTs: A study of the spiritual nature of EMS workers and its effects on perceived happiness and prayers for patients. *Prehospital and Disaster Medicine, 10*(3), 168–173.

Bedell (1997). *Yearbook of American and Canadian churches 1997.* Nashville, TN: Abingdon.

Bergin, A. E. (1991). Values and religious issues in psychotherapy and mental health. *American Psychologist, 46,* 394–403.

Bergin, A. E., & Jensen, J. P. (1990). Religiosity of psychotherapist: A national survey. *Psychotherapy, 27,* 3–6.

Blakely, B. E., & Dolon, R. (1991). The relative contributions of occupation groups in the discovery and treatment of elder abuse and neglect. *Journal of Gerontological Social Work, 17,* 183–199.

Bowker, L. H. (1988). Religious victims and their religious leaders: Services delivered to one thousand battered women by the clergy. In A. L. Horton & J. A. Williamson (Eds.), *Abuse and religion: When prayer isn't enough* (pp. 229–234). Lexington, MA: D. C. Heath.

Bowker, L. H., & Maurer, L. (1987). The medical treatment of battered wives. *Women and Health, 12,* 25–45.

Bradley, M. B., Green, N. M., Jones, D. E., Lynn, M., & McNeil, L. (1990). *Churches and church membership in the United States 1990.* Atlanta: Glenmary Research Center.

Breslau, N., Davis, G. C., Andreski, P., & Peterson, E. (1991). Traumatic events and posttraumatic stress disorder in an urban population of young adults. *Archives of General Psychiatry, 48,* 216–222.

Chalfant, H. P., Heller, P. L., Roberts, A., Briones, D., Aguirre-Hochbaum, S., & Farr, W. (1990). The clergy as a resource for those encountering psychological distress. *Review of Religious Research, 31,* 305–313.

Chinnici, R. (1985). Pastoral care following a natural disaster. *Pastoral Psychology, 33*(4), 245–254.

Clark, S. A., & Thomas, A. H. (1979). Counseling and the clergy: Perceptions of roles. *Journal of Psychology and Theology, 7,* 48–56.

Clarke, R. (1986). *Pastoral care of battered women.* Philadelphia: Westminister Press.

Craigie, F. C., Liu, I. Y., Larson, D. B., & Lyons, J. S. (1988). A systematic analysis of religion variables in *The Journal of Family Practice,* 1976–1986. *Journal of Family Practice, 27,* 509–513.

Crouse, J. S., Cobb, D. C., Harris, B. B., Kopecky, F. J., & Poertner, J. (1981). *Abuse and neglect of the elderly in Illinois: Incidence, characteristics, legislation and policy recommendations.* Springfield: Illinois Department of Aging.

Custer, C. C. (1991, September 1). The church's ministry and the coming of the aged. *Circuit Rider,* 20–23.

Cwik, M. S. (1997). Peace at home? *Journal of Psychology and Judaism, 21*(1), 7–67.

Domino, G. (1985). Clergy's attitudes toward suicide and recognition of suicide lethality. *Death Studies, 9,* 187–199.

Domino, G. (1990). Clergy's knowledge of psychopathology. *Journal of Psychology and Theology, 18*(1), 32–39.

Donahue, M. J., & Benson, P. L. (1995). Religion and the well-being of adolescents. *Journal of Social Issues, 51*(2), 145–160.

Ebaugh, H. R. (1993). The growth and decline of Catholic religious orders of women worldwide: The impact of women's opportunity structures. *Journal for the Scientific Study of Religion, 32,* 68–73.

Fergusson, D. M., Horwood, L. J., Kershaw, K. L., & Shannon, F. T. (1986). Factors associated with reports of wife assault in New Zealand. *Journal of Marriage and the Family, 48,* 407–412.

Fortune, M. M. (1991). *Violence in the family: A workshop curriculum for clergy and other helpers.* Cleveland, OH: Pilgrim Press.

Gallup, G. H. (1990). *Religion in America: 1990.* Princeton, NJ: Gallup Organization.

Gallup, G. H. (1992). *Attitude and incidence of suicide among the elderly.* Princeton, NJ: Gallup Organization.

Gallup, G. H. (1993). *Religion in America: 1992–1993.* Princeton, NJ: Gallup Organization.

Gallup, G. H. (1994). *Religion in America: 1994, Supplement.* Princeton, NJ: Gallup Organization.

Gallup, G. H., & Bezilla, R. (1992). *The religious life of young Americans.* Princeton, NJ: George Gallup International Institute.

Gil, E., & Edwards, D. (1988). *Breaking the cycle.* Santa Monica, CA: Association for Advanced Training in the Behavioral Sciences.

Gilbert, M. G. (1981). Characteristics of pastors related to pastor counseling and referral. *Journal of Pastoral Counseling, 16,* 30–38.

Golding, J. M., Siegel, J. M., Sorenson, S. B., Burham, M. A., & Stein, J. A. (1989). Social support services following sexual assault. *Journal of Community Psychology, 17,* 92–107.

Gordon, J. S. (1996). Community services for abused women: A review of perceived usefulness and efficacy. *Journal of Family Violence, 11*(4), 315–329.

Green, B. L., Lindy, J. D., & Grace, M. C. (1988). Long-term coping with combat stress. *Journal of Traumatic Stress, 1*(4), 399–412.

Gross, W. G., & Stith, S. M. (1996). Building bridges between shelters for battered women and religious organizations: Advice from victims advocates. *Pastoral Psychology, 45*(2), 107–117.

Hastings, E., & Hastings, H. (Eds.). (1994). *Index to international public opinion: 1993–1994.* Westport, CT: Greenwood.

Hill, W. S. (1993). *A mental illness awareness guide for the clergy.* Washington, DC: American Psychiatric Association.

Hohmann, A. A., & Larson, D. B. (1993). Psychiatric factors predicting use of clergy. In E. L. Worthington, Jr. (Ed.), *Psychotherapy and religious values* (pp. 71–84). Grand Rapids, MI: Baker Book House.

Horton, A. L., Wilkins, M. M., & Wright, W. (1988). Women who ended abuse: What religious leaders and religion did for these victims. In A. L. Horton & J. A. Williamson (Eds.), *Abuse and religion: When prayer isn't enough* (pp. 235–246). Lexington, MA: D. C. Heath.

Human, J., & Wasem, C. (1991). Rural mental health in America. *American Psychologist, 46*(3), 232–239.

Ingram, B. L., & Lowe, D. (1989). Counseling activities and referral practices of rabbis. *Journal of Psychology and Judaism, 13,* 133–148.

Jacob, M. (1983). Post-traumatic stress disorder: Facing futility in and after Vietnam. *Currents in Theology and Mission 10*(5), 291–298.

Jones, E. F., & Stahmann, R. F. (1994). Clergy beliefs, preparation, and practice in premarital counseling. *Journal of Pastoral Care, 48,* 181–186.

Kelly, E. W. (1994). The role of religion and spirituality in counselor education: A national survey. *Counselor Education and Supervision, 33,* 227–236.

Koenig, H. G., Bearon, L. B., Hover, M., & Travis, J. L. (1991). Religious perspectives of doctors, nurses, patients and families. *Journal of Pastoral Care, 45,* 254–267.

Koenig, H. G., & Weaver, A. J. (1997). *Counseling troubled older adults: A handbook for clergy and other religious caregivers.* Nashville, TN: Abingdon.

Lachs, M. S., & Pillemer, K. (1995). Abuse and neglect of elderly persons. *New England Journal of Medicine, 332,*(7), 437–443.

Lannert, J. L. (1991). Resistance and countertransference issues with spiritual and religious clients. *Journal of Humanistic Psychology, 31*(4), 68–76.

Larson, D. B., Pattison, E. M., Blazer, D. G., Omran, A. R., & Kaplan, B. H. (1986). Systematic analysis of research variables in four major psychiatric journals. *American Journal of Psychiatry, 143,* 329–334.

Lee, R. R. (1976). Referral as an act of pastoral care. *Journal of Pastoral Care, 30*(10). 186–197.

Lernoux, P. (1980). *Cry of the people.* Garden City, NJ: Doubleday.

Levin, J. S., Chatters, L. M., & Taylor, R. J. (1995). Religious effects on health status and life satisfaction among black Americans. *Journal of Gerontology, 50B*(3), S154–S163.

Levin, J. S., Markides, K. S., & Ray, L. A. (1995). Religious attendance and psychological well-being in Mexican Americans: A panel analysis of three-generations data. *The Gerontologist, 36*(4), 454–463.

Lowe, D. W. (1986). Counseling activities, and referral practices of ministers. *Journal of Psychology and Christianity, 5,* 22–29.

Maldonado, D. (1994). Religiosity and religious participation among Hispanic elderly. *Journal of Religious Gerontology, 9,* 41–61.

Mannon, J. D., & Crawford, R. L. (1996). Clergy confidence to counsel and their willingness to refer to mental health professionals. *Family Therapy, 23*(3), 213–231.

Martin, S. E. (1989). Research note: The response of the clergy to spouse abuse in suburban county. *Victims and Violence, 4,* 217–225.

Maton, K. I., Teti, D. M., Corns, K. M., Vieira-Baker, C. C., Lavine, J. R., Grouse, K. R., & Keating, D. P. (1996). Cultural specificity of social support sources, correlates and contexts: Three studies of African-American and Caucasian youth. *American Journal of Community Psychology, 24,*(4), 551–587.

McIntosh, J. L. (1992). Older adults: The next suicide epidemic? *Suicide and Threatening Behavior* 22(3), 322–332.

Meylink, W., & Gorsuch, R. (1987). Relationship between clergy and psychologists: The empirical data. *Journal of Psychology and Christianity, 7,* 56–72.

Millison, M., & Dudley, J. R. (1992). Providing spiritual support: A job for all hospice professionals. *Hospice Journal, 8*(4), 49–66.

Mollica, R. C., Streets, F. J., Boscarino, J., & Redlich, F. C. (1986). A community study of formal pastoral counseling activities of the clergy. *American Journal of Psychiatry, 143,* 323–328.

National Center for Health Statistics. (1993). *Vital statistics report.* Hyattsville, MD: Author.

Nichols, A. (1995). Planning and implementing a statewide collaborative gerontology education program for religious professionals in rural areas. *Journal of Religious Gerontology, 9*(2), 51–67.

Orthner, D. K. (1986). *Pastoral counseling: Caring and caregivers in the United Methodist Church.* Nashville, TN: General Board of Higher Education and Ministry of the United Methodist Church.

Osgood, N. J. (1991). Prevention of suicide in the elderly. *Journal of Geriatric Psychiatry, 24,* 293–306.

Pargament, K. I., Falgout, K., Ensing, D. S., Reilly, B., Silverman, M., Van Haitsma, K., Olsen, H., & Warren, R. (1991). The congregation development program: Data-based consultation with churches and synagogues. *Professional Psychology: Research and Practice, 22*(5), 393–404.

Pratt, C. C., Koval, J., & Lloyd, S. (1983, March). Service workers' response to abuse of the elder. *Social Casework,* 147–153.

Rowles, G. D. (1986). The rural elderly and the church. *Journal of Religion and Aging, 2,*(12), 79–98.

Rumberger, D. J., & Rogers, M. L. (1982). Pastoral openness to interaction with a private Christian counseling service. *Journal of Psychology and Theology, 10,* 337–345.

Ruppert, P. P., & Rogers, M. L. (1985). Needs assessment in the development of a clergy consultation service. *Journal of Psychology and Theology, 13,* 50–60.

Sansone, R. A., Khatain, K., & Rodenhauser, P. (1990). The role of religion in psychiatric education: A national survey. *Academic Psychiatry, 14,* 34–38.

Schindler, F., Berren, M. R., Hannah, M. T., Beigel, A., & Santiago, J. M. (1987). How the public perceives psychiatrists, psychologists, nonpsychiatric physicians, and members of the clergy. *Professional Psychology: Research and Practice, 18*(4), 371–376.

Seligman, M. E. P. (1990). Why is there so much depression today? The waxing of the individual and the waning of the commons. In R. E. Ingram (Ed.), *Contemporary psychological approaches to depression* (pp. 1–9). New York: Plenum.

Shafranske, E. P. (1996). *Religion and the clinical practice of psychology.* Washington, DC: American Psychological Association.

Shafranske, E. P., & Malony, H. N. (1990). Clinical psychologists' religious and spiritual orientation and their practice of psychotherapy. *Psychotherapy, 27,* 72–78.

Sheridan, M. J., Bullis, R. K., Adcock, C. R., Berlin, S. D., & Miller, P. C. (1992). Practitioners' personal and professional attitudes and behaviors toward religion and spirituality: Issues for education and practice. *Journal of Social Work Education, 28,* 190–203.

Sherrill, K. A., Larson, D. B., & Greenwold, M. (1993). Is religion taboo in gerontology? Systematic review of research on religion in three major gerontology journals, 1985–1991. *American Journal of Geriatric Psychiatry, 1*(2), 109–117.

Steiner-Grossman, P., & David, K. L. (1993). Involvement of rabbis in counseling and referral for genetic conditions: Results of a survey. *American Journal of Human Genetics, 53*(6), 1359–1365.

Stillion, J. M., McDowell, E. E., & May, J. H. (1989). *Suicide: Across the life span.* New York: Hemisphere.

Swain, B. J., & Domino, G. (1986). Recognition of suicide lethality and attitudes toward suicide in mental health professionals. *Omega, 16*(4) 301–308.

Tatara, T. (1995). *An analysis of state laws addressing elder abuse, neglect, and exploitation.* Washington, DC: National Center on Elder Abuse.

Tilden, V. P., Schmidt, T. A., Limandri, B. J., Chiodo, G. T., Garland, M. J., & Loveless, P. A. (1994). Factors that influence clinicians' assessment and management of family violence. *American Journal of Public Health, 84,* 628–633.

Turner, W. H. (1995). Bridging the gap: Addressing alcohol and drug addiction from a community health perspective. *American Journal of Public Health, 85*(6), 870–871.

United States Department of Labor. (1992). *Occupational outlook handbook: United States Department of Labor.* Washington, DC: Bureau of Labor Statistics.

Veroff, J., Kulka, R. A., & Douvan, E. (1981). *Mental health in America: Patterns of help-seeking from 1957 to 1976.* New York: Basic Books.

Virkler, H. A. (1979). Counseling demands, procedures, and preparation of parish ministers: A descriptive study. *Journal of Psychology and Theology, 7,* 271–280.

Walters, J., & Neugeboren, B. (1995). Collaboration between mental health organizations and religious institutions. *Psychiatric Rehabilitation Journal, 19*(2), 51–57.

Wasman, M., Corradi, R. B., & Clemens, N. A. (1979). In-depth continuing education for clergy in mental health: Ten years of a large scale program. *Pastoral Psychology, 27,* 251–259.

Weaver, A. J. (1992). The distressed family and wounded children. *Journal of Religion and Health, 31,* 207–220.

Weaver, A. J. (1993a). Depression: What clergy need to know. *Currents in Theology and Mission, 20*(1), 5–16.

Weaver, A. J. (1993b). Suicide prevention: What clergy need to know. *Journal of Psychology and Christianity, 12*(1), 70–79.

Weaver, A. J. (1995). Has there been a failure to prepare and support parish-based clergy in their role as front-line community mental health workers?: A review. *Journal of Pastoral Care, 49,* 129–149.

Weaver, A. J., Kline, A. E., Samford, J., Lucas, L. A., Larson, D. B., & Gorsuch, R. L. (in press-a). Is religion taboo in psychology? A systematic analysis of research on religious variables in seven major American Psychological Association journals: 1991–1994. *Journal of Psychology and Christianity.*

Weaver, A. J., & Koenig, H. G. (1996). Elderly suicide, mental health professionals and the clergy: A need for collaboration, training and research. *Death Studies, 20*(5), 495–508.

Weaver, A. J., Koenig, H. G., & Larson, D. B. (1997). Marital and family therapists and the clergy: A need for collaboration, training and research. *Journal of Marital and Family Therapy, 23,* 13–25.

Weaver, A. J. Koenig, H. G., & Ochberg, F. M. (1996). Posttraumatic stress, mental health professionals and the clergy: A need for collaboration, training and research. *Journal of Traumatic Stress, 9*(4), 861–870.

Weaver, A. J., Koenig, H. G., & Switzer, D. K. (1997). Pastoral care to the rural elderly: A challenge and opportunity for ministry. *United Methodist Rural Fellowship Bulletin, 57*(1), 8–10.

Weaver, A. J., Samford, J., Kline, A. E., Lucas, L. A., Larson, D. B., & Koenig, H. G. (in press-b). What do psychologists know about working with the clergy? An analysis of eight American Psychological Association journals: 1991–1994. *Professional Psychology: Research and Practice.*

Weaver, A. J., Samford, J., & Koenig, H. G. (1997). Depression awareness training and the clergy. *American Journal of Psychiatry, 154*(5), 717–718.

Weinrich, S., Hardin, S. B., & Johnson, M. (1990). Nurses response to hurricane Hugo; victims' disaster stress. *Archives of Psychiatric Nursing, 4*(3), 195–205.

Wood, N. S. (1996). An inquiry into pastoral counseling ministry done by women in the parish setting. *Journal of Pastoral Care, 50*(4), 340–348.

Wright, P. G. (1984). The counseling activities and referral practices of Canadian clergy in British Columbia. *Journal of Psychology and Theology, 12,* 294–304.

Wylie, W. E. (1984). Health counseling competencies needed by the minister. *Journal of Religion and Health, 23,* 237–249.

EDUCATION OF MENTAL HEALTH PROFESSIONALS

25

INTEGRATING RELIGION INTO THE EDUCATION OF MENTAL HEALTH PROFESSIONALS

ELIZABETH S. BOWMAN

Department of Psychiatry
Indiana University School of Medicine
Indianapolis, Indiana, 46202

In planning a curriculum to train a mental health professional, logic dictates giving emphasis to (a) topics that concern the majority of patients treated by the professional and (b) topics about which the clinician is relatively uninformed. Religious and spiritual experiences meet these criteria: The U.S. population expresses a high degree of religious concern, but mental health professionals are considerably less religious than the general population (Bergin & Jensen, 1990; Gallup, 1990) and less likely to express their spirituality via mainstream practices (Shafranske & Gorsuch, 1984). Thus, inclusion of religion and spirituality in clinical training would appear essential. However, exactly the opposite has been the case: Most clinical training programs omit or minimize training about religion or spirituality. These omissions likely reflect the general disinterest and lack of education of mental health professionals regarding religion and spirituality. The net result, however, has been a dearth of training that leaves new graduates ill-prepared to address the religious or spiritual component of their patients' life experiences.

LITERATURE REVIEW

Scientific literature on teaching mental health trainees about religion or spirituality is sparse. Training requirements mention teaching about religion but provide no details about its scope or content. The literature on religion and spirituality in mental health contains no teaching outcome research. Discussions of education in social work (Faver, 1987), nursing (Carson, Winkelstein, Soeken, & Brunins, 1986), and secular psychology (Lehr & Spilka, 1989; Shafranske & Gorsuch, 1984) have noted the dearth of interest or training in this area. Published attempts at integrating religion into psychology education have been tailored for conservative Christian programs and are not easily applied to secular training programs (Jones, Watson, & Wolfram, 1992).

A 1990 survey of 79% of psychiatry residency training programs found that only about 1 in 10 included regular exposure to didactic material on religion and two-thirds had no course on any aspect of religion. Only 20% frequently taught material about religion as a defense (Sansone, Khatain, & Rodenhauser, 1990; p. 37). One-fifth of programs frequently exposed residents to material on pastoral counseling and one-third frequently addressed patients' religious dynamics in clinical supervision. Sansone et al. concluded that "there appears to be a meaningful disparity between the public's investment in religion and the exposure of residents to the academic study of religion, particularly on a didactic level."

Before 1996, the psychiatric literature contained a single report of a program to integrate religion into training (Westendorp, 1982). In 1996, the book *Model Practice* (Larson, Lu & Swyers, 1996; hereafter referred to as the *Model Curriculum*) provided the mental health field with the only systematic or comprehensive curriculum for mental health professionals on religion and spirituality in clinical care. Written by seven psychiatric educators with experience in teaching religious and spiritual aspects of clinical care, it is specifically aimed at psychiatry residencies but its content is applicable to clinical psychologists and other mental health professionals. It is organized into two core (essential) modules and nine accessory modules for teaching special topics. The content of this curriculum is addressed in the section titled "What Should Be Taught?" of this chapter.

WHO SHOULD BE TAUGHT?

The American Psychiatric Association's (1995) *Practice Guidelines for the Psychiatric Evaluation of Adults* specifically mentions inclusion of religious and/or spiritual beliefs when obtaining a personal history and when considering the patient's individuality and cultural background. This implies that information on religion is relevant to evaluations performed by mental health clinicians who engage in clinical evaluations: psychiatrists, psychologists, social workers, psychiatric nurse clinicians, and mental health workers in emergency, inpatient, and outpatient mental health and substance abuse treatment settings. Nonpsychiatric physicians participate in the delivery of mental health care. Their medical training should include exposure to the importance of religion and spirituality in coping with illness, but discussion of this training is beyond the scope of this chapter (a primary care curriculum on religion/spirituality is currently being developed). The religious and spiritual training of pastoral counselors is not addressed in this chapter because of their unique pastoral identity (see Chapter 24).

The training requirements for psychiatrists and psychologists require didactic coverage of religion. The Accreditation Council for Graduate Medical Education's *Program Requirements for Residency Education in Psychiatry* (1995) requires all psychiatry residency training programs to include religious and spiritual factors in the didactic curriculum on human development and in instruction on cultural aspects of the patient's life, but it is not specific about scope or content. Psychology training programs explicitly require that the curriculum "includes exposure to theoretical and empirical knowledge bases relevant to the role of cultural and individual diversity" in science and practice and includes religion in the definition of "cultural and individual diversity" (American Psychological Association, 1995, pp. Iw-27, 5). The ethical guidelines for psychiatrists (American Psychiatric Association, 1990) and psychologists (American Psychological Association, 1992) each presume that clinicians will encounter religious material in treatment.

WHAT SHOULD BE TAUGHT?

I have taught a 16 to 18 hr course on religion and spirituality to Indiana University psychiatry residents since 1985. This chapter's recommendations on course content are based on that teaching experience, on Shimon Waldfogel's fourth-year psychiatry residency course at Jefferson Medical College (S. Waldfogel, personal communication), and on the previously mentioned *Model Curriculum* (Larson et al., 1996) to which Dr. Waldfogel and I were contributing authors.

Since mental health educators have only recently begun to recognize the importance of religion and spirituality to patients, the amount of training time allotted to this topic is generally severely limited. Thus, a major challenge for faculty is setting curricular priorities to maximize the use of curricular time. I suggest approaching the content of the curriculum by first determining the overall goal of teaching this material. I recommend a goal of assisting trainees in recognizing normal and pathological manifestations of religious and spiritual life and assisting them in developing ethnical and sensitive assessments and responses. This goal includes knowledge, skills, and attitudes—the three learning areas emphasized by clinical educators (Larson et al., 1996).

How do you implement this goal? If there is one law of curricular development, it is that the material always exceeds the allotted curricular time. The interaction of mental health issues with religion/spirituality is an area far to vast to be truly covered in any curriculum. In addition, trainees have limited abilities to absorb new material—and for many, religion is unfamiliar territory. I suggest approaching this "content crunch" by placing content into three categories of decreasing priority which I arbitrarily label as foundational/essential, important, and helpful. Material in the first category should be taught even if there is no time for any other material. This approach follows the suggestion of the *Model Curriculum* (Larson et al., 1996), which divides material into two core modules (overview and history gathering) and nine accessory modules (life cycle issues, consult–liaison issues, collaboration with clergy, substance abuse, women, abused persons, God images, charismatic religion, and cults). My suggestions for topics in these three areas reflect my teaching experiences and differ slightly from those of the *Model Curriculum.*

The three content categories are designed for teaching clinical trainees who are actively involved in patient care. Preclinical curricula (i.e., undergraduate psychology or social work programs) which are presumed to involve longer courses are not addressed in this chapter. However, professors in such programs can consult the *Model Curriculum* (Larson et al., 1996), which contains enough literature resources for a semester-long course.

FOUNDATIONAL OR ESSENTIAL MATERIAL

Essential content can be divided into two sections. The first section addresses general information about the relationship of religion/spirituality to mental health and illness. It places the entire topic into perspective, a necessary step before trainees can grasp the importance of this material or be interested enough to want to learn about it. The *Model Curriculum,* (Larson et al., 1996) recommends teaching an overview of five general areas on the interface of mental health and spirituality/religion: history, ethical issues, research, definitions, and the traditions and beliefs of major world religions. Due to time constraints, I have taught only three of these content areas: definitions, demographics/research, and general religious practices.

I recommend beginning with basic definitions of religion and of spirituality so that trainees understand the variable relationship between them. The ubiquitous nature of spiritual life and religious interests is emphasized to place them in perspective as part of human experience. Demographic material should cover the high level of religious interest and practices in the general population and the interest and belief gap between the general public and mental health professionals. The purpose of this material is to alert trainees to their own potential for underestimating the importance of religion and spirituality in the lives of their patients. This material (along with a historical overview) also helps them understand why patients often presume that mental health professionals are disinterested in or hostile to religion or spirituality. If the curriculum does not include a session for examination of research literature on the relationship of religious practices to mental health, a few basic findings can be included in the demographics section. This material helps dispel preconceived ideas about religious beliefs automatically conveying harm to mental health.

If possible, some material on common aspects of religious and spiritual practices and experiences should be covered. Examples include discussions of the function of religious beliefs in coping with death, grieving, and life transitions; the general structures of liberal and fundamentalist approaches to world religions; and the existential and esthetic functions of nonreligious spiritual practices. The goal of teaching this material is to build awareness of common psychological processes and needs that are addressed by diverse religions. Such material builds a foundation for looking beneath the content of belief to the process of how religion and spirituality are used by individuals.

The second area of essential material is gathering and interpreting information on a patient's religious/spiritual history. This material is essential because therapeutic responses are predicated upon taking an adequate history and understanding the psychological functions of an individual's faith. Mental health clinicians have generally received no training in asking about religious and spiritual experiences and some lack personal religious or spiritual life. Demonstration interviews can help trainees understand the dynamic richness of religious and spiritual life. Asking trainees to conduct a religious history is an efficient way to demonstrate the need to develop this interview skill and to bring them face to face with their countertransference reactions to approaching this material.

The goal is to help trainees gain enough skills and personal comfort to actually ask their patients about their religious/spiritual experiences. However, knowledge without understanding is useless at best and can be clinically dangerous. Thus, trainees need help in understanding the dynamic significance of the history. If time permits, this can be accomplished by reviewing dynamic material on correlations between images of God, self, and parents (Larson et al., 1996, pp. 80–82) and on the dynamics of religious conversion (James, 1902/1961). It is critical for trainees to understand the "differential diagnosis" of spiritual material so they recognize religious manifestations of psychopathology and avoid pathologizing mystical, spiritual, or culturally normative experiences (Barnhouse, 1986; Scotton, Chinen, & Battista, 1996). However, if the curriculum does not allow for separate consideration of this material, I recommend including it in a case discussion of religious histories.

IMPORTANT MATERIAL

I classify three topical areas as "important," i.e., their teaching is a high priority after rudimentary skills have been covered. The first and most important topic is the differential diagnosis of spiritual and religious material mentioned previously. The emphasis of this section depends on the professional discipline of the student. Psychiatrists and inpatient or emergency clinicians are most likely to encounter religious presentations of psychosis, mania, and serious depressions, whereas all types of mental health professionals need to understand distortions of religious and spiritual life related to neurosis (i.e., obsessions, anxiety, etc.) and personality disorders (Battista, 1996; Lukoff, Lu, & Turner, 1996; Meissner, 1991). Trainees should be aware of ecstatic religious experiences so these experiences are not mistaken for mania or psychosis (Larson et al., 1996, pp. 85–87). In addition to addressing religious psychopathology, trainees should be assisted in assessing the overall group process by which a faith system operates. This can assist the professional in perceiving the impact of psychologically oppressive versus life-enhancing group processes and belief systems.

The second topic involves ethical and therapeutic responses to religious issues in mental health treatment. Few topics of human discourse raise as much passion as religious beliefs. Thus, it is especially important to address the subtle interactions of therapist and patient and their basis in transference and countertransference reactions to religion (Larson et al., 1996, pp. 36–40). Using case material, trainees should be helped in understanding the common religious issues that arise in mental health treatment. These may include gender-based religious issues, spiritual implications of abuse or maltreatment, and religious resistances to dealing with therapeutic material (Larson et al., 1996, pp. 75–81): I recommend placing all this material in context by reviewing the ethical guidelines of the trainees' professional discipline about addressing religious issues (e.g., American Psychiatric Association, 1990; American Psychological Association, 1992).

The third important topic is the scientific research literature on the relationship of religion and spirituality to physical and mental health. As mentioned previously, the purpose of teaching this material is to dispel preconceived ideas about universal mental health harmfulness or helpfulness of religious beliefs. The educational targets of this material are changes in attitudes and knowledge. A subtle but important message of this section is that religion and spirituality can be studied scientifically and should not be viewed as an "untouchable" category. This section can include the explicitly spiritual focus of some substance abuse treatment programs such as Alcoholics Anonymous and their relative success rates vis-à-vis other approaches. I recommend a balanced approach that includes examination of areas in which certain types of religious approaches might harm mental health and of the scientific shortcomings of this literature. Emphasis on solely positive aspects of religious practices is neither scientifically honest nor likely to receive a positive reception from other skeptical students. Larson and Larson (1994) and the *Model Curriculum* (Larson et al., 1996, pp. 17–19) provide helpful material that shortens preparation time.

HELPFUL MATERIAL

The range of helpful topics is vast. For the fortunate professor who is allotted time to teach more material, I recommend two topics as first priority: the psychodynamics of religious/spiritual experiences and spiritual development. For other optional topics, see the *Model Curriculum* (Larson et al., 1996).

The psychodynamics of religious and spiritual experiences have been alluded to frequently and should have been touched upon in previous material. However, specific clinically relevant areas need focused attention. Clinical trainees are notoriously content bound and must be carefully taught to observe the process of interpersonal interactions and respond to the underlying dynamics or behavioral patterns. In approaching religion, the tendency to focus on and judge content is particularly salient (a human tendency that has provoked more than one religious war). The goal of teaching the psychodynamics of spiritual/religious experiences is to assist trainees in approaching this material from the content and process levels simultaneously. This approach reduces the tendency to judge belief content and potentially improves the helpfulness of clinical responses.

I suggest focusing on common clinical situations, such as the dynamics of religious conversion (James, 1902/1961), changes of religious preference, the dynamics of religious groups (cults, rule-oriented versus experientially oriented movements, etc.), and the psychodynamics of relating to deity. I have found the latter topic to be the most clinically relevant since humans tend to project their superego struggles, parental images, and self-images onto their deities (Larson et al., 1996, pp. 82–84; Rizzuto, 1979). Understanding the dynamic significance of God images assists trainees in seeing the connection between religious beliefs and personal dynamics. It can increase their willingness to respectfully listen to such material rather than avoid it as a dynamically unproductive topic.

The second topic, religion and spirituality in human development, may be the area least familiar to faculty. The purpose of teaching this material is to extend students' concept of continual human development to the spiritual/religious sphere and dispel the common misperception that spiritual development is synonymous with the development of conscience. Understanding religious and spiritual development has several clinical benefits. First, it can illuminate personal psychodynamics, such as identity development, relationship to authority figures, and individual needs and defenses. Second, it enables the clinician to tailor clinical responses to the level of the patient's spiritual development. An understanding of levels of spiritual/religious development is as critical to responding to religious material as an understanding of childhood development is to addressing the mental health problems of children and adolescents.

Spiritual and religious development can be approached in several ways. One way is to formally discuss theoretical systems such as James Fowler's (1981) *Stages of Faith,* which covers the entire life span, and/or Coles' (1990) examination of the spirituality of children. These theories can be compared with theories of conscience (Gilligan, 1982; Kohlberg, 1981; Stilwell, Galvin, Kopta, & Padgett, 1997). Fowler's stages can be examined by looking at patients' religious histories and analyzing their stage of religious development and its relationship to their clinical presentation. Material on spiritual development should not be restricted to the child and adolescent section of a clinical curriculum. A critical piece of insight for students is that spiritual development (their own included) ordinarily continues in adulthood.

The second method of teaching religious and spiritual development emphasizes the latter point by approaching the developmental uses of religion and spirituality in life stages from childhood through death (see Larson et al., 1996, pp. 45–61 for this approach and bibliographic resources). This approach easily fits into a case-focused approach and can include material on Fowler's (1981) stages. I have taught spiritual development simultaneously with religious history taking by asking psychiatry residents to construct and discuss their religious/spiritual history and to try to place themselves within Fowler's stages. Residents usually find this experience memorable and it desensitizes them to talking about religion.

WHEN SHOULD RELIGION/SPIRITUALITY BE TAUGHT?

Teaching is like an effective interpretation in psychotherapy: It is helpful only when the content and timing are both correct. In teaching, this translates into delivering relevant material at a time when the student is ready and able to utilize it. As with teaching any other clinical topic, the timing depends on the content. Teaching about religion/spirituality too early in training can result in trainees not learning the material because it is too advanced or they are unable to accommodate it in a nonconcrete fashion. Neither outcome is helpful.

Clinical trainees need to gain some understanding of general psychological theories and treatment processes and have a core mass of clinical experience before they can grasp the interaction of these topics with religious and spiritual life. How does this recommendation translate into an actual training program? A few guiding principles can inform the timing of introducing material on religion/spirituality. Very basic material on definitions, research literature on religion and mental health, and history-taking skills should be introduced fairly early to influence the student's skills and attitudes. For psychiatry residents, the end of the first year or beginning of the second year is a good time for this. Residents have enough clinical experience to understand the material and are still forming basic interviewing skills and clinical attitudes. For clinical psychologists, this material could be introduced during their preclinical curriculum and during preinternship clinical experiences.

More explicitly clinical topics, such as the differential diagnosis of religious/spiritual experiences, therapeutic responses to this material, and the psychodynamics of these experiences, are generally too advanced for students early in their clinical training. I have taught this material in a course early in the second year of psychiatry residency and have found that residents have difficulty assimilating it. When the same material is taught late in the second year or in the third year, residents' responses are richer, and their comprehension is deeper. Dr. Waldfogel's course at Jefferson is taught to fourth-year residents. I recommend trying to teach clinical topics in the third or early fourth year for psychiatry residents and at least midway in internship or the clinical practicum for psychologist or other mental health clinicians.

In teaching any topic, one faces the issue of a "multiple-dose versus single-dose" approach. I have tried both approaches, a single course and graded exposure to material at several times during training, and have found multiple exposures more effective. In light of the neurological dictum that rehearsal of material consolidates long-term memory, this is not particularly surprising. The choice of single versus multiple exposures to material on religion will probably depend on the teaching methods employed and the structure of the curriculum.

HOW CAN RELIGION/SPIRITUALITY BE TAUGHT?: TEACHING METHODS

There is no single way to teach any topic. Teaching methods for religion and spirituality should be tailored to the abilities of the professor and students. However, one principle should be considered when selecting teaching methods for mental health trainees that will maximize the effectiveness of the learning experience: Adults learn best in formats that emphasize practical applications. Lectures are the least efficient means of learning. Thus, course formats should strive to include cases and interaction such as discussion and role playing of clinical interactions. "Homework" assignments (e.g., doing a religious history with a current patient or constructing one's own history) tend to personalize and enliven learning. Faculty who intend to teach about religion and spirituality should consider gathering a collection of videotaped interviews from patients who consent to their use for education.

I have always included hospital chaplains or chaplaincy students as colearners in courses and case conferences that address religious/spiritual topics. Their presence increases cross-disciplinary exchange of knowledge and helps break down stereotypes and unhelpful transferences that mental health trainees may have about clergy. Psychiatry residents have rated their inclusion as helpful to learning. I have noted that residents increased their utilization of chaplains after such exposure.

The following sections highlight the pros and cons of common teaching methods. A more comprehensive discussion of learning formats is found in the *Model Curriculum* (Larson et al., 1996, pp. 91–99).

COURSES AND SEMINARS

A formal course on religion and spirituality has the advantage of somewhat greater exposure to the topic and more opportunity to provide exposure to clinical literature. The disadvantage of a course format is the temptation to take a didactic approach that diminishes clinical focus and utility. Unfortunately, many clinical training directors view teaching about religion and spirituality as unimportant and decline to allow more than a single session to address it (usually as part of a course on cultural and ethnic issues). In such programs, faculty need to create other opportunities to teach this topic. In other words, if you knocked at the front door and were denied entry, take a "back door" approach by offering to teach in one of the formats discussed in the following sections.

CASE CONFERENCES

This method has the advantage of clinical immediacy and relevance. Case conferences may afford an opportunity to interview a patient about religion and demonstrate clinical interaction around this topic. Their disadvantages include lack of a systematic coverage of material and "potluck" case material (unless the faculty can provide a live or videotaped patient). I recommend trying to schedule a conference for this topic so that assigned reading and solicitation of an appropriate case can be included. The disadvantage of case conferences is limited exposure to theory and literature and nonsystematic topical exposure.

GRAND ROUNDS

A grand rounds lecture or a similar departmental colloquium is an excellent way to expose trainees, supervisors, and persons from other clinical disciplines to didactic material on religion and spirituality. I recommend incorporating case material (live or videotaped) into this format whenever possible.

CLINICAL SUPERVISION

Religious and spiritual issues can be regularly addressed in individual or group clinical supervision. This method has the advantage of enabling in-depth clinical exploration and teaching clinical interventions. The disadvantage is that teaching depends on a knowledgeable and comfortable supervisor—an entity that may be as scarce as the proverbial hen's tooth. Nalini Juthani, Psychiatry Residency Training Director at Bronx–Lebanon Hospital in New York, uses the technique of teaching each resident that religious affiliation or lack of it is a basic demographic variable that must be mentioned at the beginning of each case presentation. This technique is within the reach of any supervisor and it systematically raises awareness of the need to ask basic information about spiritual history and life.

OTHER METHODS

In programs in which access to formal teaching opportunities is unavailable, a less formal approach can be adopted. Francis Lu, Clinical Professor of Psychiatry at the University of California, San Francisco, has utilized film clubs to discuss the interplay between mental health and cultural or spiritual issues. Similarly, offering to lead a journal club can provide the opportunity to examine recent literature on religion and spirituality. Inpatient personnel can offer inservice training to nurses, therapists, and occupational therapists or intentionally incorporate chaplains or discussion of religious issues in team treatment meetings in which trainees participate.

DEALING WITH RESISTANCES
TO CURRICULAR INTEGRATION

Faculty who attempt to teach mental health clinical trainees about religion and spirituality will inevitably run into some resistance from students, faculty, or program directors. Most resistance is due to ignorance or countertransference issues. Ignorance is easier to overcome: Persistent education about the ubiquity of patients' religious concerns is the antidote.

Countertransference resistances generally fall into categories of personal discomfort with the topic and unresolved religious/spiritual conflicts. These difficulties affect students and faculty alike. They occur in forms ranging from "forgetting" to address religion in case discussions to open verbal attacks on religion and the need to teach it. These resistances must be addressed on some level or teaching efforts will fail to be effective. I suggest taking an explicitly scientific approach that expresses wonderment that any other scientist would be unwilling to look at data on any clinical topic. This has the subtle effect of removing religion and spirituality from the category of "special and different" and placing it on a plane with any other clinical topic. With students, discussing countertransference reactions to religious topics early in the teaching process can help open discussion of student reactions and can defuse resistance. Unfortunately, there are some students and faculty who are unable or unwilling to examine this area. I suggest you find a way around them and teach those who are open to learning.

FUTURE DIRECTIONS: RISING INTEREST
AND DIVERSITY

Both the religious diversity of Americans and professional and public interest in religion and spirituality are increasing. The past several years have seen a rise in scientific conferences and research reports on the interface of religion and spirituality with mental and physical health. In the public sector, religious topics have recurrently made the cover of *Time* and *Newsweek*. As this trend continues, the need to teach trainees will increase as mental health clinicians confront increasingly diverse religious traditions and values.

REFERENCES

Accreditation Council on Graduate Medical Education. (1995). Program requirements for residency education in psychiatry. In *graduate medical education directory* (pp. 221, 223). Chicago: American Medical Association.

American Psychiatric Association. (1990). Guidelines regarding possible conflict between psychiatrists' religious commitments and psychiatric practice. *American Journal of Psychiatry, 147,* 542.

American Psychiatric Association. (1995). American Psychiatric Association practice guidelines for psychiatric evaluation of adults. *American Journal of Psychiatry Supplement, 152,* 64–80.

American Psychological Association. (1992). Ethical principles of psychologists and code of conduct. *American Psychologist, 47*(12), 1597–1611.

American Psychological Association. (1995). Guidelines and principles for accreditation of programs in professional psychology (pp. 5, Iw-27). In *American Psychological Association committee on accreditation site visitor handbook.* Washington, DC: Author.

Barnhouse, R. T. (1986). How to evaluate patients' religious ideation. In L. H. Robinson (Ed.), *Psychiatry and religion: overlapping concerns* (pp. 90–105). Washington, DC: American Psychiatric Press.

Battista, J. R. (1996). Offensive spirituality and spiritual defenses. In B. W. Scotton, A. B. Chinen, & J. R. Battista (Eds.), *Textbook of transpersonal psychiatry and psychology* (pp. 250–260). New York: Basic Books.

Bergin, A. E., & Jensen, J. P. (1990). Religiosity of psychotherapists: A national survey. *Psychotherapy, 27,* 3–7.

Carson, V. B., Winkelstein, M., Soeken, K., & Brunins, M. (1986). The effect of didactic teaching on spiritual attitudes. *Image: Journal of Nursing Scholarship, 18,* 161–164.

Coles, R. (1990). *The spiritual life of children.* Boston: Houghton Mifflin.

Faver, C. A. (1987). Religious beliefs, professional values, and social work. *Journal of Applied Social Sciences, 11,* 207–219.

Fowler, J. W. (1981). *Stages of faith.* San Francisco: Harper & Row.

Gallup, G. (1990). *Religion in American: 1990.* Princeton, NJ: Princeton Religion and Research Center.

Gilligan, C. (1982). *In a different voice.* Cambridge, MA: Harvard University Press.

James, W. (1961). *The varieties of religious experience.* New York: Collier MacMillan. (Original work published 1902)

Jones, S. L., Watson, E. J., & Wolfram, T. J. (1992). Results of the rech conference survey on religious faith and professional psychology. *Journal of Psychology and Theology, 20,* 147–158.

Kohlberg, L. (1981). *The philosophy of moral development.* San Francisco: Harper & Row.

Larson, D. B., & Larson, S. S. (1994). *The forgotten factor in physical and mental health: What does the research show?* Rockville, MD: National Institute for Healthcare Research.

Larson, D. B., Lu, F. G., & Swyers, J. P. (Eds.). (1996). *Model curriculum for psychiatry residency training programs: Religion and spirituality in clinical practice.* Rockville, MD: National Institute for Healthcare Research.

Lehr, E., & Spilka, B. (1989). Religion in the introductory psychology textbook: A comparison of three decades. *Journal for the Scientific Study of Religion 28,* 366–371.

Lukoff, D., Lu, F. G., & Turner, R. (1996). Diagnosis: A transpersonal clinical approach to religious and spiritual problems. In *Textbook of transpersonal psychiatry and psychology* (pp. 231–249). New York: Basic Books.

Meissner, W. (1991). The phenomenology of religious psychopathology. *Bulletin of the Menninger Clinic, 55,* 281–298.

Rizzuto, A.-M. (1979). *The birth of the living god.* Chicago: University of Chicago Press.

Sansone, R. A., Khatain, D., & Rodenhauser, P. (1990). The role of religion in psychiatric education: A national survey. *Academic Psychiatry 14,* 34–38.

Scotton, B. W., Chinen, A. B., & Battista, J. R. (Eds.). (1996). *Textbooks of transpersonal psychiatry and psychology.* New York: Basic Books.

Shafranske, E. P., & Gorsuch, R. L. (1984). Factors associated with the perception of spirituality in psychotherapy. *Journal of Transpersonal Psychology 16,* 231–241.

Stilwell, B. A., Galvin, M., Kopta, S. M., & Padgett, R. J. (1997). Moralization of attachment, a fourth domain of conscience functioning. *Journal of the American Academy of Child and Adolescent Psychiatry, 36,* 1140–1147.

Westendorp, W. (1982). The interface of psychiatry and religion: A program for career training in psychiatry. *Journal of Psychology and Theology 10,* 22–27.

26

RELIGION AND ACADEMIA
IN MENTAL HEALTH

DAN G. BLAZER

Duke University School of Medicine
Durham, North Carolina 27705

Recently, I was contacted by a writer for *Science* who was interviewing various investigators throughout the country about the research efforts of Herbert Benson to establish the efficacy of prayer as a method of healing (Roush, 1997). The responses of those persons polled were predictably diverse, but no respondent expressed surprise that these efforts were under way. Ten years ago few persons associated with academia, such as Dr. Benson (a professor of medicine at Harvard), were testing empirically the association of any overtly religious activity and a health outcome, much less a mental health outcome. As we near the end of the twentieth century, however, the academy is well aware of the recent upsurge of interest among the American public in things spiritual and the efforts of a growing number of academics to study religion as a phenomena to which the scientific method can be applied. The explorations of the interaction between religion and mental health reviewed in this book by and large reflect the interest in the scientific study of religion, the empirical approach to things spiritual. However, the empirical approach to the study of religion and mental health is but one among many applicable approaches.

The response of the academy to the scientific study of religion and mental health reflects the nature of the academy today. There is no uniform definition of the academy and therefore no one response. Perhaps even the description of a typical research university as a community of scholars with varied opinions and methods of inquiry who challenge one another in open discussion is too generous. Though periodic brush fires emerge on university campuses, such as the debates between those who expound modern versus postmodern views, most academics live within much smaller communities within the university and relate more to persons with similar interests, opinions, and methods at other universities than those in their own university. Therefore, there is no one response, nor even a typical response, to the emerging interest in religion as it impacts various aspects of our lives, such as our mental health. In fact, the academy is not only diverse in its response to areas of current interest and inquiry, such as religion and mental health, but also has been slow to recognize the impact of religion, especially evangelical Christianity, upon American society. Paul Boyer, a professor of history at the University of Wisconsin, noted in the preface to his book, *When Time Shall Be No More* (a study of prophecy belief in modern American culture) (1992), that academics have devoted little systematic attention to these widespread beliefs. Those historians of American religion who have been firmly entrenched in the academy have significantly slighted the world of modern evangelicalism and charismatic Protestantism, convinced that the influence of such beliefs collapsed under the assault of modernism, secularism, and scientific naturalism. In fact, charismatic Protestantism has had a profound impact on recent culture and politics.

Despite the diversity and relative lack of interest among academics in the increasing influence of religion upon society, approaches to inquiry and critique across the academy do inform the student of religion and mental health. I have selected six such approaches as illustrative of the diversity in academia and review earlier twentieth century precursors (works of individual scholars) of these diverse approaches to inquiry. The approaches I have selected are far from inclusive and are at best representative. Though some of the approaches have roots in antiquity, I have limited the historical review primarily to the twentieth century. The approaches include an empirical approach with Emil Durkheim as a precursor, a humanistic approach with Gordan Allport as a precursor, a postmodern approach with Sigmund Freud as a precursor, a pragmatic approach with William James as a precursor, a mechanistic biologic approach with G. Stanley Hall as a precursor, and a life cycle approach with Erik Erikson as a precursor.

EMPIRICAL APPROACH

The recent resurgence of interest in the relationship between religion and mental health in academia has been driven primarily by the emergence of empirical studies documenting the positive benefits of religious beliefs and behaviors to mental health. This approach dates at least to the pioneering work of Emil Durkheim in sociology (Durkheim, 1951). Durkheim performed ecologic studies in which he compared different rates of suicide across various European groups based on an index of social integration that contained clear religious overtones. Suicide rates were known to be higher in Protestants than Catholics, higher in the unmarried than the married, higher in soldiers than civilians, and higher during times of both economic prosperity and economic recession than during times of economic stability. He therefore suggested that the risk for suicide was greater among persons who were not integrated into group life compared to those who were. If a society lacks clear-cut norms and conduct in that society is characterized by a lack of rules (anomie), then suicide rates will be higher. To verify his theory, he found that suicide rates were higher in countries that permitted divorce, in countries during the midst of economic crisis, and among religious groups which encouraged more individuality, namely, Protestants compared to Catholics.

Durkheim moved from theory based in the importance of social control as a balance to personal independence, to practice. His methods of investigation were clearly based in empiricism, namely, gathering data about stated religious preference, laws regarding marriage, and economic indicators. Examples of recent empirical studies exploring the relationship between religion and mental health remain sparse but are increasing in number. The investigators generally begin with a hypothesis about an empirical association and attempt to test that hypothesis, usually in community-based or treatment-based studies. Ness and Wintrob (1980) studied a community-based population using standard epidemiologic procedures and found that the more frequently people engaged in religious activities, the less likely they were to report symptoms of emotional distress. Emrick, Tonigan, Montgomery, and Little (1993) performed a meta-analysis of the literature on Alcoholics Anonymous. They found that the degree to which members adhere to the movement's spiritually oriented Twelve Steps was associated with sobriety.

Empirical study of religion and mental health is but one approach to the subject in the academy, but it is a dominant approach, especially in academic health centers, in which empiricism maintains considerable status. Unfortunately, many persons pursuing empirical studies do not have an appreciation of the limits of such studies, the expression of such limits having in large part driven the current strength of the postmodern movement. Some of the limits are inherent in the method itself, so careful methodological critique will be applied to these studies as they emerge. However, other approaches in academia inform us of the limits of empiricism as well, especially the postmodern critique and the new pragmatism.

HUMANISTIC APPROACH

The humanistic approach to academic inquiry had its modern origins among the German humanistic philosophers of the nineteenth century but was reflected in American psychology earlier during the twentieth century in the writings of persons such as Gordan Allport. The humanists expressed dissatisfaction with the purely objective orientation of the empirical psychologists. In particular, Allport relied on armchair reflection rather than data collection. When he did pursue active inquiries, these inquiries were often in the form of comprehensive personality assessments rather than questionnaires (Allport, 1950). Allport focused on the construct of sentiment to designate that stable component of personality which combines both affective and cognitive factors (Wulff, 1991). The mature religious sentiment is well differentiated so that it can assimilate a wide variety of experiences; dynamic as a force in its own right; consistent in its moral consequences; comprehensive in that, unlike secular philosophies, it seeks to encompass the whole of existence; integral in that it leads to a harmonious whole; and heuristic in that, though lacking total empirical support, it is valuable in shaping research into human nature and action. Allport also emphasized the importance of development in religious maturity, a theme which will be discussed under the developmental approach. In his research methods he was a strong proponent of single-subject inquiry (though he used questionnaire methods in his investigations extensively). Allport did not concentrate on mental illness, yet he clearly emphasized the value of a mature religious faith to mental well-being and remained a devout Episcopalian throughout his career at Harvard.

Robert Bellah exemplifies the humanistic tradition of Allport, though from a different perspective, in his work on the sociology of religion (Bellah, 1970; Bellah, Madsen, Sullivan, Swidler, & Tipton, 1985). As did Allport, Bellah primarily focused on single case studies in the popular book he coauthored, *Habits of the Heart*. He emphasizes the lack of community which typifies American culture today. Even though Americans are overtly religious, they have lost their sense of religious community (if they even had such a sense of community). Bellah is also interested in religion (as well as other forces such as family and citizenship) as it contributes to a morally coherent life—to character. He notes that any discussion of character must be a discussion of the relationship of the individual to the family and community through time (much as Allport focused on the importance of development within the family in forming the religious sentiment).

These two representative scholars, one from midcentury and one current, reflect the humanistic interest in religion and its contribution to wholeness of the person. A number of well-respected scholars began their academic careers from a humanistic, holistic perspective and have moved toward the study of religion as their careers progressed. Two well-known psychiatrists fall into this category, Robert Coles and Karl Menninger. Coles won a Pulitzer prize for his study of children in poverty in the southern United States and has recently expanded his study to the religious lives of children (Coles, 1990). Menninger (1973) asked the question, Whatever became of sin? in a critique of modern culture and its contribution to psychiatric problems. Though both Coles and Menninger today may be considered at the periphery of mainstream psychiatry, they still have popular followings in academia and reflect a holistic approach to psychiatry which remains viable.

POSTMODERN APPROACH

Perhaps the most visible and controversial thrust in academia today within the humanities is the postmodern impulse. This impulse has many roots, but some have traced a major root to Sigmund Freud (Barratt, 1993). Postmodernism has no uniform definition, but in architecture, literature, and theory, postmodern studies focus on contemporary culture as a movement beyond modernism (Lundin, 1993). If the modern impulse was an effort to fill the void created by the decline in religious influence with emphasis on science and art, then the postmodern affirms the void and declares that it cannot be filled. In other words, postmodern writers challenge virtually every premise on which modern scholars sought to establish truth and reality.

Freud challenged our views of truth and reality in religion, for the very basis of psychoanalysis is that humankind has a propensity to be self-deceived regarding a transcendent power. Near the center of self-deceit is the potential to deceive ourselves regarding our faith (Freud, 1930). Freud viewed faith as based in the illusion that an idealized Father, God, can replace the lost real father who had proven fallible to the child and non longer a comfort and security. The idea that God was a projected illusion did not originate with Freud, but he certainly brought faith and religion to the center of the study of mental health and focused on how we have a propensity to deceive ourselves that we cannot naturally overcome, thus the need for psychoanalysis. Freud's solution was developing a sober and realistic view of the reality that there is no God, trusting the scientific method to further inform us of the nature of our being and the world around us, and bravely confronting the reality of the world in which we live as loving and useful citizens. This review of Freud is far too simplistic and probably does not actually represent Freud's true views, but his writings certainly supported postmodern scholars.

The postmodern impulse in modern academe has moved far beyond Freud's critique of our claims to understanding. Michael Foucault, for example, basically rejected any pretension that we can know a world of scientific fact and purposive history (Foucault, 1965, 1972). All history, all science, and all claims to knowledge are claims of either wishful thinking or, worse, the product of persons scheming to claim power in society. Modern empirical research is as suspect as religious belief. A sober and responsible life, as encouraged by Freud, is as deceitful as the religious life of the monk. The concept of madness as mental illness is a means by which persons who do not fit societal norms can be controlled by society, for example, in institutions during the early part of this century and by medications in the latter part of the century.

The current empirical study of religion and mental health would be looked on by those expounding the postmodern perspective as a means to obtain power using a frequently employed means of persuasion in modern society, the scientific method. The postmodern has moved beyond such supposed self-deceit and openly attempts to persuade and control. Therefore, one might expect clashes between those who support empirical study of religion and those driven by the postmodern impulse, but the clash will not center on the validity of the methods of study. Rather, the postmodern scholar will challenge the very project itself as manipulative and driven by desire for power within the academy and society, such as the political efforts of the religious right.

PRAGMATIC APPROACH

William James published perhaps the best known work on psychology and religion during this century, *The Varieties of Religious Experience* (1902). He was most interested in the value of religion for the life of an individual rather than the truth of a faith claim or the specific mechanisms by which religion brought value to one's life. For example, even though he was firmly grounded in medical psychology, he warned against applying a materialistic approach to the study of religion. If one knows the origin of a phenomena, that does not provide the data necessary to pass judgment on the value of that phenomenon. Though he describes in detail many individual accounts of religious experience, a type of empirical inquiry, and also considers religion within the context of both individual and historical development, he concentrates on the relative value of different religious experiences. He especially emphasized the diversity of experiences and used these diverse expressions of the religious sentiment to assist the reader to better understand human nature in general. Therefore, James' work was pragmatic to the core, both in his encouragement of society to understand and accept the religious sentiments of its members and also in his encouragement of the scientist to accept religious experiences as phenomena worthy of study.

Pragmatism has again assumed a major role in the modern university. Though not directly related to the study of religion and mental health, the work of Richard Rorty is instructive. In this book, *Philosophy and the Mirror of Nature* (1979), Rorty suggests that there is no way to account for the validity of our beliefs by examining the relation between ideas and their objects. Instead, the justification of belief is a social process through extended conversation whereby we each try to convince others of what we believe (Gardner, 1985; Rorty, 1979). Rorty rejects the idea that the mind, in any way, can be an accurate mirror of nature. Though, like James, he is in sympathy with a materialistic position, he is much less hopeful that any claim to knowledge can be radically reduced. Each area of study, such as neurology, sociology, cognitive psychology, and study of the history of philosophy, can add to our understanding of the world around us, but none gains supremacy. Rorty represents a modern pragmatism that is akin to the postmodern impulse, namely, one which sets out to prove the absolute failure of foundationalism, the idea that any knowledge is raised on a secure foundation. This leads, for example, to a loss of faith in the ability of language to mirror truth, but recognizes language for its therapeutic capacity to help us get what we desire (Lundin, 1993, p. 35). Therefore, as suggested by Stephen Carter in this book *The Culture of Disbelief* (1993), religion is not so much discriminated against as it is trivialized. The freedom to speak of one's religion within the academy might be accepted, but religious rhetoric seldom is taken seriously. Belief is taken to be no more than a harmless hobby and is expected to be primarily a private affair. If religious principles do conflict with the ongoing discourse in the academy, then these principles should give way to more universally held standards on campus, such as diversity and multiculturalism (Carter, 1993; Marsden, 1997). As Marsden has suggested, religious beliefs are not necessarily treated fairly or even pragmatically in the academy despite the plea of the pragmatist.

BIOLOGICAL MECHANISTIC APPROACH

The biological mechanistic approach to the study of religion and mental health is based on the hypothesis that all experience and behavior are grounded in bodily states and can be reduced to those states. The mechanistic orientation, however, does not subsume all investigators who call for a greater emphasis on biology, and it is important to maintain a distinction between those who are mechanistic in their explanations and those who view biology as a ground but do not subscribe to a reduction of biology to physical mechanisms. For example, Arthur Peacocke (1979) argues for a top-down approach to biology and suggests that one property "supervenes" upon another and therefore each level of understanding must be studied separately. For example, biological properties supervene on physical properties and therefore a biologist cannot describe all biological phenomena using concepts from physics. Psychological properties supervene on the biological, etc. This approach differs from the mechanistic approach in that the latter suggests that the task of scientific inquiry is to reduce all phenomena, including religious beliefs, to molecular physics.

G. Stanley Hall is a representative of the biological mechanistic approach to the study of religion and mental health from earlier in this century (Hall, 1904). He did not reduce religion to molecular biology at the turn of the century because there was no true molecular biology at that time. Nevertheless, he suggested that the religious development of the individual follows the religious development of the species (ontology recapitulates phylogeny). Therefore, the religious experience must be related to the biological development of the child. Most conversion experiences occur, for example, around the time of puberty. He also discussed the intimate relationship between religion and sexual love, such as the tendency of the lover/devotee to be fanatically dedicated to the objects of devotion. This mechanistic approach is closely related to the empirical approach because ultimately the identification of mechanisms depends on empirical verification of the association of phenomena and the causal relations between phenomena.

Modern proponents of the biological mechanistic approach are many, but perhaps the most radical is Edward O. Wilson, the father of sociobiology. In his book, *On Human Nature* (1978), Wilson suggests that scientific materialism "presents the human mind with an alternative mythology that until now has always, point for point in zones of conflict, defeated traditional religion. Every part of existence is considered to be obedient to physical laws requiring no external control" (p. 192). Wilson believes that this mechanistic approach will ultimately eliminate the study of religion as a distinct phenomena (hence the difference between Wilson's reductionism and the supervenience of Peacocke). Nevertheless, Wilson believes that religion will endure for a long time as a vital force in society until the "true Promethean spirit of science means to liberate man by giving him knowledge and some measure of dominion over the physical environment" (p. 209).

Much current neurobiological study operates under the general principle of such a reductionistic biological approach, a mechanistic approach, even though a clear statement of the philosophy underlying the approach is usually not stated. Inherent in the scientific method is the search for mechanisms and the mechanisms discovered via molecular physics and biology have been among the most important achievements of science during the twentieth century. The implications of the rapid advances of neurobiology and the discovery of genetic bases for many abnormal emotions and behaviors are profound for academics exploring the relationship of religion and mental health. One philosopher who has begun to explore the ethical implications of the new biology is Owen Flannagan (1991). He argues for an ethical reflection which is more psychologically realistic, that is, a more biologically realistic psychology of ethics. Specifically, any ethic which is to have meaning in the light of biologic mechanisms must take into account our biological variability, such as our hard-wired character traits. Many students of the psychology of religion suggest that theology should shape our approach to the study of psychology. Flannagan argues the opposite—that empirical, mechanistic biology should shape our study and, to some extent, our development of ethics. Compared to Wilson, Flannagan charts a middle course, yet it is a middle course that depends heavily on mechanistic biology. Flannagan also represents a growing number of philosophers who have a sophisticated understanding of neurobiology. Some have gone so far as to designate such studies as "neurophilosophy" (Churchland, 1986).

LIFE CYCLE APPROACH

None of the approaches described previously is mutually exclusive, either in content or in theoretical construct. The life cycle approach, perhaps more than others, shares so much with other approaches that one might suggest it provides no unique or original contribution to the study of religion and mental health. Nevertheless, the life cycle approach forces the investigator to integrate various approaches of study as applied to humankind in society. For example, a life cycle approach must consider mechanistic biology because growth and development are built into the genetic makeup and gene function of humankind. However, this genetic push to growth and development is constantly augmented and thwarted by environmental factors, both physical and social. Life cycle development also is at the core of a complete understanding of the humanistic approach because the humanistic psychologist, Gordan Allport, was most concerned with development, especially in adolescence. Human development has visibly assumed an integrative role on many college campuses through interdisciplinary certificate programs or interdisciplinary colleges within universities.

The key twentieth century figure in the study of the human life cycle was Erik

Erikson. In this classic work, *Childhood and Society* (1950), Erikson put forth what he conceived as an epigenetic approach to development. Just as each physical organ has a time to arise (and must then arise if the organism is to develop without disturbance), so also do the psychological potentials (Wulff, 1991, pp. 369–410). The eight developmental stages proposed by Erikson are well-known to most readers, identified by a bipolar formula and ranging from "basic trust versus mistrust" in infancy to "ego integrity versus despair" in old age. The ego quality to be obtained at each stage, such as trust, serves as a necessary foundation for successfully achieving the quality of the next stage, such as "autonomy," in early childhood. The environment in which the individual develops through the life cycle is critical to successful movement from one developmental stage to another.

Erikson recognized the critical role religion played in the developmental process. He suggested that the ego qualities and vital virtues (a virtue such as hope evolves from the quality basic) have been safeguarded primarily by the religious tradition of society (Erikson, 1964; Wulff, 1991, p. 379). In addition, Erikson incorporated the concept of ritualization as critical in the process of ensuring the emergence of ego qualities through life and their resultant virtues. For Erikson, ritualization was "an agreed-upon interplay between at least two persons who repeat it at meaningful intervals and in recurring contexts" (Erikson, 1966, p. 337; Wulff, 1991, p. 379). Ritual interplay in everyday life, including especially religious rituals, enhances the growth of the individual ego and brings understanding to human existence. Ritual also brings a stronger sense of community, which he views as essential for the epigenetic development of the person. For example, the ideological ritual element during adolescence: Confirmation and graduation into society imply not only the privileges but also the responsibilities of members of society and affirm a shared worldview. Just as there is a tendency for the ego qualities to not develop adequately, such as the emergence of identity confusion rather than identity during adolescence, there is the potential for the ritual element to become distorted into a maladaptive ritualism. Thus, the positive aspect of the ideological can be distorted into "totalism," a fanatic and exclusive preoccupation with what seems unquestionably ideal within a tight system of ideas (Erikson, 1977, p. 110; Wulff, 1991, p. 382).

Many scholars have built on Erikson's theories, but perhaps the best known scholar, and the one most relevant to the study of religion and mental health, is Lawrence Kohlberg (1981). Kohlberg has arguably been the most influential person in moral psychology over the past 30 years. His theories are complex and not without critics (Flannagan, 1991, pp. 181–195). His assumptions include the following: Moral judgments necessarily involve obligations; virtue is unified, not diversified; moral judgments cannot be reduced to emotive statements; and moral thinking proceeds through a series of stages which are irreversible. The latter assumption derives from Erikson's influence. These stages range from a superego model of morality (stage 1) to a stage which assumes guidance by universal ethical principles that all humanity should follow (stage 6). One can easily observe how religious development and subsequent mental health can be engrafted upon this developmental perspective of morality.

The usual critique of Kohlberg is that his scheme is too simplistic. For example, some would argue that each successive stage does not necessarily improve on the former stage. [e.g., Is guidance by a universal principle (stage 6) necessarily better than upholding the basic rights, values, and laws of a society (Stage 5)?]. Developmental biologists and psychologists attack the scheme at a more fundamental level, namely, the possibility that persons actually behave according to these progressively more developed moral standards as they develop through the life cycle (Flannagan, 1991). In other words, persons may endorse the stages of Kohlberg in the abstract, but these stages may not guide everyday behavior. Regardless, Kohlberg's theories have stimulated much discussion among theologians, psychologists, and moral philosophers, not to mention academics investigating the process of educating children and adults.

CONCLUSION

A review of the approaches to the study of religion and mental health in academia is subject to two extreme conclusions, neither of which I believe to be an accurate reflection of the academy during the latter twentieth century. The first is that such study is limited to the empirical approach, as exemplified in the biomedical science of academic health centers, in which such studies have proliferated in recent years. Though empirical science may rule supreme in some areas of the academy, it is viewed as a partial approach at best in other areas (such as among the humanists) and as a totally erroneous approach in still other portions (such as among the postmoderns). The second is that such study is so diverse as to have no connection either across disciplines or through time. In this chapter, a sampling of approaches has been reviewed. Ties across these approaches reveal that the academician must recognize that considerable overlap in interests and methods remain despite the move toward diversity and that opportunities abound for interdisciplinary conversation. In addition, most of the approaches which can be delineated on the modern university campus have historical roots at least to the earlier years of the twentieth century.

Opportunities abound for dialogue regarding religion and mental health. Unfortunately, as noted previously many academicians are so entrenched in their respective disciplines, and so focused on keeping up and getting ahead within those disciplines, that interdisciplinary conversation, much less interdisciplinary study, is sorely neglected in modern academia. No topic provides a better opportunity for such conversation than religion and mental health.

REFERENCES

Allport, G. (1950). *The individual and his religion: A psychological interpretation*. New York: MacMillan.

Barratt, B. A. (1993). *Psychoanalysis and the postmodern impulse: Knowing and being since Freud's psychology.* Baltimore: Johns Hopkins University Press.

Bellah, R. (1970). *Beyond belief: Essays on religion in a post-traditional world.* New York: Harper & Row.

Bellah, R., Madsen, R., Sullivan, W. M., Swidler, A., & Tipton, S. M. (1985). *Habits of the heart: Individualism and commitment in American life.* Berkeley: University of California Press.

Boyer, P. (1992). *When time shall be no more* (pp. 15–16). Cambridge, MA: Harvard University Press.

Carter, S. (1993). *The culture of disbelief: How American law and politics trivialize religious devotion.* New York: Basic Books.

Churchland, P. S. (1986). *Neurophilosophy: Toward a unified science of the mind/brain.* Cambridge: MIT Press.

Coles, R. (1990). *The spiritual life of children.* New York: Houghton Mifflin.

Durkheim, E. (1951). *Suicide* (G. Simpson, Trans.). Glencoe, IL: Free Press. (Original work published 1897)

Emrick, C. D., Tonigan, J. S., Montgomery, H., & Little, L. (1993). Alcoholics Anonymous: What is currently known? In B. S. McCrady & W. R. Miller (Eds.), *Research on Alcoholics Anonymous* (pp. 41–76). New Brunswick, NJ: Rutgers Center for Alcohol Studies.

Erikson, E. H. (1950). *Childhood and society* (2nd ed.). New York: Norton.

Erikson, E. H. (1966). Ontogeny of ritualization in man. *Philosophical Transactions of the Royal Society of London Series B, Biological Sciences, 251,* 337–349.

Erikson, E. H. (1974). *Insight and responsibility: Lectures on the ethical implications of psychoanalytic insight.* New York: Norton.

Erikson, E. H. (1977). *Toys and reasons: Stages in the ritualization of experience.* New York: Norton.

Flannagan, O. (1991). *Varieties of moral personality: Ethics and psychological realism.* Cambridge, MA: Harvard University Press.

Foucault, M. (1965). *Madness and civilization: A history of insanity in the age of reason.* New York: Pantheon.

Foucault, M. (1972). *The archaeology of knowledge.* New York: Pantheon.

Freud, S. (1930). *Civilization and its discontents* (standard ed., Vol. 21, pp. 57–105) (translated from German under the general editorship of J. Strachey). London: Hogarth.

Gardner, H. (1985). *The mind's new science: A history of the cognitive revolution.* New York: Basic Books.

Hall, G. S. (1904). *Adolescence: Its psychology and its relations to physiology, anthropology, sociology, sex, crime, religion, and education* (Vols. 1–2). New York: Appleton.

James, W. (1902). *The varieties of religious experience.* Cambridge, MA: Harvard University Press.

Kohlberg, L. (1981). *The philosophy of moral development: Moral stages and the ideal of justice.* San Francisco: Harper & Row.

Lundin, R. (1993). *The culture of interpretation: Christian faith and the postmodern world.* Grand Rapids, MI: Eerdmans.

Marsden, G. (1997). *The outrageous idea of Christian scholarship.* New York: Oxford University Press.

Menninger, K. (1973). *Whatever became of sin?* New York: Hawthorn.

Ness, R. C., & Wintrob, R. M. (1980). The emotional impact of fundamentalist religious participation: An empirical study of intragroup variation. *American Journal of Orthopsychiatry, 50,* 302–315.

Peacocke, A. (1979). *Creation and the world of science.* London: Clarendon.

Rorty, R. (1979). *Philosophy and the mirror of nature.* Princeton, NJ: Princeton University Press.

Roush, W. (1997). Herbert Benson: Mind–body maverick pushes the envelope. *Science, 276,* 357–359.

Wulff, D. (1991). *Psychology of religion* (pp. 580–585). New York: John Wiley.

SUMMARY AND CONCLUSIONS

Because religions beliefs and practices are so common among the patients we see, clinicians must be aware of their influences on mental health. Mental health professionals need to know something about each of the major world religions—basic information about sacred beliefs and practices and how these might influence the onset and course of mental illness, the patient's response to their mental illness, and the patient's understanding of and likelihood of complying with treatment (Chapters 13–20).

Mental health professionals also need to be aware of the growing body of scientific research that is demonstrating the enormous role that religion can play in mental health, either for better or for worse (Chapter 3). Perhaps it is not too much of an exaggeration to say that the vast majority of people in the United States and in many countries around the world use their religious faith in one way or another to understand and cope with stress, loss, and tragedy (Chapter 8). While mental health professionals have for many years ignored the spiritual or religious dimension of patients' lives, this position is no longer tenable for a competent mental health professional moving into the third millennium (Chapter 2). We simply know too much about the positive effects that religious beliefs and practices can have in preventing mental illness or facilitating recovery to eliminate them from consideration when treating patients with depression, anxiety, or even major psychotic disorders (Chapters 9–12).

There is no question that certain aspects of religious belief and practice may constrict or limit healthy mental functioning, and we must learn about these pathological influences, the situations in which they occur, how they exert their negative effects, and what to do about them. We must also realize that what we may be interpreting as a belief or behavior that is limiting or impairing the mental health of our patient may only be a result of our own limited knowledge about and unfamiliarity with that person's faith tradition. Thus, such judgments should be made cautiously and perhaps after consultation with someone knowledgeable in the patient's faith tradition. The clinician must also remember that mental illness itself may distort and pervert healthy religious expression, and wounded people in desperate attempts to cope with their pain may manipulate religious beliefs and practices to justify also sorts of actions or disguise rage and hatred. Even when religion is used in this seemingly maladaptive manner, the sensitive clinician must learn to proceed cautiously, helping the patient recognize his or her maladaptive use of faith by delicately and sensitively questioning and challenging that use.

The mental health influence of religious beliefs and practices—particularly when imbedded within a long-standing, well-integrated faith tradition—is largely a positive one (Chapters 3, 8). Most major world religions promote and enhance social cohesion and build "social capital" which has been associated with better mental health and even greater economic growth (Kawachi, Kennedy, & Lochner, 1997). Religions guide and structure our personal and social lives and provide time-tested ways of thinking, making decisions, living with and cooperating with each other, and ultimately combating the normless anomie that can easily creep into our lives as we lose our vertical and horizonal connections (Chapter 4). Religion provides a belief system that helps people make sense of the world around them, the uncontrollable forces that affect their lives, and the sometimes intolerable feelings that well up from within. Religion can often provide an external structure and sense of cohesion when an individual's personal life and world is falling apart.

Thus, for the most part, the religious beliefs and traditions that people hold are resources. These resources, then, can be used to complement and enhance the powerful psychotherapies and psychopharmacological treatments that modern medical science has now provided us (Chapter 22). Neither religion nor modern psychotherapeutics can be replaced without losing something in the process. Before psychotherapeutic approaches were developed for treating mental illness, many persons with deep and devout religious faith had to suffer the agonizing pains of depression, paralyzing anxiety, or psychotic disorganization. As we have come to depend on our secular armamentarium of treatments, we have neglected to care for that vital component of the person—the spirit. The time has now come to utilize and maximize the benefits of both religious and secular approaches to help relieve the turmoil, loneliness, and confusing pain that our patients experience.

We have a long way to go, though, to integrate religious and secular therapies to maximize health and healing. There are both personal and professional barriers that stand in the way of this goal. Our personal beliefs and experiences invariably influence how we approach and deal with the religious beliefs of our patients and how we use those beliefs to enhance and complement our secular therapies. Because of the intensely personal nature of religious belief, we must develop sensitive and respectful ways of inquiring about and taking advantage of the patient's religious resources, keeping our focus on the patient's needs and beliefs and away from our own needs and prejudices. While advances have been made to educate mental health professionals in this area (Larson, Lu, & Swyers, 1996), this is only the first step. There are no fast and easy rules that can be applied in every situation, and how one proceeds will depend on the individual therapist, the individual patient, and the individual situation. We have tried in this book to provide some broad guidelines in this regard (Chapter 22). There also remain major resistances at the academic level which make the integration of secular and religious therapies challenging, in terms of both training and research (Chapters 7, 25, 26). These barriers, however, are slowly beginning to fall.

Finally, mental health professionals without religious or spiritual training must approach spiritual topics with some degree of humility and recognition of limitation. Religious professionals typically have knowledge, training, and years of experience that have prepared them to address spiritual problems (Chapters 23, 24). For example, a hospital chaplain will typically have 4 years of college, 3 years of divinity school, 2 or 3 years of clinical pastoral education, and often additional training in areas of special expertise. An uninformed secular therapist who delves into sensitive religious issues that he or she has little knowledge about or experience in may easily become the proverbial "bull in the china closet." At times, the most sensible, sensitive, and respectful intervention that a nonreligious professional can make is to appropriately refer the patient. At other times, however, referral may not be an option because the patient refuses or because religious professionals are not immediately available. In those cases, the therapist may need to make the effort to consult a religious professional of the patient's faith to obtain advice on how to proceed. At other times, the situation and timing may be such that the therapist must take advantage of the moment and simply intervene in a reasonable manner to the best of his or her ability. Communicating honestly with the patient about one's lack of expertise and trepidation about proceeding, yet the desire to see the patient get help and be relieved of his or her suffering, can often accomplish a great deal; if nothing else, it will let the patient know that the therapist recognizes how important these areas are in the patient's life and their need for attention.

REFERENCES

Kawachi, I., Kennedy, B. P., & Lochner, K. (1997), (November/December). Long live community: Social capital as public health. *The American Prospect, 35,* 56–59.

Larson, D. B., Lu, F. G., & Swyers, J. P. (Eds.). (1996). *Model curriculum for psychiatry residency training programs: Religion and spirituality in clinical practice.* Rockville, MD: National Institute for Healthcare Research.

INDEX

children
after Second Vatican Council, 217–218
before Second Vatican Council, 214–216
Mormon beliefs, 230
pastoral counselors, 342–343
reeducative therapies, 330–331
Educational material, religious
essential, 370–371
important and helpful, 371–374
Ego, Eriksonian view, 387
Egypt, Muslim death anxiety, 152–159
Elder abuse, need for clergy–mental health
worker collaboration, 356–357
Elderly
organizational involvement, 42
pastoral care and depression and suicide,
354–355
religion and anxiety, 148–149
religious coping, 56–57
religiousness, 129–130
Emmanuel movement, psychology of, 13
Emotions
experienced by schizophrenics, 165–166
positive, engendered by worship, 40–41
subserved by limbic system, 81
Epidemiologic research, religious involvement
and mental health outcomes, 35–36
Equality, Islamic conception, 284–285
Ergotropic system, balance with trophotropic
system, 80–81, 91
Erikson, Erik, ego quality, 387
Eternal progression, Mormon tenet, 228, 230
Ethics
medical, Islamic, 288
psychiatric care: secular and Christian, 314
in therapeutic responses to religious issues,
372
Ethnicity, Catholicism in context of, 218–219
Ethnic minorities, importance of clergy and
mental health professionals, 357–358
Etiology
mental illness, from religious discipline,
52–54
psychoses, 162–163
Europe
Renaissance medical literature, 6–7
view of spirituality and mental disorders,
7–9
Evangelism, in Mormon tradition, 235
Evolution, *see also* Neuroevolution
brain structures, 75
medical terms, in Unity students' thinking,
247

Expectations, about treatment, held by Protestants, 207–208
Experience
mystical, extrovertive and introvertive,
84–85
religious
effect on personal belief systems, 161–162
in schizophrenia, 166–168
understanding subjective nature of, 87–88
spiritual
methods of attainment, 77–79
neuroevolution, 76–77
psychodynamics, 372–374
in psychological practice, 90–91
Experiential model, substance use–religiousness
relationship, 185

Faith
communities
liaisons with, 341–342
and role of mental health brokers, 344–345
declaration, in Islam, 283
Freud's view, 383
importance to Americans, 349–350
Mormon Articles of Faith, 229
optimism and hope generated by, 41–42
Family
Islamic tradition, 288
Jewish, changing nature, 259
Jews as, 256
of mentally ill, responses to illness, 55–56
Mormon values, 231–232
practice of Catholicism, 218–219
violence, and pastoral counseling, 355–356
Fantasies, clinical implications for Catholics,
220
Fear
physiological effects, according to Nemisius,
5–6
psychiatric probing of religious values, 271
Feelings, negative
confronted by Mormon client, 239
experienced by therapist, 334
Females
American and Egyptian
death anxiety scale, revised, 156
intrinsic religious motivation, 154
Mormon, special issues, 233–234
non-Pentecostal African Americans, smoking,
181–182
seeking help from clergy and mental health
professionals, 359